Register Now for Online Access to Your Book!

P9-CCK-787

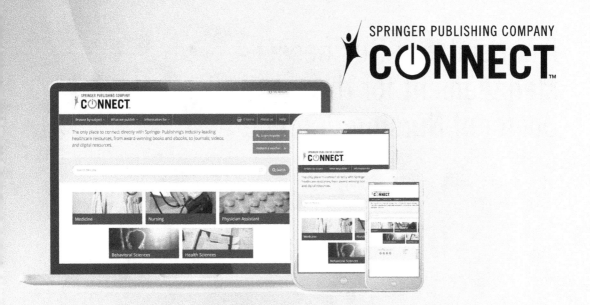

SPRINGER PUBLISHING COMPANY
CONNECT™

Your print purchase of *Financial and Business Management for the Doctor of Nursing Practice, Second Edition,* **includes online access to the contents of your book**—increasing accessibility, portability, and searchability!

Access today at:

**http://connect.springerpub.com/content/book/978-0-8261-2209-4
or scan the QR code at the right with your smartphone
and enter the access code below.**

NHCJT3V6

*Scan here for
quick access.*

LS

SPRINGER PUBLISHING COMPANY
View all our products at springerpub.com

Financial and Business Management for the Doctor of Nursing Practice

KT Waxman, DNP, MBA, RN, CNL, CHSE, CENP, FAAN, is a nurse leader with more than 30 years of experience in health care and corporate settings. She has held positions as chief nursing officer, chief operating officer, vice president for Patient Care Services, and senior manager in a large consulting firm. In 2009, Dr. Waxman made the leap to academia. Currently she is an associate professor in the School of Nursing and Health Professions at the University of San Francisco where she directs the Executive Leadership Doctor of Nursing Practice (DNP) program and teaches advanced financial management. She created and implemented the California Simulation Alliance (CSA) at HealthImpact, a 4,000-member virtual alliance serving the health care simulation community, where she serves as director. An internationally known speaker and author, Dr. Waxman is also a past president and past board member of the Association of California Nurse Leaders (ACNL). She served on the executive board and as treasurer for the American Organization of Nurse Executives (AONE) from 2013 to 2015, and she has served on the strategic planning and education committees for AONE. Dr. Waxman is a fellow in both the Society for Simulation in Healthcare and the American Academy of Nursing.

Financial and Business Management for the Doctor of Nursing Practice

Second Edition

KT Waxman, DNP, MBA, RN, CNL, CHSE, CENP, FAAN

Editor

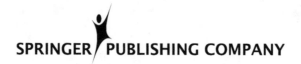

SPRINGER PUBLISHING COMPANY

Springer Publishing Company, LLC
11 West 42nd Street
New York, NY 10036
www.springerpub.com

Acquisitions Editor: Margaret Zuccarini
Senior Production Editor: Kris Parrish
Compositor: Westchester Publishing Services

ISBN: 978-0-8261-2206-3
ebook ISBN: 978-0-8261-2209-4
Instructor's Manual ISBN: 978-0-8261-2465-4
Instructor's PowerPoints ISBN: 978-0-8261-2474-6

Instructor's Materials: Qualified instructors may request supplements by emailing textbook@springerpub.com

17 18 19 20 / 5 4 3 2 1

Library of Congress Cataloging-in-Publication Data

Names: Waxman, KT, editor.
Title: Financial and business management for the doctor of nursing practice / [edited by] KT Waxman.
Description: Second edition. | New York, NY : Springer Publishing Company, [2018] | Includes
    bibliographical references and index.
Identifiers: LCCN 2017034450 | ISBN 9780826122063 (hardcopy : alk. paper) |
    ISBN 9780826122094 (ebook)
Subjects: | MESH: Economics, Nursing | Nursing Services—economics
Classification: LCC RT86.7 | NLM WY 77 | DDC 610.73068—dc23 LC record available at
    https://lccn.loc.gov/2017034450

Printed in the United States of America by Gasch Printing.

This book is dedicated to those nurse leaders who have made the decision to continue their education and obtain a doctoral degree, and to my colleagues and friends for their encouragement and support during the writing of this text—they know who they are!

Contents

PART I. THE BIG PICTURE OF HEALTH CARE FINANCE

PART II. BUDGETING FOR ACUTE AND AMBULATORY CARE

PART III. QUALITY, DATA ANALYSIS, AND LEGAL/ETHICAL ISSUES

Contributors

Carlton Abner, DNP, RN-BC, Associate Vice President, Talent Strategies, Lenexa, Kansas

Marjorie Barter, EdD, RN, CNL, CENP, Professor Emerita, Health Care Systems Leadership, School of Nursing and Health Professions, University of San Francisco, San Francisco, California

Tim Bock, DNP, MBA, Director of Patient Care Services, Salmon Creek Medical Center, Legacy Health, Vancouver, Washington

Fay L. Bower, DNSc, FAAN, Retired Professor, Holy Names University, Oakland, California; Consultant, Nursing Education

Elena Capella, EdD, MSN, MPA, RN, CNL, CPHQ, LNCC, Assistant Professor, School of Nursing and Health Professions, University of San Francisco, San Francisco, California

Lisa Gifford, DNP, RN, CHPCN, CHPCA, Assistant Professor, School of Nursing and Health Professions, University of San Francisco, San Francisco, California

Carol A. (Reineck) Huebner, PhD, RN, CENP, FAAN, NEA-BC, Professor Emerita, University of Texas Health Science Center, San Antonio School of Nursing, San Antonio, Texas

Judith Lambton, EdD, MS, RN, Professor Emerita, School of Nursing and Health Professions, University of San Francisco, California; Adjunct Professor, Rafic Hariri School of Nursing, American University of Beirut, Beirut, Lebanon

Mary Lynne Knighten, DNP, RN, PN, NEA-BC, Independent Hospital and Healthcare Consultant, Knighten Consulting, Los Angeles, California

Lisa J. Massarweh, DNP, RN, PHN, NEA-BC, CPHQ, CCRN-K, Executive Director, Patient Care Services, Performance & Workforce Strategy, Kaiser Foundation Hospitals, Northern California; Robert Wood Johnson Foundation Executive Nurse Fellow (2006–2009)

Juli Maxworthy, DNP, MBA, RN, CNL, CPHQ, CPPS, CHSE, FSSH, Assistant Professor, School of Nursing and Health Professions, Past Chair, Healthcare Leadership and Innovations Department, Director, BSN to DNP Program, University of San Francisco, San Francisco, California; CEO, WithMax Consulting; Secretary, Society for Simulation in Healthcare; Region One Coordinator, Sigma Theta Tau International, San Francisco, California

Anna Mullins, PhD, RN, Adjunct Faculty, School of Nursing, University of California, San Francisco; Healthcare Consultant, San Francisco, California

Kathleen M. Nakfoor, EdD, MBA, MSIS, RN, Principal, Nak4Health Consulting; Adjunct Faculty, School of Nursing and Health Professions, University of California, San Francisco, California

Susan J. Penner, RN, MN, MPA, Dr.PH, CNL, Adjunct Faculty, Graduate Programs, School of Nursing and Health Professions, University of San Francisco, San Francisco, California

Susan Prion, EdD, RN, CNE, CHSE, Professor, School of Nursing and Health Professions, University of San Francisco, San Francisco, California

Mikhail Shneyder, MBA, RN, President and CEO, Nightingale College, Salt Lake City, Utah

Michael D. Spencer, MBA, Retired Adjunct Professor, University of California, San Francisco, San Ysidro, California

Joanne Spetz, PhD, FAAN, Professor, Philip R. Lee Institute for Health Policy Studies; Associate Director of Research, Healthforce Center, University of California, San Francisco, California

Chrys Marie Suby, RN, ANP, MS, President and CEO, Labor Management Institute, Bloomington, Minnesota

Karen Van Leuven, PhD, FNP, Associate Professor, School of Nursing and Health Professions, University of San Francisco; Primary Care Provider, Spherical Medical Group, San Francisco, California

KT Waxman, DNP, MBA, RN, CNL, CHSE, CENP, FSSH, FAAN, Associate Professor, School of Nursing and Health Professions; Director, Executive Leader DNP Program, University of San Francisco; Director, California Simulation Alliance at HealthImpact, Oakland, California

Foreword

This definitive update to the first edition is geared to nursing professionals who need to know about health care financing in non-CPA (certified public accountant) terms. Dr. Waxman has organized excellent authors who are knowledgeable about their topics and address the issues using real-life examples that make sense to nursing professionals. The book is deductive, beginning with the big picture of health care financing and then applying a financial management perspective to nursing practice and general health care issues.

Part I effectively covers the complexity inherent in reimbursement and insurance coverage. This is necessary in order to understand the source of health care financing, as well as how financing is used to deliver patient care. Doctor of nursing practice (DNP) students will gain an excellent overview of health care economics, insurance coverage, and reimbursement.

Part II lays the foundation for students to acquire budgeting skills and to prepare to make executive-type financial decisions at the macro and micro levels. Understanding budgeting as a plan rather than as the core to finance is critical for nurse practitioners, whether they work in acute care settings or independently. The focus on independent practitioners is timely. The inclusion of this content makes this one of the most forward-thinking books in today's market to assist practitioners in becoming entrepreneurs. Advanced practice registered nurses (APRNs) and DNPs will gain a great deal of skill in understanding and applying budgeting for both short-term operations and long-term strategies, including capital budgeting. This section concludes with a timely update of strategic planning, another necessary skill.

Part III emphasizes business skills for DNPs. It points out the fiscal and ethical responsibility of all providers of care to ensure that data are appropriately used to support the cost of care and the importance of data to provide quality. This section stresses that quality must be an outcome of services and that financial managers cannot ethically take shortcuts that may benefit the profit margin at the cost of quality outcomes. Having taught many classes in financial management, I am encouraged to note how all of these facets are synthesized by energizing the reader to use the learned skills applied to business management. A new chapter on the efficient hospital helps DNPs understand the inner workings of a streamlined hospital.

Part IV wraps up with entrepreneurship and the future. This section includes being an entrepreneur, writing a business plan, financial management in academia, and ultimately the issues behind global health care financing.

I am thrilled that Dr. Waxman has used her knowledge and skills to revise this book, keeping it up to date on reimbursement issues and challenges in the financial milieu. The book provides faculty with the information they need to integrate financial concepts into nursing practice, as opposed to translating content that either is not applicable or was written to inform accounting or business majors. The key takeaway is that a useful book about finance for professional nurses is finally here! Congratulations to Dr. Waxman and her excellent authors. I look forward to using this book in my future financial management classes.

Roxane Spitzer, PhD, MBA, RN, FAAN
Editor-in-Chief Emerita, Nurse Leader
Board of Directors Ensemble
Professional Role-Based Practice Solutions
Stuart, Florida

Preface

It has been exciting to complete the second edition of this book. In the 4 years since it was first published, there has been increased awareness and commitment to providing nurses with the financial and business skills they need. The American Organization of Nurse Executives (AONE) launched two key programs to address this need: the Certificate in Advanced Health Care Financial Management in conjunction with the Healthcare Financial Management Association (HFMA), and the finance and business skills course for nurse leaders. As we move into the next era of health care leadership, which will look different than it does today, nurse executives and doctors of nursing practice (DNPs) need to be able to "talk the talk" with both chief financial officers and staff.

When I graduated from the first DNP program in California at the University of San Francisco, in 2008, I felt a need to further communicate the role and degree to the nursing community. As a nurse executive, former chief nursing officer, and now academic, I learned the importance of nurse leaders understanding the business acumen and financials of health care. As nurses, we do not receive adequate training in this subject, even though we may be held accountable for the budget of our area(s). We need more textbooks and tools to assist nurse leaders in acquiring the skills they need for success. I have had a passion for teaching nurses to be savvy in finance since the late 1980s when I was a nursing director with budgetary responsibility. My education in finance and business skills was "on the job"—I worked at a for-profit health care system in which numbers guided our lives!

This second edition has been updated to reflect the latest tools and trends in health care. Critical thinking exercises have been added to each chapter for use in the classroom. Also, a new chapter (13) on the efficient hospital of the future has been added. The book is laid out in four sections and begins at the national level with the economics of health care, insurance coverage, reimbursement, and policy. The chapter authors are all experts in their topics, and you will gain a wide perspective from reading the chapters.

Part I The Big Picture of Health Care Finance provides background information regarding the big picture of health care. This section includes discussion of hospitals and health systems as businesses, the economics of health care, and insurance coverage and reimbursement in both acute and nonacute settings. It is important to have this information as a basis for managing the finances in your organization.

Part II Budgeting for Acute and Ambulatory Care focuses on budgeting for these areas, and there is also a specific chapter for DNPs on building their own businesses. Understanding the financial indicators, acronyms, and formulas is essential to being able to build and manage a budget. The section concludes with a robust chapter on strategic planning and capital budgeting, with new tools and tips that are critical for the DNP who may be "at the table" contributing to key decisions regarding the organization's goals and objectives.

Part III Quality, Data Analysis, and Legal/Ethical Issues builds the financial case for quality, reviews financial statements, and presents more terminology. The first chapter, which focuses on quality, is critical for helping students understand the cost of quality, how the organization defines quality, and the implications around tracking and monitoring. The updated data analysis chapter provides new formulas and examples and the legal/ethical chapter has been updated to address our current political environment. Skills such as project management and grant writing are also critical for the DNP, and these chapters have added new tools and information.

Part IV Entrepreneurship and the Future focuses on what the hospital and health system of the future may look like as well as business skills for the DNP, including a sample business plan. If you are in academia, Chapter 15 will assist you in creating a feasibility study for a new program. Part IV ends with a global perspective on health care finance and the DNP.

I hope that this book will be useful in helping you speak a new language: the language of finance. This updated book serves as both a foundation for those students who have not had financial education, and a review and validation for those with experience in health care finance. Ultimately, readers will be able to "talk the talk" with the financial department, build a case, and stand up for what they need to bridge the clinical agenda with the financial agenda. **Qualified instructors may obtain access to ancillary materials, including an instructor's manual and PowerPoints, by emailing textbook@springerpub.com.**

At the time of this publication, the American Association of Colleges of Nursing (AACN) website (http://www.aacnnursing.org/News-Information/Fact-Sheets/DNP-Fact-Sheet) reports that 303 DNP programs are currently enrolling students at schools of nursing nationwide, and an additional 124 new DNP programs are in the planning stages (58 postbaccalaureate and 66 post-masters programs). DNP programs are now available in 50 states and the District of Columbia. The states with the greatest number of programs (10 or more) are California, Florida, Illinois, Massachusetts, Minnesota, New York, Ohio, Pennsylvania, and Texas. From 2015 to 2016, the number of students enrolled in DNP programs increased from 21,995 to 25,289. During that same period, the number of DNP graduates increased from 4,100 to 4,855.

In 2008, the Robert Wood Johnson Foundation (RWJF) and the Institute of Medicine (IOM) launched a 2-year initiative to respond to the need to assess and transform the nursing profession. The IOM appointed the committee on the RWJF Initiative on the Future of Nursing to produce a report that would make recommendations for an action-oriented blueprint for the future of nursing. Through its deliberations, the committee developed four key messages:

1. Nurses should practice to the full extent of their education and training.
2. Nurses should achieve higher levels of education and training through an improved educational system that promotes seamless academic progression.
3. Nurses should be full partners, with physicians and other health care professionals, in redesigning health care in the United States.
4. Effective workforce planning and policy making requires better data collection and information infrastructure.

The United States has the opportunity to transform its health care system, and nurses can and should play a fundamental role in this transformation. However, the power to improve the current regulatory, business, and organizational conditions does not rest solely with nurses; government, businesses, health care organizations, professional associations, and the insurance industry all must play a role. Working together, these many diverse parties can help ensure that the health care system provides seamless, affordable, quality care that is accessible to all and leads to improved health outcomes (IOM, 2010).

From the key messages noted, eight recommendations are included. In five states, it is recommended: *double the number of nurses with a doctorate by 2020.* Schools of nursing, with support from private and public funders, academic administrators, university trustees, and accrediting bodies, should double the number of nurses with a doctoral degree by 2020 to add to the cadre of nurse faculty and researchers, with attention to increasing diversity (IOM, 2010). With health care reform on the horizon, it is imperative that nurses have a clear understanding of the financial health of their organizations. Speaking the language of finance, being able to clearly articulate their financial impact when building their case for change, and being able to read financial statements are key skills DNPs need to do their jobs effectively. This text is designed to provide DNP students with the knowledge and skills needed to practice at a doctoral level. Congratulations on making the decision to obtain a doctoral degree in nursing practice!

KT Waxman

REFERENCE

Institute of Medicine. (2010). *Future of Nursing report.* Retrieved from http://www.nursingworld.org/Main MenuCategories/ThePracticeofProfessionalNursing/workforce/IOM-Future-of-Nursing-Report-1

Acknowledgments

I want to thank my colleagues and mentors for making this book a reality. Thank you to all the finance professors around the country who used the first edition in their courses; to Dr. Susan Penner, who recommended me to Springer Publishing Company and had faith in my ability to actually complete the task; to Dr. Marjorie Barter, my mentor, who provided support and encouragement to me during the writing process of this book; to the chapter authors, not only for their expertise and contributions, but also for adhering to timelines and weaving the *DNP Essentials* into each chapter. Working with this group of professional colleagues has been a joy!

Thank you to my family for their support of my work and me over the years: Steve, my husband of over 30 years, who has supported me through three degrees, culminating with my DNP; my daughters Ashley and Samantha; my son-in-law Brian; and granddaughter Olive.

1

The Economic Context of Nursing Practice in the United States

Joanne Spetz

demand	insurance	production
economics	nursing shortage	supply
health reform		

The provision of health care services occurs within the context of the health care system. Regardless of whether you are a nurse practitioner (NP), physical therapist, pharmacist, or home health assistant, the way you work is affected by how health care is financed and organized. The health care system of the United States has evolved over centuries, shaped by a combination of market economics and public policy decisions. In order to understand how health care financing and organization influence nursing care, one must understand the underlying economics of health care, as well as the legislative and regulatory policies that have shaped our system.

It is essential for the doctor of nursing practice (DNP) to understand health economics, in order to serve as a policy advocate, to provide leadership, to foster evidence-based practice, and to fully know the scientific underpinning of practice. The patients who seek care from NPs and other health professionals are affected by the economic system in which they live. Economic factors such as the price of healthy food, the link between education and pay, and the cost of transportation influence the jobs your patients have, the choices they make about diet and exercise, and whether they seek health care when they need it. Understanding human behavior and developing care plans for patients must take these factors into consideration—economics thus is a part of the scientific underpinnings of good practice. Moreover, evidence-based practice involves delivering not only the care that has been proved most effective, but also the care that uses resources most efficiently and cost-effectively. The DNP role also provides leadership to improve the quality of care. To be successful, a leader must adapt to the organizational culture and economic context of the nursing practice environment. And, to be an effective advocate for improved health policy, one must understand the economics that drive not only the U.S. health care system but also all other countries' health care systems.

This chapter explains the economic context of nursing practice, focusing on the organization and financing of the U.S. health care system. It begins with a discussion of the basic principles of economics and how decisions are made by comparing marginal costs with marginal benefits. Then, health care is connected to this economic framework, with a focus on why some aspects of a "free market" economic system do not apply to health care. This leads to a discussion of the fundamental economic problem that all health care systems must address. The chapter concludes by considering how the United States is responding to its health care problems, including the effects of policy changes since 2010.

WHAT IS HEALTH ECONOMICS?

PRINCIPLES OF ECONOMICS

The discipline of economics involves the study of how resources are allocated. There are three key principles embedded in this definition. The first is that resources are scarce. In this sense, "scarce" does not mean that there are insufficient resources for people to survive. It simply means that no resource is infinite. A group of people might have access to only a certain land area, expect limited rainfall, enjoy only 24 hours in a day, and have a fixed nutrient base in the soil.

The second principle of economics regards the fact that resources can be used for multiple purposes, and decisions must be made about how to use them. Land can be used for housing, farming, or factories; waking hours can be used to work or for leisure pursuits. Individuals and communities must make decisions about how to allocate resources and time. Whether and how a resource is used can impinge upon the possibility of making another choice—for example, using land to grow a crop can preclude using that scarce land for grazing cattle or building houses. The lost value of what cannot be done once a decision is made is called the *opportunity cost*. So, using land to grow corn has the opportunity cost of the value of using that same land to raise cattle.

The third key principle of economics is that people's preferences differ. Although one person might prefer to use land to grow apples, another person might dislike apples and want to grow pears. Heterogeneity of preferences—meaning peoples' differences in preferences—is important because it creates competition and debate about how resources should be used, and because it creates opportunities for trade between people.

WHY TRADE OCCURS

Trade is motivated by people having different resources available to them, different skills for using those resources, and different preferences. Variation in resources and skills leads to variation in productivity, which makes it logical for people (or communities) to specialize their production. One person might be a skilled cattle rancher and have access to large amounts of grazing land, whereas another person might excel at growing tomatoes and have a smaller plot of rich soil. The person with the grazing land will be much more productive as a cattle rancher than as a tomato farmer, and vice versa. Both people will be better off if they specialize in the pursuit where they have the productive advantage, and then trade cattle and tomatoes with each other.

Similarly, an NP has specialized skills in providing health care services, and a farmer has different skills. They each are better off working in their area of expertise, and then trading health care for food and vice versa. Money is a mechanism through which trade is facilitated—the NP receives money for providing health care services, which then is given to the farmer for food.

THE ROLE OF PREFERENCES

People's preferences also affect decisions about consumption and trade. Not only is there variation in preferences across people, but also there is variation based on how much has already been consumed. For example, you might get a lot of pleasure from drinking a cup of coffee in the morning, and be willing to trade $3 for that coffee. But, after finishing that first cup of coffee, the second cup of coffee might not be quite as valuable to you. At some point, you will have had so much coffee that you are not willing to part with $3 to get another cup.

Economists often use the generic term *utility* to refer to the pleasure, value, or usefulness of something that is consumed or experienced. In this example, then, you are making a decision about whether the utility of another cup of coffee is greater than the utility of having those $3 to spend on something else. Utility can refer to the pleasure you get from playing with your children, or from sleeping, or from feeling satisfied with the quality of your work.

MARGINAL UTILITY AND MARGINAL COSTS

This example illustrates the fact that people make decisions about consumption based on a comparison of the utility and costs of a product. But, people do not simply make decisions based on the *average* utility and cost of a product. Decisions are made based on the *marginal* costs and utility. The *marginal utility* is the value of one more, given that a certain amount has already been consumed. As illustrated in Figure 1.1, the utility of each cup of coffee is lower than that of the previous cup. In other words, the marginal utility of coffee is declining. In fact, the utility of coffee can be negative—meaning it makes you worse-off—when you have had a lot of it. You might get the jitters and feel nauseous, so even if the coffee were free, you would stop drinking it when the marginal utility of the next cup is negative.

The marginal cost of consumption can also vary—in fact, sellers often price their products so that there is a discount for purchasing larger volumes. If T-shirts are sold as "1 for $10 or 2 for $15," the marginal cost of the first T-shirt is $10, and the marginal cost of the second T-shirt is $5. The average cost if you buy two T-shirts is, of course, $7.50. When buying T-shirts, then, you are deciding whether the second T-shirt will give you $5 worth of additional utility, after you already have purchased one T-shirt. Figure 1.2 illustrates this decision. The marginal utility of one T-shirt

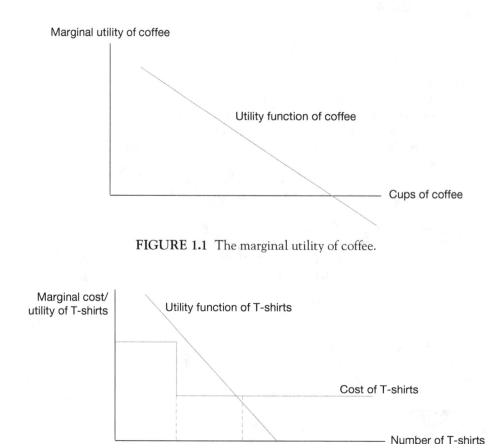

FIGURE 1.1 The marginal utility of coffee.

FIGURE 1.2 Comparing marginal costs and utility.

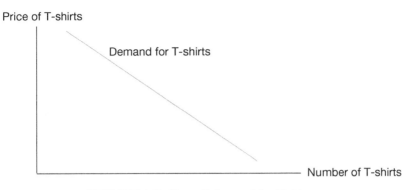

FIGURE 1.3 Overall demand for T-shirts.

is higher than the marginal cost of that T-shirt ($10). But, the marginal utility of the second T-shirt is lower than the marginal cost of $5. Thus, you will buy only one T-shirt.

In general, people will consume something until the marginal cost and marginal utility are equal to each other. If the marginal utility of the next item is greater than the marginal cost, then it is more valuable to you to consume one more item—and thus you will consume one more. If the marginal utility of the next item is lower than the marginal cost, then you will not consume it. As noted, this idea applies to both things you might purchase and ways you might spend your time. If the marginal utility of sleeping 8 hours instead of 7 hours is greater than the cost of missing one additional hour of work or leisure time, you will sleep 8 hours. But, if the marginal utility is lower than the cost of missing your favorite TV show, then you will sleep only 7 hours.

For most products, the decision rule of balancing marginal cost and marginal utility will mean that as the price increases, people will demand less of the product. If the price of a cup of coffee rises, fewer people will find that the marginal utility of another cup of coffee is greater than the marginal cost and thus less coffee will be demanded. Thus, if the marginal utility line slopes downward, as in Figure 1.2, the overall demand will also slope downward, as in Figure 1.3.

PRODUCTION DECISIONS

People or companies that produce goods and services make production decisions according to comparisons of marginal costs and benefits. Production costs can include expenses for factories, workers, and supplies. In many cases, the marginal costs of production decline as the quantity produced increases. For example, a company that makes aspirin may find that as the number of pills it makes increases, it can purchase the chemicals used to make the pills in bulk quantities and thus at lower prices. As illustrated in Figure 1.4, the change in cost of making aspirin declines as larger quantities are produced. Thus, the average cost of making a small amount of aspirin is higher than the average cost of making a greater number of pills. When a producer faces decreasing marginal costs, we say there are "economies of scale"—in other words, there is a lower cost per item to produce a large quantity than a small quantity. The relationship between the amount produced and the cost of production is called the "production function."

The demand for a product will exhibit a relationship between price and quantity, as described in Figure 1.3. In general, as the price rises, the quantity demanded falls. This relationship also matches the marginal revenue that the producer can receive for the product. At low quantities, the producer might be able to charge a relatively high price, and thus the marginal revenue for each item sold will be high. But, as the quantity produced increases, the producer must charge a lower price to sell all of the product, thus receiving a lower marginal revenue.

A producer will have an incentive to produce more of a product any time the marginal revenue is greater than the marginal cost. If the aspirin manufacturer can sell another 1,000 pills for

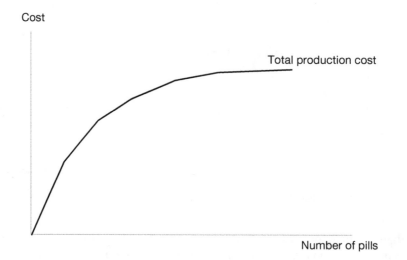

FIGURE 1.4 The total cost of producing pills: Diminishing marginal costs.

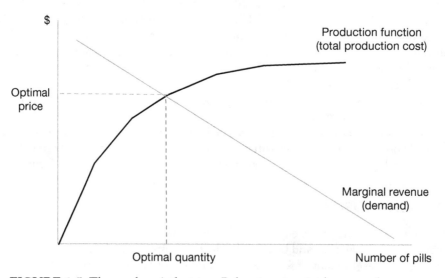

FIGURE 1.5 The producer's decision: Balancing marginal costs and revenues.

$1 each, but it costs only 80 cents to make each of those pills, the manufacturer can earn 20 cents profit per pill and will clearly want to do so. But, if the aspirin company needs to drop the price to 70 cents to sell those next 1,000 pills, then the money received would be lower than the cost of production, and the company will not make more. Figure 1.5 illustrates this point. The optimal point of production and price is the equilibrium point where the production function and the demand (marginal revenue) intersect. This is the price and quantity we will see in the market.

This general principle applies to all goods and services that are produced or traded, whether by an individual or a company. It applies to employment decisions as well. An individual will make choices about how much to work based on the marginal revenue of work and the marginal cost. The revenue is the total compensation one receives for work, which can include both salary and satisfaction. The cost is the value of other things that are traded for working hours—in other words, the opportunity cost of work is the utility of leisure time. When a person can receive higher pay per hour, or finds that each hour of work provides greater satisfaction, that person is more likely to find that the marginal revenue of work is greater than the marginal cost of lost leisure time, and thus will work more. In this way, employers can increase the number of hours of work supplied to them by offering higher wages and better working conditions.

EQUILIBRIUM IN A MARKET

The interaction between consumption and production creates a market. The market for nurses provides an example in Figure 1.6. The supply of nurses will increase as the wages offered to them rise, because the marginal value of work will exceed the marginal cost for a greater number of nurses. This is the line labeled "supply." The demand for nurses will decline as their wages rise, because the marginal revenue that can be generated by nursing labor will be less likely to exceed the marginal cost of nurses—this is the "demand" line in the figure. Wages and the number of working nurses will be balanced where the supply and demand lines intersect, shown as W* and N* in Figure 1.6. If the wage is too low, such as at W_1, then the demand for nurses will be greater than the supply of nurses. Employers will be willing to offer a higher wage, because the marginal revenue generated from more nursing work is greater than the wage. Thus, wages will rise. As wages rise, nurses will be willing to work more, because the marginal revenue of work will be greater than the marginal cost. Similarly, if the wage is too high, the imbalance between supply and demand will tend to push wages down, until the equilibrium of W* and N* is reached.

CHANGES IN EQUILIBRIUM

Because we live in a changing world, it is rare that the equilibrium point of balanced price and quantity is stable over time. Changes in production technology, preferences, and other factors can cause shifts in supply or demand that lead to changes in prices and quantities. It is important to understand these changes because they help us predict what might happen as conditions change.

Figure 1.7 illustrates what happens when there is a change in the demand–price relationship. In this example, demand declines so there are fewer nurses demanded at any given wage. This type of change could occur if there is an increase in the availability of other workers who substitute for nurses, which then would reduce hospitals' willingness to pay for nurses. Or, if the revenue from hospital care drops, hospitals can earn less money for each patient and thus their demand for nurses might drop. When the demand line shifts, there is greater supply than demand

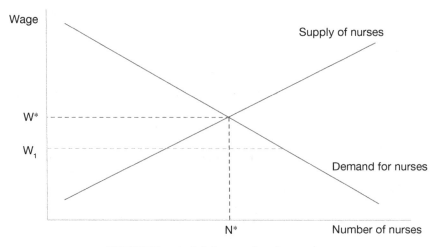

FIGURE 1.6 A labor market for nurses.

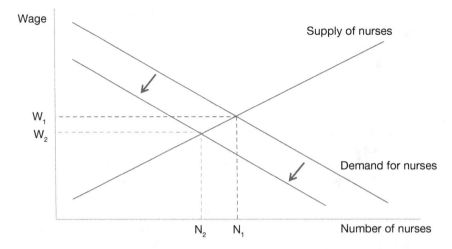

FIGURE 1.7 Change in equilibrium when there is a decline in demand.

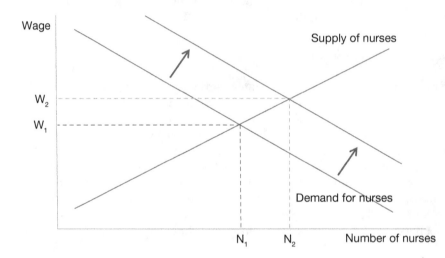

FIGURE 1.8 Change in equilibrium when there is an increase in demand.

at the old price of W_1. As a result of the excess supply, wages will decline, and the end result will be lower wages (moving from W_1 to W_2) and lower employment (from N_1 to N_2).

Demand can also increase, as in Figure 1.8. This can occur if, for example, hospitals decide that employing more registered nurses will lead to higher quality, and thus will help to bring more business to the hospital. At the same wage, hospitals will want to employ more nurses; this is represented by an upward shift in the demand line. The old wage W_1 is "too low," and hospitals will push wages upward as they compete against each other to hire nurses. As the wage rises to W_2, more nurses will choose to work, and the market will reach a new equilibrium at W_2 and N_2.

Supply shifts occur in labor markets as well. If there is a large influx of nurses, such as when nursing schools expand rapidly, there are more nurses available to work at the same wage. This is depicted in Figure 1.9 as a shift to the right of the supply line. Employers will find that they can hire the number of nurses they want at a lower wage, so wages will drop. And, when the wage is lower, employers will want to hire more nurses. Thus, the wage will decline from W_1 to W_2, and the number of employed nurses will rise from N_1 to N_2.

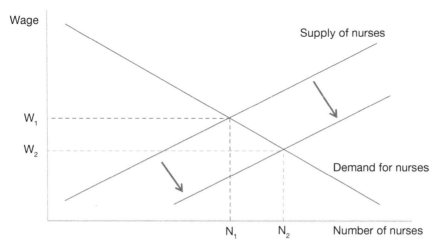

FIGURE 1.9 Change in equilibrium when there is an increase in supply.

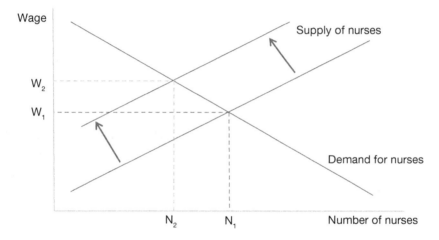

FIGURE 1.10 Change in equilibrium when there is a decrease in supply.

A drop in the supply of nurses—such as a large wave of retirements—would move the supply line in the opposite direction. Figure 1.10 illustrates this scenario. At the wage W_1, there is greater demand for nurses than supply, and thus wages will be pushed upward to W_2. At this higher wage, employers will not be able to afford to hire as many nurses, so the employment of nurses will drop.

When predicting the effects of changes in the labor market, one must be careful to not confuse changes that occur along existing supply and demand relationships with changes that occur due to shifts in supply and demand. If there has not been a fundamental change in the number of nurses who are willing to work at a certain wage, or in the number that employers want to hire at that wage, the market could still be out of equilibrium if wages are too high or low. This could occur if, for example, a union negotiates a better benefits package, so that overall compensation rises. As depicted in Figure 1.11, this would move the "wage" (or total compensation) from W_1 to W_2, and at W_2 there are more nurses willing to supply their work than demand. Over time, the employer will strive to reduce overall compensation—perhaps by limiting wage increases or reducing other benefits—until the total compensation has returned to W_1 and the market is in balance again.

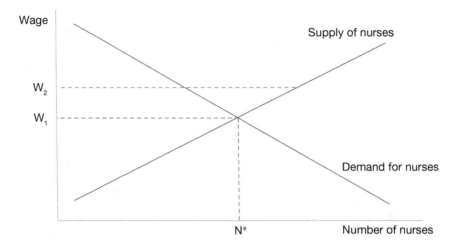

FIGURE 1.11 Change in equilibrium when there is not a fundamental change in supply or demand.

THE CONCEPT OF A "PERFECT MARKET"

When there is an imbalance between demand and supply, the price of the product or service will adjust to rectify the imbalance. In the examples, shortages or surpluses of nurses pushed wages higher or lower, which would end the shortage or surplus. When this type of adjustment can occur naturally, the market is described as "perfectly competitive" or a "perfect market." For a market to be perfect in this sense, the market needs to have several attributes.

First, there needs to be many buyers and sellers of the product or service. When there are many nurses willing to work, and wages are too high, some of those nurses will be willing to accept a lower wage to get a job—and if they do not, then another nurse will get the job. Similarly, if there are many employers, and wages are too low, then at least one employer will raise wages in order to attract more nurses—and other hospitals will follow suit. But, if there is only one employer, the employer may (correctly) believe that he or she does not need to raise wages to compete against other employers, and instead will permanently report they cannot find enough nurses to work.

Second, sellers and buyers of products or services need to be able to enter or exit the market freely. If it is difficult for a person to start selling a product, then it will be difficult for the supply to rise even if the price increases. Similarly, if it is difficult to become a buyer, then even if prices drop, there may not be an increase in demand.

Third, the product or service being exchanged in the market needs to be homogeneous—in other words, the quality and characteristics of the product need to be identical. If products have different quality, then price differences can emerge and this can affect overall movements of wages.

Finally, buyers and sellers need to have perfect information about the attributes of products, prices, and effect of the product on their own marginal utility. If such information is not well known, then buyers and sellers might inadvertently estimate that the price should be higher or lower than what would create equilibrium.

▦ HEALTH CARE IN THE ECONOMIC FRAMEWORK

Although a large body of economic theory and research focuses on perfect markets, most health economists believe that perfect markets do not exist in most aspects of health care. First, there often are not many buyers or sellers in a health care market. In our nursing labor market example, we know that nurses must be licensed to practice registered nursing, and there are a limited number of people who have met the qualifications for licensure. Health care settings that employ nurses, such as hospitals, require large capital investments, licensure, and a sufficient demand from potential patients to continue their operations. Thus, there are a limited number of employers able to purchase nursing labor. In the long term, the number of nurses can increase, as can the number of employers, but in the short term the market is not perfectly competitive.

Second, there is not free entry or exit in the health care market. People do not demand most health care services on a whim, and thus demand for things such as surgery or oncology does not rise or fall much as prices change. In fact, the need for services has a random component, which is why people seek health insurance. Those who offer health care products and services, such as physicians and hospitals, cannot choose to do so at any time. They must go through licensing, training, construction, or other processes that inhibit entry into the market. Pharmaceutical products and medical devices are patented, so companies that might want to sell a drug or device must go through a product licensing and regulatory process to enter the market as a seller.

Third, the products and services provided in the health care sector are not homogeneous. NPs, RNs, physicians, and other professionals have unique skills and each offers somewhat different products. One NP might be an excellent communicator, whereas another might excel at diagnosis. Artificial joints have different qualities, which creates different, smaller markets that are less competitive. And, those who demand health care services and products—patients—are not homogeneous. Each patient has different needs, and different preferences. Patients respond differently to pharmaceuticals, they recover differently from surgery, and they make different choices about end-of-life care.

Fourth, health care is rife with imperfect information. People do not know when they might be diagnosed with an illness or have an accident that requires medical care. There is often uncertainty about diagnosis and the best course of treatment. Patients can find it difficult to get accurate information about the quality of care provided by health professionals, hospitals, nursing homes, and other care providers. Across nearly every dimension of health care, there is a lack of information that inhibits markets from functioning well.

IMPERFECT COMPETITION IN NURSING LABOR MARKETS

Many of the problems that affect the market for health care in general can be found in the nursing labor market. As discussed earlier, there are a limited number of employers of nurses, and there are restrictions on the entry of nurses into the profession. Licensure requirements cause delays between increases in wages and increases in supply, which can cause a shortage to persist for several years. Thus, if there is an increase in demand, as in Figure 1.8, the adjustment to the new wage W_2 may take several years, and during that interim shortages will be reported. This is thought to be an important explanation for recurrent shortages in the RN labor market (Brewer, 1996; Buerhaus, 1991; Yett, 1975).

Moreover, employers can be slow to react to changes in the labor market. When there is a shortage, employers should increase wages to induce more nursing supply. However, employers' ability to raise wages is often tied to annual budgeting processes, so they might be slow to offer higher compensation. They also may be in multiyear contracts with unions, and feel that they should wait until the next contract negotiation to make changes to wages. These delays in wage increases further slow the adjustment of the labor market.

When employers increase wages in response to a shortage of nurses, they should also reduce their demand for nurses. However, they may be unwilling or unable to adjust staffing (Spetz & Given, 2003). They may believe that good staffing is important for securing and maintaining insurance contracts and a steady flow of patients. They also may face regulations that prevent

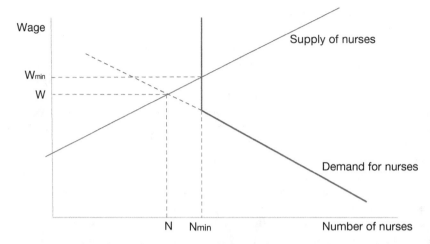

FIGURE 1.12 The effect of minimum staffing regulations on the nurse labor market.

them from reducing staffing, such as in California where there are minimum nurse-to-patient staffing regulations. This scenario is depicted in Figure 1.12. The supply line appears as it is in the classic model, but the demand line is kinked, so that demand is never lower than N_{min}. If demand were not regulated, the market would be in equilibrium at wage W and number of nurses N. However, because demand cannot go below the minimum, demand is stuck at N_{min}. This forces the wage to be W_{min}, which is higher than the competitive wage. Research on California's minimum staffing regulation has found that RN wages in California rose more rapidly compared with other states after the regulation was implemented, which would be predicted by this model (Mark, Harless, & Spetz, 2009).

When there is a surplus of nurses, such as in Figure 1.11, wages are even slower to decline. It is rare for employers to force a reduction in wages on employees. What occurs more often is stagnant or slow wage growth, which is outstripped by increases in the cost of living. Thus, over time, inflation-adjusted wages gradually decline. This was observed in the mid-1990s, when demand for nurses dropped as managed care health insurance expanded. RN wages did not keep up with inflation, so that between 1993 and 1997 average inflation-adjusted wages had declined (Spetz, 2004).

THE ROLE OF HEALTH INSURANCE

Health insurance plays an important role in the health care system of the United States. In order to understand how insurance impacts the economics of health care, one must first consider the purpose of insurance. All types of insurance are intended to protect people from risks, primarily financial risks. People purchase insurance for their homes so that they do not suffer an enormous financial loss if there is a fire, and auto insurance protects them from the cost of repairing their car and paying medical bills in the event of an accident. Note that insurance does not normally cover the cost of regular home or car maintenance, nor does it prevent calamities. It simply provides financial protection.

Insurance is a normal market response to uncertainty and risk, and naturally will occur in a competitive market when such uncertainty exists. However, the existence of insurance can change people's behavior in important ways. If a person has auto insurance, he or she may be less concerned about whether he or she is parking his or her car in an area prone to auto burglaries. Similarly, if a person has health insurance, he or she may be less concerned about certain health-related risks, because the cost of care is covered.

More importantly, many health insurance plans cover not only the costs associated with major health events, but also the costs of routine care. The addition of routine care coverage to insurance probably has its roots in both an effort by insurance companies to compete for customers and the belief that paying for routine care might prevent higher cost care in the future. But, when people have insurance coverage for every visit they might make to the doctor, the price of seeking care has dropped for each visit. In other words, the *marginal cost* of seeing the doctor is lower. This will lead people to seek more care than if they had to pay the full cost directly, because the marginal cost is more likely to be below the marginal benefit. Even if the price of the health insurance plan more than makes up for the cost of each office visit, the prepaid nature of insurance changes behavior on the margin. Economists call this "moral hazard."

THE FUNDAMENTAL PROBLEM OF HEALTH CARE POLICY

The combination of health insurance and moral hazard creates a problem that every nation with a developed economy faces. Insurance is a natural response to uncertainty and risk, such as exists in health care, and thus it is a normal product in a developed economy. Insurance, however, creates moral hazard. Figure 1.13 illustrates this. The diagonal line is a stylized depiction of the marginal benefit of health care. For most types of health care services, as with most other products, the marginal benefit to the patient declines and the quantity consumed rises. The first visit to the NP can have very high value to the patient, but the 10th visit has much less value, on the margin. In this example, the true cost of care is the same for all levels of consumption, at C_1, which reflects all the costs of the personnel, equipment, and supplies used to deliver health care. In truth, there might be economies of scale, so the marginal cost of providing health care is declining, but for this example we assume the marginal cost is constant.

If there was not health insurance, patients would pay the true economic cost, C_1, and they would thus demand health care at the point where the marginal cost and marginal benefit are equal—at Q_1. However, people do have health insurance. Even if health insurance requires the patient to pay a portion of the cost of care—such as a 10% co-payment—the marginal cost the patient pays for each service, C2, is well below the true cost of C_1. And, at this lower marginal cost, the patient will demand much more care, at Q_2. This is not only more care than the individual would otherwise demand, but it is more care than is optimal for the economy as a whole. The full marginal cost to society is C_1, but with patients demanding Q_2 care, there is a large difference between the social optimum and the actual consumption. This places a large opportunity cost

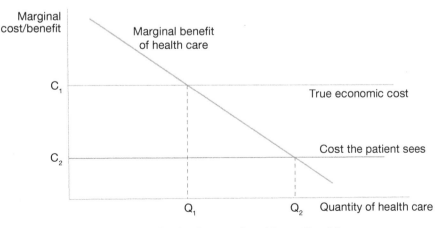

FIGURE 1.13 The fundamental problem of health care.

on society, with resources diverted in a suboptimal way from other things—such as schools, parks, and personal purchases—toward health care.

Whether a nation has a single-payer health care system, with the government controlling nearly all health care services and financing the system through taxes, or a nation has a multi-payer, market-based system such as in the United States, it will face this problem. Nations with highly controlled and centrally financed health care systems often try to address this problem by establishing controls over how much care people can receive. This might involve explicit ration-ing or implicit controls such as limiting the number of hospital beds available in a community. In nations with less coordinated health care systems, it can be harder to address this problem. In these countries, the public is generally unwilling to accept strict rationing or government con-trol, and insurance companies have little need to control expenditures because they can simply charge higher annual premiums to make up the difference.

U.S. HEALTH FINANCING AND REFORM

HOW HEALTH CARE IS FINANCED IN THE UNITED STATES

Health care spending in the United States reached $3.2 trillion in 2015, amounting to 17.8% of the nation's gross domestic product (GDP; Martin et al., 2017). Growth in health care spending was more than 6% per year from 2000 to 2007, and then dropped to lower levels from 2009 to 2013 ranging between 2.9% and 4.1%, as shown in Figure 1.14. However, spending growth increased again in 2014, at 5.3%, and again in 2015, at 5.8% (Martin et al., 2017). The slowdown in health spending growth followed the economic recession that began in December 2007, coinciding with a slow economic recovery. The uptick after 2014 occurred as there were expansions in health insurance coverage due to the Affordable Care Act of 2010 (ACA), which was designed to expand health insurance coverage for poor adults, near-poor individuals and families, early retirees, young adults, the self-employed, and those working in small businesses that do not offer health insur-ance to employees. This legislation is discussed in more detail next.

The U.S. health care system is financed through a mix of public (government) and pri-vate payments (Figure 1.15). The main government programs that support health care are the

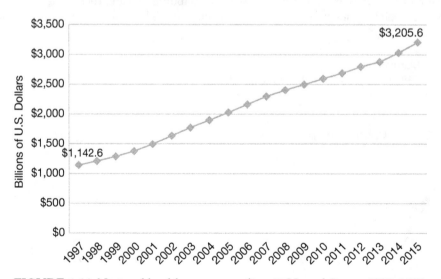

FIGURE 1.14 National health care expenditures, United States, 1997–2015.

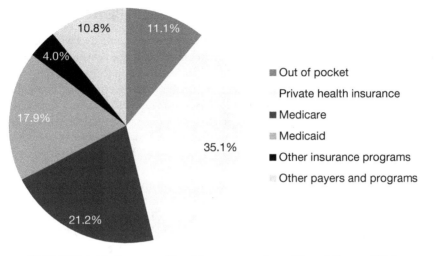

FIGURE 1.15 Sources of health care spending, United States, 2010.

Medicare program, which provides health insurance for the elderly and disabled, and Medicaid, which offers health insurance to people and families with low incomes and/or disabilities. Medicare was established in 1965 to provide hospital and outpatient insurance for people 65 years and older, as well as those who are disabled. The portion of Medicare that covers hospital care is fully funded by the federal government with automatic enrollment. Medicare insurance for outpatient care and pharmaceuticals is voluntary, partially subsidized by the government and partly paid by enrollee insurance premiums.

Medicaid also was established in 1965, and is a partnership between the federal and state governments. The federal government offers funds to participating states, at a rate that varies according to the state's poverty rate and other characteristics. A related program called the State Children's Health Insurance Program was created in 1997 to provide health insurance to children in households who do not qualify for Medicaid, but have low household incomes, making private insurance difficult to purchase. Together, these programs insured 39% of children in 2015 (Kaiser Family Foundation, 2017).

Private health insurance accounts for about 35% of health spending (Martin et al., 2017). About 56% of nonelderly adults and children receive health insurance provided by employers (Barnett & Vornovitsky, 2016), although this share has dropped from 67% in 1999 (Long, Rae, & Claxton, 2016). Employer-sponsored health insurance has its origins during World War II, when employers faced wage controls but could compete for scarce labor by offering better benefits. A small but growing share of people purchase health insurance independently. Most insurance plans require that patients pay a portion of costs out of pocket, through deductibles, co-payments, and coinsurance. Most employers also require that their employees pay a portion of health insurance premiums.

Many Americans do not have any type of health insurance, and rely on a mix of publicly funded community and public health programs, charity care, and self-payment to support medical care. The elderly are guaranteed insurance through Medicare, but 22% of nonelderly adults and 8% of children were uninsured in 2010. The number of uninsured nonelderly Americans declined precipitously between 2010 and 2015 as the ACA was implemented, to 13% of adults and less than 5% of children (Ward et al., 2016). The uninsured usually receive some medical care services, particularly if they have an urgent need. However, their ability to obtain primary and preventive care services is usually limited (Hoffman & Paradise, 2008).

WHY MIGHT CHANGES IN THE U.S. HEALTH SYSTEM BE NEEDED?

The health care system of the United States fares poorly when compared with other developed nations in the areas of cost, equity, and health outcomes. First, the costs of the U.S. health system exceed those of other countries by a wide margin, measured both in per capita terms and as a share of GDP. Growth in health care costs has routinely exceeded overall economic growth, raising concern that the health care system will consume a greater share of our national economic activity. The sustainability of this trend is uncertain. Second, many Americans do not have health insurance and rely on a mix of poorly coordinated public and private services to obtain minimal care. The inequity in access to basic health care services, and impact of this inequity on public health, is viewed by many as worrisome.

Finally, despite having the most costly health system in the world, numerous studies find that the U.S. system performs poorly relative to other countries (Banks & Smith, 2011; Davis, Schoen, & Stremikis, 2010; Docteur & Berenson, 2009). The United States does not do well in the areas of quality, efficiency, or overall population health. Life expectancy in the United States is at or below the average of other developed countries (Docteur & Berenson, 2009), and the United States has the highest rate of deaths for conditions that could be prevented or treated successfully.

THE HISTORICAL CONTEXT OF HEALTH REFORM

Significant changes to the U.S. health care system have been considered for decades. The establishment of Medicare and Medicaid in 1965 was a response to problems among the elderly and poor in purchasing health insurance and receiving needed health care services. In 1972, President Nixon proposed national reform that would have mandated that employers offer health insurance to all their employees. President Clinton again proposed an employer mandate in the 1990s, to address the inequity of access to care. He also recommended other changes to control health care costs through market-based approaches. The intention of those changes was to increase people's sense of the true economic costs of health care, so that there would be movement toward the social optimum depicted in Figure 1.13. Finally, in 2010, the ACA was passed and signed by President Obama. However, there remained substantial resistance to the ACA among the Republican Party and, after the election of President Trump, efforts have been redoubled to repeal the ACA and implement different health system policies.

To understand why the situation of the U.S. health care system has been viewed as needing reform, one must understand how the system arrived at its present state. As noted earlier, Medicare and Medicaid were established to address inequities for seniors and the poor. In the years following their establishment, health care expenditures in the United States grew more rapidly than anybody had forecasted. With the majority of the population insured, there was no limit to the amount and types of health care that could be demanded, because most people did not see the true marginal cost of care. Throughout the 1960s and 1970s, insurance had no price controls, no lists of preferred providers, and no formulary. A patient could go to any doctor they wanted, and the doctor could bill Medicare or another insurer whatever she or he wanted. The same was true for hospital care. With no controls on the bills submitted to insurers and Medicare, new treatments and technologies were developed to address an ever-broadening array of ailments.

By the early 1980s, the federal and state governments began to act to address rampant cost growth in health care. California and other states passed laws that allowed for the growth of managed care insurance plans, in which insurance companies could develop their own networks of providers and restrict patients' choice of doctors and hospitals. In theory, insurance companies would bargain with doctors and hospitals to keep costs down, and employers would prefer these insurance plans because they lowered the cost of providing health benefits to their employees. Also in the early 1980s, Medicare introduced the first in a series of reforms that changed the fee-for-service payment system to one of prospectively determined payment rates, based on patient diagnoses and services provided.

After these changes, insurance companies rapidly developed networks of physicians and hospitals that were willing to accept lower payments for services. Occupancy rates at hospitals dropped because hospitals had an economic incentive to treat patients in the outpatient setting or with shorter hospital stays. Cost savings during the 1980s largely came through lower payments to hospitals and physicians, and most people who signed up for a health maintenance organization (HMO) in the 1980s found little restriction in their choice of doctor or hospital.

By the early 1990s, these easy cost reductions had been tapped; in order to further control costs, insurance companies became more aggressive, and health care providers consolidated. Physicians joined medical groups and independent practice associations (IPAs) so they could better manage their contracts with insurance companies. Hospitals joined multihospital systems so they could purchase supplies in bulk and bargain with insurers as a group. Some of these hospital organizations joined forces with physicians' groups, either through loose alliances or outright purchases. As these large groups negotiated with insurance companies, insurers continued to establish contracts with the lowest priced physician groups and hospital systems. National health expenditures grew in the 1990s at the lowest rates seen in over 30 years.

However, patients did not like the restrictions of these "managed care" insurance plans. They found their choice of doctors and hospitals more limited, and many patients complained that their insurance companies were micromanaging their medical care. By the end of the 1990s, the focus on reducing health care costs had waned substantially, and incentives to control utilization of health services lost favor. The insistence of patients that they receive better access to their doctors, quicker services from laboratories and hospitals, and unfettered use of the newest and best technologies led to the return of double-digit increases in health care costs, but little improvement in health outcomes. By the late 2000s, national health reform returned as an issue in the presidential election, and Congress passed and the president signed the ACA in 2010.

THE AFFORDABLE CARE ACT

The ACA was based on the previous mix of financing of health insurance in the United States (Kaiser Family Foundation, 2010). The main impact of the ACA was in the area of extending health insurance to nearly all Americans, using a variety of strategies. A centerpiece of the ACA was a mandate that all U.S. citizens and legal residents have health insurance. The intention of this mandate was to prevent people from choosing to not buy insurance, and then later getting care that would be paid for by the government and other payers. The ACA enacted a mix of policies to make health insurance affordable for various populations. An employer mandate (for employers with more than 50 full-time employees) was intended to lead more people to obtain health insurance through their workplaces. Small businesses that offer health insurance would receive tax credits to purchase health insurance for their employees (Kaiser Family Foundation, 2013).

States were given the opportunity to expand Medicaid to a larger number of lower income people, offering the program to all people with incomes up to 133% of the federal poverty level, with at least 90% of the cost paid by the federal government (Kaiser Family Foundation, 2013). Existing State Children's Health Insurance Programs also expanded. However, despite the significant financial incentive to expand Medicaid, only 32 states elected to do so (FamiliesUSA, 2016). It has been estimated that an additional 6.2 million people would have had health insurance in 2016 if all states had expanded Medicaid (FamiliesUSA, 2016).

Finally, states were expected to develop "health insurance exchanges" to make shopping for individual and small-group insurance easier (Kaiser Family Foundation, 2013). By grouping individuals and small groups together, the exchanges created purchasing pools similar to those of large businesses that buy health insurance for their employees. They also made it easier for individuals and small businesses to compare health insurance plans. Finally, and most importantly, they provided a mechanism for offering federally funded subsidies to individuals and families who did not qualify for Medicaid, but who might find health insurance unaffordable because their incomes are relatively low. States could elect to develop their own exchange or rely on a federal exchange. Eleven states and the District of Columbia established their own exchanges, 18 states relied entirely on the federal exchange, and the remainder worked with varying state–federal partnership strategies (The Commonwealth Fund, 2015).

Various protections were provided to Americans through the ACA, including prohibitions on insurance companies discontinuing policies of those who become ill, guaranteeing that insurance would be offered to those with preexisting conditions, and elimination of limits on the lifetime benefits received by enrollees. Families were permitted to enroll children in their health plans until age 26. Health insurance plans offered to individuals, small groups, and through the exchanges were required to offer a minimum set of benefits, including ambulatory care, emergency services, hospitalization, pregnancy/maternity care, mental health and substance use disorder services, prescription drugs, rehabilitative services and devices, preventive and wellness services, and pediatric dental and vision care. Most private health insurance plans will be required to provide preventive services without cost sharing by enrollees. In order to further expand access to care for the poor and people living in communities with low access to health services, there was greater funding to community health centers, school-based health centers, and nurse-managed health clinics.

COST CONTAINMENT

The insurance and access expansions of the ACA addressed concerns about inequity in the U.S. health care system, but the ACA did less to address controlling costs. The cost containment mechanisms of the ACA were generally framed as efforts to improve overall efficiency or increase the value of the health services received. Some of these approaches encouraged innovations and pilot projects, whereas others accelerated Medicare's movement into *value-based purchasing* (VBP). In VBP, health care providers are given financial incentives to improve the quality of care they provide—either a loss of funds for poor-quality care, or greater payment for high-quality care. The fee-for-service payment approach historically used in the United States gives health care providers an incentive to focus on the volume of care they deliver rather than the value of care. In this context, value is often described as outcomes such as quicker recoveries, fewer readmissions, lower infection rates, and fewer medical errors. Changes in the organizational and financial incentives health care providers face are anticipated to achieve better outcomes at a lower cost (Cosgrove, 2013).

Medicare had already implemented some VBP programs prior to passage of the ACA (Lindenauer et al., 2007; Mehrotra, Damberg, Sorbero, & Teleki, 2009). One of the early Medicare programs was the Hospital Inpatient Quality Reporting Program, which was established in the Medicare Prescription Drug, Improvement, and Modernization Act (MMA) of 2003. The Centers for Medicare and Medicaid Services (CMS) was authorized in this legislation to pay hospitals more if they reported selected quality measures and eventually to penalize them if they did not report (CMS, 2013). In 2008, CMS stopped reimbursing hospitals for adverse events and conditions occurring during hospital stays, such as surgical site infections, serious pressure ulcers, and blood transfusion incompatibility (National Conference of State Legislatures, 2008). These programs evolved into the CMS Hospital Value-Based Purchasing (HVBP) program, which provides incentive payments to hospitals based on how well they perform with respect to a selected set of outcomes, and/or how much improvement they achieve toward those outcomes (CMS, 2015b). Outcomes include measures of the process of care, patient experiences as measured through surveys, and patient outcomes such as heart failure mortality rates and hospital-acquired infections.

The ACA had two main provisions to advance VBP. One was the establishment of the Center for Medicare and Medicaid Innovation within CMS. This center funds projects to test, evaluate, and expand innovative payment structures and care delivery approaches with the threefold aim of improving quality, improving health, and controlling costs. The second provision was the creation of the Medicare Shared Savings Program, which was intended to encourage the development of "accountable care organizations" (ACOs). An ACO is an organization of health care providers that is accountable for the quality, cost, and overall care of patients. If ACOs meet quality performance standards and generate financial savings, they will be able to share those savings with CMS (2015a).

Through the Innovation Center, CMS launched a national pilot program to evaluate offering "bundled payments" for patient care, which provide a fixed payment for an "episode of care" that begins prior to a hospitalization and continues through 30 days following discharge from a hospital. Multiple health care settings share these payments in order to streamline transitions between ambulatory and outpatient care, hospitals, and postacute care. The program tested four different models of payment, and included 48 "episodes of care" such as acute myocardial infarction, cervical spinal fusion, and gastrointestinal hemorrhage (CMS, 2016). The evaluation data have shown some reductions in Medicare payments, and in early 2016 CMS made bundled payments for hip and knee replacements mandatory in selected cities. In July 2017, bundled payment programs were scheduled to begin for bypass surgery, acute myocardial infarction treatment, and surgeries for hip and femur fractures in 98 markets but their implementation was delayed by President Trump's administration.

The ACA includes some additional cost control measures. Medicare cost growth will be limited for some types of care, payments to Medicare Advantage plans will be reduced, and fraud will be handled more aggressively. Private insurance plan rate increases will be reviewed, and these plans must dedicate 85% of insurance premiums to patient care. Administration costs will be reduced in part by establishing electronic billing standards that will reduce paperwork.

The degree to which the ACA had a role in the slower health spending growth observed in the United States between 2009 and 2013 is unknown. Most provisions of the ACA had not yet been implemented, and it is likely that lower spending was associated with the recession and slow economic recovery rather than the ACA. During the first 2 years of ACA implementation, cost growth returned to the level seen prior to the recession, likely due to the expanded number of people with health insurance. Whether the ACA might have controlled health care costs in the long term may never be learned.

CHANGES AFOOT

The Republican Party opposed the ACA when it was debated in Congress, and continued to oppose it throughout its implementation. The House of Representatives voted to repeal the ACA six times, and also worked to reduce funding allocations for programs authorized by the ACA. With the election of President Trump and Republican majority control of both houses of Congress, repeal or significant modifications of the ACA appear inevitable.

President Trump proposed several health care reforms during his campaign, including allowing individuals to deduct the full amount of premiums for individual health plans from their federal tax returns, providing block grants to finance state Medicaid programs, and allowing insurers to sell insurance across state lines. Independent analysis of these proposals, when combined with repeal of the ACA, estimate that there would be an increase in the number of uninsured individuals by 16 million to 25 million relative to the ACA (Saltzman & Eibner, 2016).

Several representatives and senators also proposed health reforms in 2016 (Kliff, 2016). Representative Paul Ryan's plan would focus on tax credits as an incentive for individuals to purchase health insurance. It would eliminate the minimum benefits requirements but require that all insurance plans offer insurance that covers preexisting conditions. Insurers would be allowed to charge a higher premium if a person allowed the insurance coverage to lapse. Perhaps more importantly, the proposal would shift Medicaid from offering federal matching funds to states to a block grant program, in which states would receive a fixed amount of money to offer Medicaid to residents. Supporters of block grants argue that this approach would give more control to states to create Medicaid programs that meet their local needs; however, opponents worry about analyses that suggest that 18 million people would lose Medicaid coverage. Senator Orrin Hatch offered a proposal that is similar to that of Representative Ryan in many ways but offered poorer people higher subsidies. Tom Price, who was appointed by President Trump to lead the U.S. Department of Health and Human Services, introduced a bill when he was a representative with fewer protections than Representative Ryan's, and Senator Ted Cruz's proposal left Medicaid intact but repealed much of the ACA's private insurance market reforms. Congress will likely spend a large part of President Trump's first term trying to develop, refine, and implement new health care reforms, whether or not they fully repeal the ACA.

■ CONCLUSION

The economics, organization, and financing of health care have important effects on the work of all health professionals. The disjointed payment system in the United States has made it difficult for policy makers or payers to address the root cause of escalating health care expenditures. The ACA attempted to tackle these issues through a variety of payment reforms and pilot programs. Other possible strategies include making patients more responsible for the costs of their care, while continuing to provide health insurance for the most expensive medical and health care. Within any health care organization, nurses—including advanced practice registered nurses (APRNs)—have multiple opportunities to improve both the quality of care and its efficiency. It is essential that nurses play a central role in defining and evaluating these changes.

CRITICAL THINKING EXERCISES

1. In 2011, it was reported that there was a surplus of registered nurses in many parts of California (Bates, Keane, & Spetz, 2011). Identify possible explanations of the emergence of a surplus. What might have changed in the labor market? How can you depict this in a chart? What changes would switch the labor market to a shortage in the future?
2. Medicare rules pay NPs 85% of the fee paid to physicians for ambulatory care. The ACA offers full payment to NPs for providing preventive services in an outpatient setting. How might this change affect the quality of care? Access? Costs?
3. A growing share of health insurance plans have high deductibles, so that an individual must spend up to $6,450 before insurance begins to pay for services. What problem(s) are these insurance plans trying to solve? Answer this question using economic terminology related to health insurance. For what reasons might these plans be successful? In what ways might these plans backfire?
4. The fundamental problem of health policy is presented in Figure 1.13. Countries that have single-payer or other universal health insurance systems, such as Canada and Germany, face this problem, as does the United States. How might health policy try to address the fundamental problem in the context of universal health insurance? Identify specific programs or strategies that might be used, and consider their potential benefits and drawbacks.

REFERENCES

Banks, J., & Smith, J. P. (2011, October). *International comparisons in health economics: Evidence from aging studies* (RAND Labor and Population Working Paper Series). Santa Monica, CA: RAND Corporation. Retrieved from http://www.rand.org/content/dam/rand/pubs/working_papers/2011/RAND_WR880 .pdf

Barnett, J. C., & Vornovitsky, M. S. (2016). *Health insurance coverage in the United States: 2015.* Washington, DC: U.S. Census Bureau. Retrieved from https://www.census.gov/content/dam/Census/library/publi cations/2016/demo/p60-257.pdf

Bates, T., Keane, D., & Spetz, J. (2011). *Survey of nurse employers in California, Fall 2010.* San Francisco: Philip R. Lee Institute for Health Policy Studies, University of California, San Francisco.

Brewer, C. S. (1996). The roller coaster supply of registered nurses: Lessons from the eighties. *Research in Nursing and Health, 19*(4), 345–357.

Buerhaus, P. I. (1991). Dynamic shortages of registered nurses. *Nursing Economic$, 9,* 317–328.

Centers for Medicare and Medicaid Services. (2013). Hospital inpatient quality reporting program. Retrieved from https://www.cms.gov/medicare/quality-initiatives-patient-assessment-instruments/hospitalquali tyinits/hospitalrhqdapu.html

Centers for Medicare and Medicaid Services. (2015a). Accountable care organizations. Retrieved from https://www.cms.gov/Medicare/Medicare-Fee-for-Service-Payment/ACO/index.html?redirect=/aco

Centers for Medicare and Medicaid Services. (2015b). Hospital value-based purchasing. Retrieved from https://www.cms.gov/Outreach-and-Education/Medicare-Learning-Network-MLN/MLNProducts/ Downloads/Hospital_VBPurchasing_Fact_Sheet_ICN907664.pdf

Centers for Medicare and Medicaid Services. (2016). Bundled payments for care improvement initiative. Retrieved from https://www.cms.gov/Newsroom/MediaReleaseDatabase/Fact-sheets/2016-Fact-sheets -items/2016-04-18.html

The Commonwealth Fund. (2015). *The Affordable Care Act's health insurance marketplaces by type.* New York, NY: Author. Retrieved from http://www.commonwealthfund.org/interactives-and-data/maps -and-data/state-exchange-map

Cosgrove, T. (2013, September). Value-based health care is inevitable and that's good. *Harvard Business Review.* Retrieved from https://hbr.org/2013/09/value-based-health-care-is-inevitable-and-thats-good

Davis, K., Schoen, C., & Stremikis, K. (2010). *How the performance of the U.S. health care system compares internationally.* Washington, DC: The Commonwealth Fund. Retrieved from http://www.common wealthfund.org/~/media/Files/Publications/Fund%20Report/2010/Jun/1400_Davis_Mirror_Mirror _on_the_wall_2010.pdf

Docteur, E., & Berenson, R. A. (2009). *How does the quality of U.S. health care compare internationally?* Wash- ington, DC: The Urban Institute. Retrieved from http://www.urban.org/uploadedpdf/411947_ushealth care_quality.pdf

FamiliesUSA. (2016). *A 50-state look at Medicaid expansion.* Washington, DC: Author. Retrieved from http:// familiesusa.org/product/50-state-look-medicaid-expansion

Hoffman, C., & Paradise, J. (2008). Health insurance and access to health care in the United States. *Annals of the New York Academy of Sciences, 1136,* 149–160.

Kaiser Family Foundation. (2010). *Summary of the new health reform law.* Menlo Park, CA: Author. Retrieved from http://www.kff.org/healthreform/upload/8061.pdf

Kaiser Family Foundation. (2013). *Summary of the Affordable Care Act.* Menlo Park, CA: Author. Retrieved from http://kff.org/health-reform/fact-sheet/summary-of-the-affordable-care-act

Kaiser Family Foundation. (2017). *Health insurance coverage of children 0–18.* Menlo Park, CA: Author. Retrieved from http://kff.org/other/state-indicator/children-0-18/?currentTimeframe=0&sortModel=% 7B%22colId%22:%22Location%22,%22sort%22:%22asc%22%7D

Kliff, S. (2016, November 17). What we know about how Republicans might replace Obamacare. *Vox.* Retrieved from http://www.vox.com/2016/11/17/13626438/obamacare-replacement-plans-comparison

Lindenauer, P. K., Remus, D., Roman, S., Rothberg, M. B., Benjamin, E. M., Ma, A., & Bratzler, D. W. (2007). Public reporting and pay for performance in hospital quality improvement. *New England Jour- nal of Medicine, 356,* 486–496.

Long, M., Rae, M., & Claxton, G. (2016). *Trends in employer-sponsored insurance offer and coverage rates, 1999–2014.* Menlo Park, CA: Kaiser Family Foundation. Retrieved from http://kff.org/private-insurance/issue-brief/trends-in-employer-sponsored-insurance-offer-and-coverage-rates-1999-2014

Mark, B., Harless, D., & Spetz, J. (2009). California's minimum-nurse-staffing legislation and nurses' wages. *Health Affairs, 28*(2), w326–w334. doi: 10.1377/hlthaff.28.2.w326

Martin, A. B., Hartman, M., Washington, B., Catlin, A., & the National Health Expenditure Accounts Team. (2017). National health spending: Faster growth in 2015 as coverage expands and utilization increases. *Health Affairs, 36*(1), 166–176.

Mehrotra, A., Damberg, C. L., Sorbero, M. E. S., & Teleki, S. S. (2009). Pay for performance in the hospital setting: What is the state of the evidence? *American Journal of Medical Quality, 24,* 19–28.

National Conference of State Legislatures. (2008). *Medicare nonpayment for medical errors.* Washington, DC: Author. Retrieved from http://www.ncsl.org/Portals/1/documents/health/MCHAC.pdf

Saltzman, E., & Eibner, C. (2016). *Donald Trump's health care reform proposals: Anticipated effects on insurance coverage, out-of-pocket costs, and the federal deficit.* New York, NY: The Commonwealth Fund.

Spetz, J. (2004). Hospital nurse wages and staffing, 1977–2002: Cycles of shortage and surplus. *Journal of Nursing Administration, 34*(9), 415–422.

Spetz, J., & Given, R. (2003). The future of the nursing shortage: Will wage increases close the gap? *Health Affairs, 22*(6), 199–206.

Ward, B., Clarke, T. C., Nugent, C. N., & Schiller, J. S. (2016). Early release of selected estimates based on data from the 2015 National Health Interview Survey. Retrieved from https://www.cdc.gov/nchs/data/nhis/earlyrelease/earlyrelease201605.pdf

Yett, D. (1975). *An economic analysis of the nurse shortage.* Lexington, MA: Lexington Books.

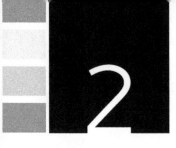

2

Insurance Coverage and Reimbursement in Acute and Nonacute Settings

Carol A. (Reineck) Huebner

". . . health insurance is not insurance in the conventional sense. Rather, it is a system for the collective, long-term prepayment for the costs of health services that each member of the group of people covered will, on average, use during the time period for which he or she is covered. Furthermore, the term is a misnomer in the sense that not much 'health insurance' money actually pays for the maintenance and promotion of health. Rather, most of it goes to cover the costs of care during sickness."

(Goldsteen, Goldsteen, & Goldsteen, 2017, p. 230).

At the time of this writing (2017), landmark changes are happening in health insurance programs. Despite significant legislative uncertainty, fundamental principles remain—primarily value, integration, and quality—on which reimbursement for health care services is increasingly based. This chapter addresses those principles as well as trends and suggestions for doctors of nursing practice (DNPs) navigating an uncertain insurance coverage and reimbursement future.

This chapter is essentially about where the money comes from and where it goes. *Insurance* is one way that health care is reimbursed. "*Reimbursement* is how hospitals and care systems describe payment received for services they have already provided" (Goldsteen et al., 2017, p. 130). Insurance and reimbursement take place within an economic market. As markets go, health care is an imperfect economic market and does not conform to the conventional economic theory of supply and demand.

How is the health care sector so different? Arrow (1963), in his classic work, described these differences as uncertainty, asymmetry of information, and nonmarketability of risks inherent in medicine and medical practice. For example, knowledge is exploding at an exponential rate, yet our understanding remains limited in many areas. With regard to asymmetry, patients often know more about their own history, yet providers know more about disease processes and treatment modalities. A caveat to this, however, is that many consumers are becoming more Internet savvy and come to their appointments equipped with suggestions, questions, and challenges! Finally, nonmarketability of risk means that people behave differently in the health care marketplace when they are insured. This is also termed *moral hazard*. Therefore, in large part based on these three differences—uncertainty, asymmetry of information, and nonmarketability of risk—the financing mechanism in health care represents only one component of health systems. Unlike other countries, the health care financing mechanism in the United States is not centralized from any single source; hence, the complexity.

Health systems have five components (Goldsteen et al., 2017), one of which is the focus of this chapter—the financing mechanism. The other four components of health systems are the facilities; the workforce; the providers of health care therapeutics, including pharmaceuticals and medical equipment; and the educational and research institutions that train the workforce and produce knowledge. Students in DNP and other professional doctoral programs form an integral part of the health care system because they are studying in educational institutions and assimilating new knowledge about how to translate evidence into practice. Again, there is no single national structure dedicated to paying for health care. The focus of this chapter is to organize the complexity surrounding insurance and reimbursement.

▦ OVERVIEW

DNP ESSENTIAL RELATED TO REIMBURSEMENT

The American Association of Colleges of Nursing (AACN) developed essential elements for nursing education curricula at various levels. *DNP Essential II* pertains to organizational and systems leadership for quality improvement and systems thinking (AACN, 2006). Knowledge of business and finance principles, including those related to health insurance and reimbursement, will equip the DNP to collaborate on an interprofessional basis to design systems that optimize reimbursement. Knowledge of payers, documentation, billing and coding processes, and the prospective payment system (PPS) complement the clinical and scientific knowledge base the DNP has developed.

This chapter begins with a focus on *acute care* settings, starting with a discussion of the context in which health insurance operates. Historical foundations of the financing mechanism, followed by a review of relevant *DNP Essentials*, give the reader an understanding of why this is relevant for DNP students. The discussion then proceeds at the macrosystem and presents the view from the executive level in health care organizations and systems. This discussion includes emerging trends as the health sector moves from volume to value, requiring evidence of quality. Experience with the Patient Protection and Affordable Care Act (ACA) of 2010 paves the way for understanding the political dialogue currently underway. Third-party collection in the diagnosis-related groups (DRGs) reimbursement framework for advanced practice nursing is detailed, followed by essential aspects required to optimize reimbursement. Health insurance and reimbursement in *nonacute care* settings follows. Nonacute settings include long-term care, rehabilitation, and several emerging or "revitalized" settings. With the most recent (2016) U.S. presidential election bringing likely repeal of previous health care legislation, current legislative and political issues in health care that are driving reimbursement as well as the role of the DNP in the financing mechanism complete the chapter. A legislative update toward the end of this chapter in the section on Current Issues points to the political difficulty facing health care reform. Knowing where the money comes from and how the money is paid will equip the DNP graduate to appreciate the intricacies involved in transferring payment from consumers to health care providers, organizations, and systems.

ENVIRONMENTAL SCAN

The 2017 Environmental Scan of the American Hospital Association (AHA, 2016, special insert) outlined current and future trends that have an impact on the payment mechanism for health care. This scan is relevant because health care reimbursement does not take place in a neat and orderly system. Rather, payments operate in a vortex of forces, including providers, government, consumer, the economy, technology, workforce, and quality and safety requirements. For example:

- *Providers*—Providers may not be aware that performance measurement for the Medicare Access and CHIP Reauthorization Act (MACRA) payment models begins in 2017 and that fee-for-service payments will be frozen beginning in 2019.
- *Government*—The percentage of reimbursement to providers from Medicare based on quality and value of service, rather than volume, is expected to increase.
- *Consumers*—If only 65% of individuals achieved normal values in prominent areas of health, chronic diseases would be reduced by 80% to 90%, resulting in a savings of $600 billion in health care spending per year. Currently, only 3% to 4% of the U.S. population entering Medicare meets those levels, according to Future Scan 2016–2021.
- *Economy*—Private health care spending continues to increase faster than the economy and is now at 17.4% of the gross domestic product (GDP). That is, nearly 18% of all goods and services produced in the United States are health care related.
- *Technology*—Health care economists estimate that 40% to 50% of annual health care cost increases can be traced to new technologies or the intensified use of old ones. According to Callahan (2008), "Patients expect it, doctors are trained primarily to use it, companies make billions of dollars selling it, and the media love to write about it" (pp. 79–82).
- *Workforce*—The rapid growth in the supply of advanced practice registered nurses (APRNs) and the increased role these clinicians play in patient care delivery are lowering projected shortfalls of physicians.
- *Quality and safety*—Today, a typical health system accepts patients from dozens of payers. Each of these payers has its own measures for evaluating performance. There is an astounding proliferation of quality measures . . . numbering more than a thousand . . . and we will see a renewed effort to align and simplify the measurement cacophony (DeVore, 2015). The quality and safety challenge extends beyond the acute care arena. "Inpatient procedures are shrinking and outpatient procedures are growing at double-digit rates" (Beasley, 2015, p. 23). The quality, cost, and value imperatives form the Triple Aim driving reimbursement (Institute for Healthcare Improvement [IHI], 2017) and require measurement and reporting.

HEALTH INSURANCE

APRNs and advanced specialty nurses are becoming more aware of the need to bill independently for their services. The problem, as cited by Dontje and Forrest (2006), is "when insurance companies either do not recognize Nurse Practitioners (NPs) as providers or reduce reimbursement to a percentage of that allowed to physicians for the same services" (p. 101). The most important take-home point is for APRNs to work toward independent billing and to recognize the strong ties to quality and customer satisfaction that are imperatives in value-based insurance systems.

Reimbursement varies by the source of payment, one of which is health insurance. A health insurance policy is an agreement between a person and an insurance company that lists medical benefits. The insurance company agrees to cover the cost of certain benefits, called "covered services" (FamilyDoctor.org, 2015). Although a certain medical condition may lead a provider to indicate that treatment is needed (medical necessity), the treatment may or may not be covered by insurance. Insurance companies decide what services they will cover. Insurance companies study populations and develop actuarial tables, which are predictions about what kinds of medical conditions may surface among different groups depending on factors including age and health-related behaviors such as smoking.

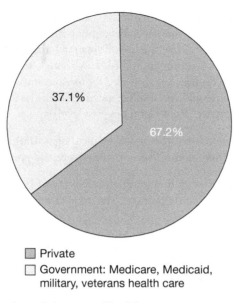

FIGURE 2.1 Percent of people by type of health insurance coverage in the United States.

Note: Percentages exceed 100% because some individuals carry both types of insurance.

Source: Barnett and Vornovitsky (2016).

The main sources of health insurance are the federal government, state governments, commercial insurers, and self-insurance (U.S. Census Bureau, Current Population Survey, 2016 Annual Social and Economic Supplement). The U.S. Census Bureau (2016; report based on 2015 data) reported that of those who are insured, 78.4% had one coverage type and 21.6% had multiple coverage types. Of those with a private plan (67.2%), most (55.7%) are employment based. More than 37% of people carry some sort of government insurance. Among those with any type of coverage, more than 67% have a government plan, primarily Medicare (16.3%), Medicaid (19.6%), military (4.7%), or veterans health care (see Figure 2.1).

The following terms are important fundamental information about health insurance.

Benefit—The amount the insurance company pays when the insured suffers a loss.

Benefit period—The amount of time involved in an individual claim. In the case of hospitalization, this includes the first day of the hospital stay through the day of discharge and often up to 60 days after release from the facility.

Cafeteria plan—Offers a choice between two or more benefits or a choice between a benefit or cash.

Claim—A request to the insurance company to pay benefits for a loss.

COBRA—A federal law (Consolidated Omnibus Budget Reconciliation Act) that allows employees to continue their coverage, through self-pay, after they leave employment.

Co-payment—A small charge the insured pays at the time service is received.

Deductible—The amount of covered expenses the insured must pay out of pocket before the insurance company pays.

Federal poverty level (FPL)—Poverty thresholds are the dollar amounts used by the U.S. Census Bureau to determine *poverty* status. Each person or family is assigned one out of 48 possible poverty thresholds that vary according to the size of the family and the ages of the members. The same thresholds are used throughout the United States. *Poverty* thresholds are updated annually for inflation by the U.S. Bureau of Labor Statistics, using the Consumer Price Index for All Urban Consumers (CPI-U). Although the *poverty* thresholds in some sense reflect a family's needs, they are intended for use as a statistical yardstick, not as a complete description of what people and families need to live. The FPL for one person in 2017 is $11,880 (www.obamacare.net/2017-federal-poverty-level).

Health maintenance organization (HMO)—A medical organization providing a wide range of services for a specified group of enrollees for a fixed, prepaid premium.

Managed care—Coordination of financing and delivery of health care services to produce quality yet affordable health care coverage. Managed care puts limits on the use of services and the charges of providers.

Out-of-network care—Medical services obtained by managed care plan members from non-contracted health care providers.

Preferred provider organization (PPO)—Managed care arrangement consisting of a group of hospitals, physicians, and other providers contracted with an insurer, employer, or other group to provide health care services to covered persons in exchange for prompt payment and higher patient numbers.

Preapproval—The requirement set forth by an insurance company to approve certain care before it is provided.

Denying the claim—When an insurance company does not pay a bill because the service was not covered, or because preapproval or other conditions were not met.

Additional terms and definitions about health insurance coverage and an example at the individual level are available at www.dol.gov/sites/default/files/ebsa/laws-and-regulations/laws/affordable-care-act/for-employers-and-advisers/SBCUniformGlossary.pdf

MAJOR TRENDS

Health care reimbursement continues its shift from a volume-based to a value-based system. The ACA of 2010 resulted in several new payment models that drive this shift toward greater emphasis on quality. The U.S. Department of Health and Human Services (DHHS) aims to tie 50% of payments to these new models by 2018 (Beasley, 2015). Selected alternative payment models (APMs) are introduced as follows:

- Accountable care organizations (ACOs) are groups of health care providers and hospitals that jointly provide coordinated care of the patient population with the goal of delivering higher quality care more efficiently. ACOs rely on health information technology (IT) to measure and report quality indicators.
- The patient-centered medical home (PCMH) moves away from illness-based, episodic care to a system of coordinated primary care.
- Bundled payment, or episode-based payment, ties provider reimbursement to clinically defined episodes of care. It is a "middle ground" between fee-for-service reimbursement and capitation. An overview of the bundled payment model, with inherent risks and rewards, is described further in Table 2.1.
- Hospital Value-Based Purchasing (HVBP) and Hospital Readmissions Reduction Program: By 2018, it is anticipated that 90% of Medicare payments will be tied to quality or value.

The MACRA establishes two separate tracks for physicians and provider organizations to capitalize on their strengths and weaknesses. The two tracks are APMs and merit-based incentive programs (MIPs). An APM is a payment approach that provides additional incentives to clinicians to provide high-quality and cost-efficient care. The MIP is a pay-for-performance (P4P) system (Kaplan, 2016; Van Dyke, 2017), which will include approximately 90 performance measures that will go into effect by 2019. APRNs will be included in MACRA by that time. APMs are growing rapidly and include non–fee-for-service payment structures including ACOs and bundled payment models. MACRA imposes penalties if data are not submitted, up to 9% by 2022. For more information, visit www.qpp.cms.gov.

The Centers for Medicare and Medicaid Services (CMS) estimates that more than 90% of eligible clinicians will be in the MIPs in 2017 versus the APMs. To avoid MIP penalties or to earn bonuses, hospitals and providers will benefit from starting with these steps (Van Dyke, 2016):

1. Recognize the financial impact of bonuses and penalties.
2. Educate clinicians. A MACRA 101 video series is available at www.aha.org/advocacy-issues/ physician/macra-video-series.shtml.
3. Assess current performance on quality, improvement activities, and advancing health information.
4. Create synergies that integrate reporting activities for various requirements.
5. Choose a pace that will include reporting some data, such as one quality measure, to avoid a penalty in 2019.
6. Decide on reporting mechanisms. Some are using electronic health records; others use qualified clinical registries.
7. Report as individuals or a group. Under MIPs, providers can report as individual clinicians or as part of a group practice.
8. Establish clear roles. Establish who is going to do what to ensure Quality Payment Program (QPP) compliance.
9. Prepare for 2018 and beyond. Engage clinicians in improvement activities and decrease variation in practice. Data and analytics need not be the first step.

It should be noted that some health care financial management professionals think that there may be some retraction on MACRA. This remains to be seen.

THE ACA EXPERIENCE

From 2014 to 2017, during the implementation of the ACA of 2010, several unintended consequences arose, which led to the 2017 new presidential administration aiming to repeal and replace this legislation. These unintended outcomes included (a) employers pushing rising costs of health insurance onto employees, creating a shift toward high-deductible plans; (b) increased out-of-pocket expenses; and (c) bad debt and uncollectible balances leading to increased write-offs. The ACA of 2010 aimed to reduce the number of the uninsured. The next section covers this population.

THE UNINSURED

Employers are under significant financial pressure due to high costs and increasing regulation. This results in many employers shifting the burden of health insurance to the employee by either stopping health insurance benefits completely or increasing the share of premiums borne by the employee. Still, 55.7% of employees had health insurance benefits from their employer in 2015 (Barnett & Vornovitsky, 2016). More employees are leaving their employer's plans behind because they have become too expensive. With more uninsured, reliance on the government has increased. An especially vulnerable group within the uninsured is the group of children younger than 18. The ACA aimed to help the uninsured find affordable coverage in insurance exchanges that began in 2014. Health insurance coverage was mandated at that time. This was called the individual mandate.

In 2015, 9.1% of the population, or 29 million people, were uninsured. Three groups make up the bulk of the uninsured: foreign-born residents who are not U.S. citizens, young adults aged 19 to 25, and low-income families with an annual household income of less than $25,000. A provision in 2010 allowed parents to keep their children on their health insurance policy until they are 26 years old. This is one feature that remains popular as new legislation is written.

In a September 2011 report by the AHA, the authors stated, "Economic Futurist Ian Morrison believes that as the payment incentives shift, health care providers will go through a classic modification in their core models for business and service delivery. He refers to the volume-based environment hospitals currently face as the *first curve* and the future value-based market dynamic as the *second curve*. Progressing from the *first curve* to the *second curve* is a vital transition for hospitals" (AHA Committee on Performance Improvement, 2011, p. 3). The top four priorities in the report were (a) hospital physician/provider alignment across the continuum of care, (b) evidence-based practice to improve quality and safety, (c) improved efficiency through productivity and financial management, and (d) development of integrated information systems (AHA Committee on Performance Improvement, 2011, pp. 4–5). The U.S. health care system is now well into the second curve—the *value-based* market dynamic.*

Suppose a patient had joint replacement surgery at Total Quality Hospital (TQH). Under a volume-based paradigm (now obsolete), hospitals and physicians were reimbursed differently based on the number and coding of surgeries, office visits, implants, and related services. Complications sometimes led to more payments to the provider. In contrast, as reimbursement shifts to a value-based paradigm, integrated TQH physician/APRN teams share payment and are penalized for readmissions and complications. In return, these integrated care networks may be rewarded for shared savings, quality improvements, and use of best practices. Potential partnerships with health plans may form to share savings and keep populations healthier.

▨ REIMBURSEMENT

NATIONAL HEALTH EXPENDITURES

Reimbursement to providers takes place in the economic macrosystem involving national health expenditures. How much money are we talking about? In 2013, the United States spent more than $2.919 trillion on health services. This amounted to about 17.4% of the GDP (Goldsteen et al., 2017). The GDP is the total of all the goods and services produced in the country. Unlike countries with a single payer, in the United States all the money paid for health services comes essentially from the general population. How does the money travel from the population to those providing health services? There are three pathways: (a) via government, (b) via insurance and managed care companies, and (c) direct out-of-pocket payment (Goldsteen et al., 2017; Jonas, Goldsteen, & Goldsteen, 2007).

Money from the government, insurance companies and managed care companies, and individual payers goes to different recipients each year—32% to hospitals and 20% to physicians and clinics. The remaining recipients are pharmaceutical and medical nondurable sectors, dental services, and nursing care facilities and continuing care retirement communities (USDHHS,

---

*Insurance Scenario Illustrating Morrison's Volume-Based and Value-Based Curves (Adapted From AHA Committee on Performance Improvement, 2011, p. 8).

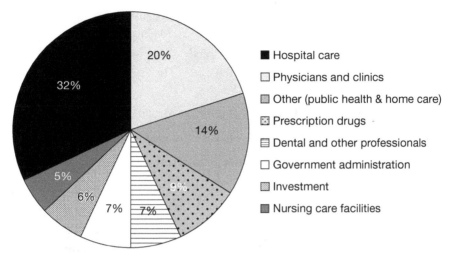

FIGURE 2.2 Distribution of national health expenditures by type of service, 2013.
Source: USDHHS (2014).

2013; see Figure 2.2). Only 3% of the nation's health care dollars go to government public health activities. The United States, unfortunately, still pays more for sick care than preventive care.

THE MACROSYSTEM-THE PROMINENCE OF GOVERNMENT

Nelson, Batalden, Godfrey, and Lazar (2011) view the macrosystems as the "outside in" (p. 332). The most prominent aspect of the macrosystem with regard to financing health care is government. Federal, state, and local governments participate in financing in three ways (Goldsteen et al., 2017).

1. *Direct payment for its own programs*, such as the Department of Veterans Affairs, Department of Defense Military Health System, and municipal hospitals serving the poor. The U.S. DHHS operates more than 100 different programs in 11 operating divisions. The CMS is one of the 11 DHHS divisions (DHHS, 2017).

   State governments also play a role in health care financing, most especially mental illness treatment services and Medicaid operations. Local governments pertain to geographical areas such as a county, city, town, parish, or village.

   To summarize the macrosystem, a classic passage from Dr. Richard Remington (Institute of Medicine [IOM], 1988) poses lingering questions about the proper role of government:

   > But what is the most appropriate nature of that governmental presence? How should government's role relate to that of the private sector? How should governmental responsibility for public health be apportioned among local, state, and federal levels? Should government be the health care provider of last resort or does it have a greater responsibility? Should public health consist only of a necessary residuum of activities not met by private providers? How should governmental activities directed toward the maintenance of an environment conducive to health be apportioned among various agencies? But above all, just what is public health? What does it include and what does it exclude? Based on an appropriate definition, what kinds of programs and agencies should be constructed to meet the needs and demands of the public, which is often resistant to an increasing role, or at least an increasing cost, of government? (IOM, 1988, pp. v–vi in Institute of Medicine 1988 [as cited in Jonas et al., 2007, p. 110]).

2. *Grants and contracts* for biomedical research and medical education.
3. *Payment to providers for delivering care to patients* (e.g., Medicare and Medicaid). These government programs are described in the next section.

The Medicare program is administered by the CMS. The CMS Payment Taxonomy Framework organizes payments into four categories (Beasley, 2015):

Category 1—Fee for service with no link of payment to quality

Category 2—Fee for service with a link of payment to quality

Category 3—APMs built on a fee-for-service architecture

Category 4—population-based payment

More than 50 years old, Medicare has four parts:

1. Hospital insurance (Part A). Part A covers hospital care; limited care in a skilled nursing facility (SNF); and hospice and home health care. Part A is funded mostly from social security taxes.
2. Supplementary medical insurance (Part B). Part B covers physician and certain other health professional services, hospital outpatient care, and certain other services. Part B is funded from general revenues and enrollee premium payments.
3. Medicare + Choice (Part C). Part C permits Medicare beneficiaries to enroll in managed care organizations.
4. Medicare Prescription Drug Coverage (Part D). Part D is funded through premiums.

DRG-BASED REIMBURSEMENT

Although the financing mechanism consists of no single payer, the payment system in the United States today is the PPS. The PPS operates based on DRGs. Financing refers to funding source, whereas payment refers to the method used to move money from consumers to providers. The payment system is prospective in that defined reimbursement for services is set forth first, before the services are provided. The defined reimbursement is detailed in a system of thousands of what are termed DRGs. The hospital receives a preset flat rate for the DRG, regardless of the volume or type of services provided to the patient. The DRG system of codes is described later in this chapter. Entire new occupational specialties are now required to translate clinical care into codes upon which payment is based. Most often, payment is made by an intermediary or "third party."

THE VIEW FROM THE C-SUITE

Uncertainties exist as to how health care reform in the United States will take shape. A 2015 survey by the American College of Healthcare Executives (ACHE) revealed that financial challenges ranked number one on the list of hospital CEO's top concerns (ACHE, 2016). Enhancing quality while managing cost will be closely linked in one form or another to payment, and therefore be of critical interest to health care executives. Three strategies for success in health care organizations were recommended by the Healthcare Financial Management Association (HFMA, 2011b) in its *Education Report* and are still relevant today.

1. Develop structure for clinical–financial collaboration.
2. Create structures that support collaboration across the continuum of care.
3. Focus on improving case management—that is, paying attention to avoiding readmissions and avoidable complications.

THIRD-PARTY COLLECTION IN MANAGED CARE ENVIRONMENTS: PAYER MIX

Payer mix refers to the proportions of payments received from each kind of payer—federal, state, private, or self-pay.

Federal: Medicare—Medicare provides access to care for individuals 65 years of age and older, those younger than 65 with long-term disabilities, and those with end-stage renal disease.

State: Medicaid—Medicaid is a government program serving 70 million people, jointly funded by states and the federal government. "A growing number of states are sharply limiting hospital stays under Medicaid to as few as 10 days per year to control rising costs of the health insurance program for the poor and disabled" (Galewitz & Kaiser Health News, 2011, p. A1). Medicaid, under enormous financial pressure driven by high enrollment and medical costs, is designed to meet the health care needs of children, people with disabilities, and the elderly (DHHS, 2017). Galewitz continues, "To deal with the higher costs, states are pushing Medicaid recipients into managed-care plans run by private insurers, cutting reimbursement rates to hospitals and doctors and reducing benefits" (p. A3). Included in the 70 million Medicaid recipients are 17 million who enrolled since the ACA was instituted in 2010.

Private insurance and self-pay—These constitute the remaining main types of payers. Private insurance companies are trying to merge in some cases, to maintain financial viability.

APRN REIMBURSEMENT

Provider reimbursement can be considered along a continuum representing the financial risk borne by the buyer (patient) and the risk borne by the seller (provider). Any risk not borne by the buyer or the provider is borne by the third-party payer (see Figure 2.3; Goldsteen et al., 2017, p. 134).

"The involvement of the Advanced Practice Registered Nurse (APRN) in the reimbursement process depends on whether the APN is allowed by the applicable state and federal regulations to practice and bill independently and is able to obtain direct reimbursement for those independently delivered services" (Hamric, Spross, & Hanson, 2009, p. 570). Current information about APRNs billing Medicare is available at www.cms.gov/Outreach-and-Education/Medicare-Learning-Network-MLN/MLNProducts/Downloads/Medicare-Information-for-APRNs-AAs-PAs-Booklet-ICN-901623.pdf. The state practice environment is variable with respect to the best environments in which to practice and seek reimbursement for services. Information is available at www.aanp.org/legislation-regulation/state-legislation/state-practice-environment.

TYPES OF PROVIDER PAYMENT

There are six basic types of payments to providers: cost/cost plus, time and materials, fee for service, fixed price, capitation, and value. Providers generally prefer cost/cost plus. Patients and other third-party payers generally prefer value. Figure 2.3 shows that when there is alignment between what kind of payment the patient wants to use and what kind the provider wants, a third-party payer is not necessary because of this alignment. Unfortunately, in the health care market, this alignment is not often realized; hence, the complexity. Each type of payment is briefly defined.

Cost/cost plus—The provider organization is reimbursed for actual costs plus an additional percentage of those costs to generate a margin.

Time and materials—This is an hourly payment method often used when the scope of work is not clear to either party.

Fee for service—When the scope of work is more clear, this is a method most common for the "other professional services" category in the national health expenditures data. A set fee is billed

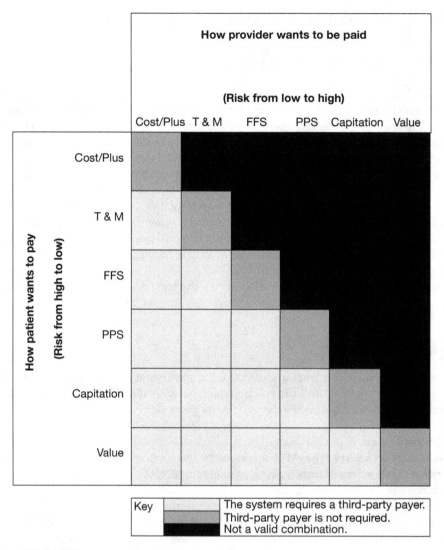

FIGURE 2.3 Provider and patient risk matrix.

FFS, fee for service; PPS, prospective payment system; T & M, time and materials.

Source: Goldsteen et al. (2017).

at the risk of additional services being required at the time of treatment. The local market drives the rates that patients are willing to pay. This method of payment is becoming less frequent as value-based systems of reimbursement become more common.

Fixed price—This approach focuses on a fixed price for treating a certain disease condition. This is the category in which the DRG system falls. The provider is rewarded for efficiency. The dangers of this approach include (a) fraudulent "up-coding" to maximize reimbursement, (b) seeking healthier patients, and (c) paying low priority to prevention. Disease classification determines the amount of payment that will be received (Goldsteen et al., 2017).

Capitation—In this payment arrangement, the provider is paid a fixed amount per member of a health plan per month. The amount is called a capitated rate. This is the common way of paying for Veterans Administration hospitals, state mental hospitals, and local health department clinics (Goldsteen et al., 2017).

TABLE 2.1 Value-Based Reimbursement Options: Overview, Risks, and Rewards of Payment Models

Reimbursement Option	Overview	Risk	Rewards
Pay-for-performance (P4P)	P4P establishes, measures, and reports clinical quality benchmarks. It is emerging as the most commonly used model.	Reduction of unnecessary services may not occur.	Robust information technology (IT) expenditures can be avoided.
Shared savings	This Medicare program rewards providers who reduce total health care spending. Savings are shared between the health care system and CMS.	This model requires upfront IT costs. APRN services may not be covered.	Providers receive a bonus when they reduce costs, but there is no penalty if they fall short.
Bundled payments (BP)	BPs are contracts through which providers are given a budget to cover the estimated costs associated with all the care needed by a patient for a given condition or procedure. Total hip replacement is an example.	Actual costs may exceed negotiated cost.	Providers are automatically rewarded for less costly episodes of care.
Shared risk	In this model, payers and providers determine a budget. Providers receive performance-based incentives.	Providers are liable for a portion of the costs if targeted costs are exceeded.	All stakeholders are motivated to work together to reduce costs.
Global capitation	This is a payment-per-person plan, originated in the 1990s, in which providers accept members for a certain set price. IT advances are helping this model overcome its previous negative reputation.	Providers have significant financial exposure and actuarial risk.	Providers are incentivized to keep members healthy through preventive care.
Provider-sponsored health plans (PSHPs)	In PSHPs, providers assume 100% of the risk by directly collecting insurance premiums from members and providing care.	Health care systems in this model have full power to decide how patients are cared for.	PSHPs may garner increased market penetration and control over population health.

APRN, advanced practice registered nurse; CMS, Centers for Medicare and Medicaid Services.
Source: Adapted from Henkel and Maryland (2015).

Value—Value is the payment model in which the organization providing the services is rewarded for the value delivered. The federal government is increasingly defining value in terms of quality and safety. Hospitals will not be reimbursed for care resulting from avoidable falls, errors, infections, and other adverse events such as readmissions for the same diagnosis within 30 days of discharge. Nelson et al., in their book, *Value by Design* (2011), describe the full scope of value and steps to create it. The authors propose that, going forward, one guiding principle is to change the payment system. They state, "modify health care payments to reward high performing health systems who take responsibility for delivering and improving value and provide incentives for people who take actions to promote health, prevent illness, and intelligently self-manage illness and injury" (p. 325). Nelson et al.'s suggestion is now reality in that payments are currently based on value.

Henkel and Maryland (2015) described six value-based reimbursement options. These options are collectively termed *fee for value* and it is likely that health care systems will experiment with a combination of these models depending on their specific markets. Table 2.1 summarizes the options, provides an overview of each, and gives associated risks and rewards.

Henkel and Maryland (2015) add that health care systems and providers have many value-based models to choose from. These include P4P, shared savings, bundled payments, shared risk, global capitation, and PSHPs. These alternative payment methods are consistent with what the U.S. DHHS (2015) established as a goal—shifting 50% of Medicare payments to alternative models by the end of 2018.

OPTIMIZING REIMBURSEMENT

More than 13,000 diagnostic codes have been developed by CMS. In 2009, the secretary of the U.S. DHHS released a final rule calling for the adoption of a new edition of the *International Statistical Classification of Diseases and Related Health Problems (ICD)* standards known as the 10th edition using Clinical Modifications (CM) and the Procedure Coding System (PCS). *ICD-10-PCS* codes are strictly intended for use by hospitals to report inpatient procedures and would not be used for outpatient or physician billing (AHA, 2009). The codes in *ICD-10* are much more specific than in previous revisions. CMS is no longer being lenient and is scrutinizing codes more carefully (McCarty & Swanson, 2016).

Documentation—To bill for services, insurance companies require the use of specific medical documentation guidelines, classifications, reimbursement codes, and, in the case of the APRN, evidence of current credentials. There is a standard language that is used to record and classify care (Hamric et al., 2009):

1. The evaluation and management (E&M) services guidelines, which have seven components (nature of presenting problem, history, physical examination, medical decision making, counseling, coordination of care, and time)
2. ICD-10-CM codes
3. The *Current Procedural Terminology (CPT)* codes. CPT codes are used for outpatient procedures.

Billing and coding—The structure of ICD-10 codes is more expansive than the ICD-9 codes. ICD-10 codes are three to seven characters in length for coding diagnoses and seven alphanumeric characters for coding procedures. ICD-10-CM codes are used for all inpatient and outpatient diagnoses. ICD-10-PCS codes are used for the hospital inpatient setting only.

Example of *ICD-10* diagnostic code: S12-9XX A

Key to deciphering the code format:

S12 = Category

9XX = Etiology, anatomic site, severity

A = Added code extension (seventh character) for obstetrics, injuries, and external causes of injury

(AHA, 2009, p. 23)

Example of *ICD-10-PCS* Structured Format Procedure Code (Medical/Surgery): 1 2 3 4 5 6 7

Key to deciphering the code format:

1 = Section

2 = Body system

3 = Root operation

4 = Body part

5 = Approach

6 = Device

7 = Qualifier (AHA, 2009, p. 23)

Technology—Payers recognize the need for data to inform them if levels of quality and cost are in an acceptable range. The electronic health record is far from being pervasive in the United States. DNPs will serve an important role to help design and implement these systems, use the systems for data collection to answer empirical questions, and improve the interface between the systems and the people who use them.

HEALTH INSURANCE AND REIMBURSEMENT IN NONACUTE CARE SETTINGS

Nonacute care settings are referred to collectively as alternate care by the Association for Health Care Resource and Materials Management. Alternate care includes:

- Long-term care
  - Skilled nursing, intermediate care, and subacute services
  - Assisted living
  - Community service agencies
- Dialysis or rehabilitation
- Physician offices
  - Primary care
  - Specialty care
  - Owned/managed care
  - Self-operated care
- Home health
- Behavioral health
- Hospice care
- Social services agencies
  - Adult day care
- Other
  - Dental, optometry
  - Schools
  - Correctional facilities

A contemporary (2016) organizing framework for the postacute and complex care settings simply views these settings as either (a) traditional or (b) revitalized. Traditional settings include an acute inpatient rehabilitation facility (IRF), long-term acute care hospital (LTACH), short-stay SNF, home health care, or hospice. Revitalized settings include provider-based house calls, assisted living (AL) adaptation for short-stay joint rehabilitation, complex care coordination clinics, complex care PCMHs, new long-term care insurance products that promote and provide services to age in place, and care transition models (Health Dimensions Group, 2016). Reimbursement for care delivered in these settings is shifting from traditional fee for service toward population health ACO models. The shift is clear—toward increasing value and accountability in which DNPs play a central role.

Issues affecting care in primary care settings include reimbursement, regulatory requirements such as the Health Insurance Portability and Accountability Act (HIPAA), cost increases due to malpractice insurance, the educated consumer, and safety compliance. In long-term care, issues include but are not limited to reimbursement, staffing, compliance reviews, occupancy, and liability.

Most long-term care services are paid for by the government. Medicare and Medicaid together pay for the majority of long-term care. Because Medicaid is funded by both state and federal government, and because state budgets vary, there is significant variation, adding to the overall complexity of services. Ng, Harrington, and Kitchener (2010) referred to this state of affairs as "piecemeal developmental history and shared federal-state responsibility" (p. 22), which confuses both providers and patients. They asserted that the system of long-term care needs structural reform.

When there are multiple payers in health care, this introduces conflicting incentives for providers, which may have negative implications for cost containment, service delivery, and the quality of care (Glazer & McGuire, 2002). Grabowski (2007) described dual-eligible patients caught in this economic confusion. "Many persons who are dually eligible for both Medicare and Medicaid require both extensive acute and long-term care services. However, because Medicare covers relatively few long-term care services, Medicaid must cover the bulk of these expenditures for dual eligibles" (p. 580). The result is that neither government program takes full responsibility for care management. Grabowski (2007) suggested policy options including capitation, P4P, and "federalization," in which the federal government would assume Medicaid's costs for dual eligibles.

A state-by-state scorecard, available at www.longtermscorecard.org, ranks states and the District of Columbia in four areas of long-term care: affordability and access, the choice of settings and providers, quality of life and quality of care, and support for family caregivers. Forty-three percent of discharges receive postacute care, making it necessary for acute care systems to partner with postacute care settings to ensure the care coordination that reimbursement systems increasingly require (Health Dimensions Group, 2016).

The ACA (Public Law 111-148) is the official name for health care reform. Section 3502 of the ACA authorized Medicare "Medical Homes," which are community-based interdisciplinary, interprofessional teams to support primary care practices within a certain area. "Such health teams may include nurses, nurse practitioners, medical specialists, pharmacists, nutritionists, dieticians, social workers, and providers of alternative medicine. Under the program, a health team must support patient-centered medical homes, which are defined as a mode of care that includes personal physicians, whole-person orientation, coordinated and integrated care, and evidence-informed medicine" (American Nurses Association [ANA], 2010, p. 5).

The Independence at Home Program (Section 3024) created a program for "chronically ill Medicare beneficiaries to test a payment incentive and service delivery system that utilizes physician and nurse practitioner-directed home-based primary care teams aimed at reducing expenditures and improving health outcomes. Section 2951 authorized states to establish evidence-based nurse home visitation programs for maternal, infant, and early childhood purposes among high-risk populations" (ANA, 2010, p. 5).

The Health Care and Education Reconciliation Act of 2010 included Section 4101 on School-Based Health Clinics that serve a large population of children eligible for Medicaid (ANA, 2010, p. 6). Legislation concerning long-term care includes Section 6103 Nursing Home Transparency–Nursing Home Compare (www.medicare.gov/nursinghomecompare/search.html?); Section 6105 Whistleblower Protection; and Sections 6101 through 6121 Staffing Accountability (ANA, 2010, p. 7). Section 5208 "established nurse-managed health clinics (centers operated by

APRNs that provide comprehensive primary care and wellness services to underserved or vulnerable populations)" (ANA, 2010, p. 8). Section 10325 addresses Resource Utilization Groups, which are payment rules for skilled nursing facilities (ANA, 2010, p. 9).

CMS issued a new 700-page rule in late 2016, commonly referred to as either "The Final Rule" or "Rules of Participation," a series of guidelines and requirements for long-term care facilities that receive Medicare or Medicaid funding. The new regulations, to be implemented in three phases, represent the most comprehensive update in decades. The new regulations move the long-term-care industry from a fee-for-service system to one that is quality based (Granger, 2017).

■ CURRENT ISSUES

VALUE-BASED PURCHASING

As the AHA states, "the terms P4P and value-based purchasing (VBP) are used to identify various methods that link payments to some measure of individual, group, or organizational performance. An increasing number of purchasers and payers of health care services, including CMS, are embracing P4P/VBP strategies to improve the quality and cost-effectiveness of care while achieving high value for their health care dollars and thereby promoting high value health care" (ANA, 2010, p. 4). The ANA presents 10 principles to guide the nurse in any pay-for-quality discussion (ANA, 2010, p. 10).

Dall, Chen, Seifert, Maddox, and Hogen (2009) reported that "payers are raising reimbursement rates for facilities that provide higher levels of care" (p. 103). The conclusion from their literature synthesis on the economic value of professional nursing is that improved staffing leads to decreased risk and decreased length of stay, which, in turn, result in medical cost savings, improved productivity, and lives saved.

HEALTH CARE REFORM

The Federal Register (www.federalregister.gov) is a comprehensive resource for pending legislation. In a major step forward, legislation in 2016 permitted the Department of Veterans Affairs to allow nurse practitioners (NPs), clinical nurse specialists (CNSs), and certified nurse midwives (CNMs) to practice to the full extent of their education. Read more at www.federalregister.gov/documents/2016/12/14/2016-29950/advanced-practice-registered-nurses.

At the time of the writing of this chapter, five plans competed to be a replacement for the ACA. Their backers promise no disruption in coverage for the 20 million newly insured through Medicaid expansion in 31 states and the health care marketplaces in states. The name given to the new legislation is the American Health Reform Act (2017). Keckley (2017) offers these suggestions for hospital boards and management until this new legislation is enacted or until budget reconciliation takes place: (a) plan on continuation of bundled payments; (b) accelerate cost reduction; (c) manage the triple aim of lowering costs, improving quality, and managing patient experiences through skillful clinical leadership; (d) manage capital and cash; (e) develop systems of health; (f) take care of employee stress; and (g) engage with local, state, and national lawmakers. These coping mechanisms may be helpful for organizations because it is not certain when new legislation will be enacted, appropriated, and implemented. The American Health Care Act of 2017 is a congressional bill to partially repeal the Patient Protection and Affordable Care Act, also known as Obamacare. The Senate vote to amend and move forward the House resolution failed. Had legislation passed the Senate, it would have renamed the legislation as the Better Care Reconciliation Act of 2017, Obamacare Repeal Reconciliation Act of 2017, or Health Care Freedom Act of 2017. Political wrangling continues.

Under BCRA, both the individual and the employer mandate are repealed, premium subsidies are replaced with means-tested tax credits, a "State Stabilization Fund" is established, coverage is preserved for preexisting conditions, and Medicaid expansion would end by 2024. Political wrangling between the major political parties and within the parties prevented a vote on BCRA at the time of this writing. Separating the "repeal" from the "replace" was suggested as a way to increase the likelihood of passage, but that, too, met with disagreement for fear of the uncertainty that would ensue. DNP students may learn more updates from the Kaiser Family Foundation at www.kff.org/health-reform/issue-brief/how-the-senate-better-care-reconciliation-act-bcra-could-affect-coverage-and-premiums-for-older-adults.

ACCOUNTABLE CARE ORGANIZATIONS (ACOs)

ACOs are "groups of doctors, hospitals, and other health care providers, who come together voluntarily to give coordinated high quality care to their Medicare patients. The goal of coordinated care provided by an ACO is to ensure that patients, especially the chronically ill, get the right care at the right time, while avoiding unnecessary duplication of services and preventing medical errors" (USDHHS, 2013). The concept was introduced in the ACA. "Under this model, a network of providers is responsible for quality, cost and overall care of Medicare beneficiaries. The network uses shared savings to promote structural changes in the delivery of care, especially coordination of care across the continuum of care providers. Among its requirements, an ACO must define processes to promote evidence-based medicine and patient engagement, report on quality and cost measures, and coordinate care" (HFMA, 2011b, p. 2). Implementation experiences and rural participation in the ACO concept were explored in a pilot study (Bagwell, Bushy, & Ortiz, 2017). Three themes emerged: (a) ACOs are growing in size and number; (b) there is an expanding emphasis on preventive primary care and chronic disease management; and (c) there is a need for improved IT integration with clinical services and financial systems.

POLITICAL AND ECONOMIC ENVIRONMENT

The National Organization of Nurse Practitioner Faculties (NONPF) is a member organization of the Nurse Practitioner Roundtable. This collaborative includes the American College of Nurse Practitioners (ACNP), the National Association of Pediatric Nurse Practitioners (NAP-NAP), the American Academy of NPs (AANP), the Gerontological Advanced Practice Nurses Association (GAPNA), and the National Association of Nurse Practitioners in Women's Health (NPWH). The Nurse Practitioner Roundtable (2010) advances policy issues and made the following recommendations:

- Support efforts that increase patient access to the full primary care provider workforce and allow for patient choice in provider selection.
- Reengineer reimbursement systems to reflect the true costs of care to ensure that all practice settings, including primary care practices, nurse-managed health centers, and emerging delivery models, can be self-sustaining.
- Promote reimbursement based on services provided.
- Track provider-specific services and outcomes; linking outcomes to specific providers will promote accountability in care.
- Recognize outcomes of care as critical indicators in effective reimbursement models.
- Include NP-led practices and NPs as full partners in medical homes, ACOs, insurance exchanges, and other developing innovations.
- Continue to remove the outdated legislative and regulatory barriers that impede the utilization of NPs to the top of their education and abilities in addressing patient care needs.

Stuart Butler (2016) of the Brookings Institution suggested six aspects of the ACA that need rethinking considering disappointing enrollment in the ACA exchanges and the growth in premiums and out-of-pocket expenses. First, subsidies to make coverage more affordable and understandable need revision. Second, the fact that health insurance expenses cannot be deducted from taxes is troubling and regressive from economists' perspective. Third, the employer and individual mandates to offer or carry health insurance, respectively, need a relook at the state level, with the goal of giving clearer guidance to states regarding use of waiver authority. Fourth, lackluster enrollment in exchange plans needs to be reversed by turning Medicaid into a private option that is a subsidy for purchasing private plans on the exchanges. Fifth, the Independent Payment Advisory Board (IPAB) should be replaced to help contain the Medicare budget. And, finally, sixth, the ACA should promote health rather than simply making health services and insurance more available. "In the future, blending health, housing, transportation, social services, and other budget streams are essential to improve health while reducing the need for costly medical services" (Butler, 2016, p. 496).

The ACA features that have been well received include coverage for preexisting conditions and subsidies for those at the FPL (Mathews & Radnofsky, 2017). The AHA sent a letter (AHA, 2017) to the president of the United States and members of Congress outlining AHA's top priorities as the future of the ACA is being deliberated. The priorities included their requests to (a) ensure continuous coverage during the transition, (b) restore and avoid further reductions to hospitals and health systems, (c) treat Medicaid-expansion and nonexpansion states in an equitable manner, (d) address regulatory reform, and (e) move to fee-for-value-based payment that provides incentives for clinically integrated coordinated care.

INTERPROFESSIONAL IMPLICATIONS: THE IDEAL INTEGRATED DELIVERY SYSTEM (IDS)

Nearly 20 years ago, Shortell, Gillies, Anderson, Erickson, and Mitchell (1999) suggested that an ideal health care system would be fully integrated in an IDS. That is, an IDS would be one in which patients, providers, and payers are well aligned. It is only now that all features of this vision are finally driving reimbursement. The following features characterize Shortell et al.'s (1999) IDS:

1. Serves a defined population.
2. Provides a defined set of services/benefits.
3. Integrates services, administratively and clinically, and has an integrated information system covering all the services offered.
4. For the most part, pays providers on a capitated basis.
5. Has hospital beds and one or more long-term care services.
6. Pools funds coming in from several sources.
7. Has a shared mission, philosophy, and vision.
8. Has centralized and joint planning and management.
9. Provides an organized continuum of care, through health care teams.

Building on the aforementioned view from nearly a generation ago, while looking to the future, Dr. Don Berwick, a former acting administrator at CMS, advocates for a new era in health care, toward a model based on cooperation and prevention versus competition and treatment (O'Connor, 2016). In future IDSs, DNPs will play an important role on the team, especially related to optimizing reimbursement through quality care. To explain, "Clinically integrated systems of care are designed to collect and share data from all participating providers. This process fosters interdependence and collaboration among physicians and other clinicians that can lead to quality improvements and enhanced cost-effectiveness" (Henkel & Maryland, 2015, p. 6). Hallmarks of an IDS are "evaluation, continuous clinical performance improvement, reduction of unnecessary services, and management and support for high-cost and high-risk patients" (Henkel & Maryland, 2015, p. 6).

DNP ROLE RELATED TO REIMBURSEMENT

The DNP is in a strategically important position to optimize reimbursement through effective clinical leadership to promote clinically effective, evidence-based care. The IOM imperatives (IOM, 2001, p. 1) are to provide care that is safe, timely, effective, efficient, equitable, and patient centered. All imperatives require clinical leadership.

Safe—Patient safety is defined by the IOM as "freedom from accidental injury; ensuring patient safety involves the establishment of operational systems and processes that minimize the likelihood of errors and maximizes the likelihood of intercepting them when they occur" (IOM, 2000, p. 211).

Timely—Timely care is provided to align length of stay with reimbursable arrangements. Optimizing patient flow and reducing waiting times and delays for both providers and patients are aspects of timely care (HFMA, 2011a).

Effective—Care that produces the desired or intended results. For example, hospitals intend treatment to be accomplished without infection. Preventing infection is challenging, but imperative. The financial cost of infection is staggering. Approximately 2 million patients acquire a nosocomial infection each year, resulting in 80,000 deaths and adding $5 billion to the U.S. health care costs every year (IOM, 2000). Data from the Centers for Disease Control and Prevention (CDC, 2016) suggest that nosocomial infections are declining in both acute care and nonacute care settings, but more improvement is needed. DNPs who focus on infection control play a significant role in this daunting area of concern. Knowledge of how to enhance organizational adherence to infection control guidelines is a key capability of DNP graduates. The federal government and most insurers will no longer reimburse for days of stay resulting from preventable infections.

Efficient—Care that reduces quality waste (e.g., unnecessary tests) and reduces administrative or production costs (e.g., multiple entries, complex classification, layers of control).

Equitable—To improve health status and to do so in a manner that reduces health disparities.

Patient centered—"Encompasses qualities of compassion, empathy, and responsiveness to the needs, values, and expressed preferences of the individual patient" (IOM, 2001, p. 48).

Patients may be confused with their insurance coverage and billing, and will look to the DNP to listen to their concerns. Lankford (2017) states that the Alliance of Claims Assistance Professionals (www.claims.org) offers free consultation and basic advice. Help with billing, coding, and coverage questions is available at www.medicalclaimshelp.org. Patients may also experience health literacy challenges. The Kaiser Family Foundation identified three concerns: (a) people's ability to determine their coverage eligibility and navigate the enrollment system; (b) the broad choice of plans and people's ability to compare insurance plans and coverage; and (c) once people are enrolled, it is a challenge for them to use their coverage to connect to the care they need (National Academy of Science, 2016).

Cost reduction is a key role of the DNP. Cost reduction involves (a) reducing variation by standardizing protocols; (b) removing unnecessary care by reducing errors, preventable readmissions, avoidable conditions, and unnecessary tests; (c) restructuring costs to use the lowest cost setting and provider possible for each service; and (d) adopting a system of care strategy such as medical homes and disease management that will reduce the overall need for hospital services. The DNP is a key leader to standardize protocols, minimize unnecessary care, advocate for the lowest cost setting and provider, and focus on chronic disease management (Larkin, 2011).

The DNP plays a crucial role in chronic care management. RPG Group's Bill Bellenfant stated, ". . . the greatest opportunity to derive added value from health care today is in how we treat those with chronic conditions. How strong are our programs for managing diabetes? What are we doing for patients with hepatitis? The key is to get consensus from your clinical staff on optimal practices and standardize these treatments. Mine your data—identify the better patient outcomes, the shorter length of stay (LOS), the good financial outcomes, the lower infection rates. And then replicate those protocols across your patient populations" (HFMA, 2011b, p. 6). Highly collaborative care—especially for patients with complex medical needs—notably during care transitions is an important strategy to help reduce costly hospital admissions and readmissions.

Jason Dinger, CEO of MissionPoint (Henkel & Maryland, 2015, pp. 13–14), and his team see health care evolving on three primary fronts: (a) health care as an internet of things, (b) broader proliferation of video, and (c) a better focus on social determinants of health. These factors form yet another, albeit positive, triple overlay on an already complex health care reimbursement landscape described in this chapter.

CONCLUSION

The federal government makes the rules that apply to health care reimbursement. The reimbursement conditions and rules operate in an imperfect economic market within a vortex of environmental factors. Health care entities receive reimbursement in a prospective method from government and private insurers, who increasingly require quality measures to certify that the health care delivered is of sufficient value. This is a marked change from prior eras when straightforward volume drove reimbursement. DNPs are in an excellent position to drive health care quality, which will not only ensure that patients are safely and effectively treated but also that optimum reimbursement for services is realized. At the time of this writing, legislation is once again proposed to develop a new national program—successor to the ACA—to increase access to care while reducing costs and avoiding unexpected consequences. The name of the pending legislation is the American Health Care Act. One thing remains constant: clinically integrated, quality, efficient, and effective coordinated care is paramount. Both consumers and payers expect no less.

CRITICAL THINKING EXERCISES

1. List three ways the DNP provides leadership in helping a health care entity optimize reimbursement from insurers.
2. Considering factors in today's health care environment, draw from Remington's lingering questions about the proper role of government. Select one question and propose a response.
3. Choose two preferred financial and patient care outcomes from the following list and describe two ways to achieve each of them:
   a. Reduction in overall hospital admissions
   b. Reduction in average length of stay
   c. Reduction in avoidable hospital readmissions
   d. Reduction in high-tech imaging services
   e. Reduction in CMS-paid amount per beneficiary.
4. Can the kind of care proposed in an IDS be provided in a system that has a primary focus on either provider or corporate incomes and profit accumulation?

5. Why is it financially important for hospitals to institute effective discharge planning programs?
6. Partnerships between acute care and community-based settings improve continuity of care. How do these partnerships influence reimbursement for health systems?

ADDITIONAL READINGS

Buppert, C. (2005). Capturing reimbursement for advanced practice nurse services in acute and critical care. *AACN Clinical Issues, 16*(1), 23–35.
Kutzleb, J., Rigolosi, R., Fruhschien, A., Reilly, M., Shaftic, A. M., Duran, D., & Flynn, D. (2015). Nurse practitioner care model: Meeting health care challenges with a collaborative team. *Nursing Economic$, 33*(6), 297–304.

ADDITIONAL RESOURCES

www.commonwealthfund.org (The Commonwealth Fund)
www.healthinsuranceproviders.com/health-insurance-association-of-america-hiaa (America's Health Insurance Plans)
www.hfma.org/dollars (Healthcare Financial Management Association)
www.intalere.com (Operational Excellence in Health Care)
www.kff.org (Kaiser Family Foundation)

REFERENCES

American Association of Colleges of Nursing. (2006). *The essentials of doctoral education for advanced nursing practice.* Washington, DC: Author. Retrieved from http://www.aacnnursing.org/Portals/42/Publications/DNPEssentials.pdf
American College of Healthcare Executives. (2016). Survey: Healthcare finance, safety, and quality cited by CEOs as top issues confronting hospitals in 2015. Retrieved from http://www.ache.org/pubs/releases/2016/top-issues-confronting-hospitals-2015.cfm
American Health Reform Act of 2017, H.R. 277, 115th Cong. (2017–2018). Retrieved from https://www.congress.gov/bill/115th-congress/house-bill/277
American Hospital Association. (2009). HIPAA code set rule: *ICD-10* implementation—An executive briefing. Retrieved from http://www.aha.org/aha_app/issues/HIPAA/index.jsp
American Hospital Association. (2016, November). Environmental scan: 2017. *Hospitals & Health Networks* (Special Insert). Retrieved from https://www.hhnmag.com/articles/7616-aha-2017-environmental-scan
American Hospital Association. (2017, January 27). Letter to the president of the United States. Retrieved from http://www.aha.org
American Hospital Association Committee on Performance Improvement. (2011). Hospitals and care systems of the future. Retrieved from http://www.aha.org
American Hospital Association's Society for Healthcare Strategy and Market Development and American College of Healthcare Executives. (2016). Future scan 2016–2021. Retrieved from http://www.aha.org/presscenter/pressrel/2016/160128-pr-futurescan.shtml
American Nurses Association. (2010). *Principles of pay for quality.* Silver Spring, MD: Author.
Arrow, K. (1963). Uncertainty and the welfare economics of medical care. *American Economic Review, 53*(5), 941–973.
Bagwell, M., Bushy, A., & Ortiz, J. (2017). Accountable care organization implementation experiences and rural participation. *Journal of Nursing Administration, 47*(1), 30–34.
Barnett, J., & Vornovitsky, M. (2016). *Health insurance coverage in the United States: 2015* (Current Population Reports, P60-257[RV]). Washington, DC: U.S. Government Printing Office.

Beasley, D. (2015, August 1). Alternative payment models: A changing landscape. *Medical Laboratory Observer*, 20–23.

Butler, S. (2016). The future of the Affordable Care Act: Reassessment and revision. *Journal of the American Medical Association*, 316(5), 495–497.

Callahan, D. (2008). Health care costs and medical technology. In M. Crowley (Ed.), *From birth to death and bench to clinic: The Hastings Center bioethics briefing book for journalists, policymakers, and campaigns* (pp. 79–82). Garrison, NY: The Hastings Center. Retrieved from http://www.thehastingscenter.org/wp-content/uploads/Health-Care-Costs-BB17.pdf

Centers for Disease Control and Prevention. (2016). Executive summary on healthcare related infections. Retrieved from https://www.cdc.gov/hai/pdfs/progress-report/exec-summary-haipr.pdf

Dall, T., Chen, Y., Seifert, R., Maddox, P., & Hogan, P. (2009). The economic value of professional nursing. *Medical Care*, 47(1), 97–104.

DeVore, S. (2015, December 30). Six big trends to watch in healthcare for 2016. *Health Affairs Blog*. Retrieved from http://healthaffairs.org/blog/2015/12/30/six-big-trends-to-watch-in-health-care-for-2016

Dontje, K., & Forrest, K. (2006). Third-party reimbursement. In J. Nagelkirk (Ed.), *Starting your practice: A survival guide for nurse practitioners* (Chap. 6). St. Louis, MO: Elsevier.

FamilyDoctor.org. (2015). Health insurance: Understanding what it covers. Retrieved from https://familydoctor.org/health-insurance-understanding-covers

Galewitz, P., & Kaiser Health News. (2011). States to limit hospital stays. *USA Today*, p. A1.

Glazer, J., & McGuire, T. (2002). Multiple payers, commonality, and free-riding in health care: Medicare and private payers. *Journal of Health Economics*, 21, 1049–1069.

Goldsteen, R. L., Goldsteen, K., & Goldsteen, B. Z. (2017). *Jonas' introduction to the U.S. health care system* (8th ed.). New York, NY: Springer Publishing.

Grabowski, D. (2007). Medicare and Medicaid: Conflicting incentives for long-term care. *The Milbank Quarterly*, 85(4), 579–610.

Granger, B. (2017, January 19). Focusing on patient care: The final rule. *South Texas Healthcare Financial Management Association Newsletter*. Retrieved from http://stxhfma.org/focusing-patient-care-final-rule

Hamric, A., Spross, J., & Hanson, C. (2009). *Advanced practice nursing: An integrative approach* (4th ed.). St. Louis, MO: Saunders Elsevier.

Healthcare Financial Management Association. (2011a). Educational report: Creating value for patients for business success. Retrieved from http://www.digitalhealth.net/includes/images/Document_Library0365/HFMA-Leadership-2011-Spring-Summer-Clairvia.pdf

Healthcare Financial Management Association. (2011b). Strategies for value-based healthcare. Retrieved from http://www.hfma.org

Health Dimensions Group. (2016, March 14). Optimizing your operational and financial performance. Retrieved from http://www.healthdimensionsgroup.com

Henkel, R., & Maryland, P. (2015). The risks and rewards of value-based reimbursement. *Frontiers of Health Services Management*, 32(2), 3–16.

Institute for Healthcare Improvement. (2017). Triple aim for populations. Retrieved from http://www.ihi.org/Topics/TripleAim/Pages/default.aspx

Institute of Medicine. (1988). In R. Remington (Ed.), *The future of public health* (pp. v–vi). Washington, DC: National Academies Press.

Institute of Medicine. (2000). *To err is human: Building a safer health system*. Washington, DC: National Academies Press.

Institute of Medicine. (2001). *Crossing the quality chasm: A new health system for the 21st century*. Washington, DC: National Academies Press.

Jonas, S., Goldsteen, R., & Goldsteen, K. (2007). *Jonas' introduction to the U.S. health care system* (6th ed.). New York, NY: Springer Publishing.

Kaplan, A. L. (2016, November). Alternative payment models "how you win under MACRA." *Urology Times*, 44(12), 23.

Keckley, P. (2017, January). The imperatives for hospitals while the repeal dust settles. *Hospitals & Health Networks*. Retrieved from http://www.hhnmag.com/articles/8019-the-imperatives-for-hospitals-while-the-repeal-dust-settles

Lankford, K. (2017). Hire help to handle hefty medical bills. *Kiplinger's Retirement Report.* Retrieved from http://www.kiplinger.com/article/retirement/T027-C000-S004-hire-help-to-handle-hefty-medical-bills.html

Larkin, H. (2011, October). Smart money management. *Hospitals & Health Networks.* Retrieved from http://www.hhnmag.com/articles/4508-smart-money-management

Mathews, A., & Radnofsky, L. (2017, January 13). Health care's bipartisan dilemma. *The Wall Street Journal,* A1, A6.

McCarty, J., & Swanson, N. (2016). Diving into the new *ICD-10* codes. *American Speech-Language-Hearing Association (ASHA) Leader, 21,* 28–30.

National Academy of Science. (2016, December). Health insurance and insights from health literacy: Helping consumers understand: Proceedings of a workshop—in brief. Retrieved from https://www.nap.edu/read/24613/chapter/1

Nelson, E., Batalden, P., Godfrey, M., & Lazar J. (Eds.). (2011). *Value by design: Developing clinical microsystems to achieve organizational excellence.* San Francisco, CA: Jossey-Bass.

Ng, T., Harrington, C., & Kitchener, M. (2010). Medicare and Medicaid in long-term care. *Health Affairs, 29*(1), 22–28.

Nurse Practitioner Roundtable. (2010). *Nurse practitioner perspective on health care payment.* Washington, DC: Author. Retrieved from https://www.aanp.org/images/documents/federal-legislation/NPPerspectiveonHCPmt.pdf

O'Connor, M. (2016, September). Don Berwick imagines a new era of health care. *Hospitals & Health Networks.* Retrieved from http://www.hhnmag.com/articles/7633-don-berwick-imagines-a-new-era-of-health-care

Shortell, S. M., Gillies, R. M., Anderson, D. A., Erickson, K. M., & Mitchell, J. B. (1999). Working toward an ideal system. In J. A. Russell (Ed.), *Managed care essentials: A book of readings* (p. 8). Chicago, IL: Health Administration Press.

U.S. Census Bureau. (2016). Figure 3. Health insurance coverage in the U.S. Retrieved from http://www.census.gov/content/dam/Census/library/publications/2016/demo/p60-257.pdf

U.S. Department of Health and Human Services. (2013). Accountable care organizations. Retrieved from http://www.cms.gov/medicare/medicare-fee-for-service-payment/ACO/index.html?redirect=/ACO

U.S. Department of Health and Human Services. (2015). Better, smarter, healthier: In historic announcement, HHS sets clear goals and timeline for shifting Medicare reimbursement from volume to value. Retrieved from http://www.hhs.gov/news/press/2015pres/01/20150126a.html

U.S. Department of Health and Human Services. (2017). HHS organizational chart. Retrieved from https://www.hhs.gov/about/agencies/orgchart/index.html

U.S. Department of Health and Human Services, Centers for Medicare and Medicaid Services, Office of the Actuary. (2014). National health expenditures by type of service, 2013: NHE web tables. Retrieved from http://www.cms.gov/research-statistics-data-and-systems/Statistics-Trends-and-Reports/NationalHealthExpendData/NationalHealthAccountsHistorical.html

Van Dyke, M. (2016, December). Make way for MACRA. *Hospitals & Health Networks, 90*(12), 27–31.

Van Dyke, M. (2017, January). MACRA and the rural provider. *Hospitals & Health Networks, 91*(1), 16–21.

3

Hospital Utilization, Staffing, and Financial Indicators

Susan J. Penner and Michael D. Spencer

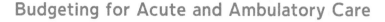

KEY TERMS

admissions, discharges, and transfers (ADTs)

boarder

capacity

census

cycle time

encounter

full-time equivalent (FTE)

microsystem

outlier

patient days

utilization

Pacific Hospital needs to increase its profitability and to position its priorities and resources from trends such as new technologies and an aging population. Pacific Hospital executives face uncertainty about funding and reimbursement related to anticipated but unspecified changes in health reform legislation. The chief nursing officer (CNO), an executive leadership doctor of nursing practice (DNP) graduate, builds a team of clinical care DNPs, nurse managers, and clinical nurse leaders (CNLs) from the emergency department (ED), ICUs, perioperative services, outpatient clinics, and other areas of the hospital to help determine what steps can be taken by nurse leaders to proactively manage this situation.

Imagine that you are the CNO or a team member. Where would you begin? How would you pinpoint sources of high costs and revenue shortfalls? How would you know if these problems are related to patient utilization or nursing productivity? What information would you use to guide your proposals for strategies to address these concerns? What steps would you take to plan for change in your institution or your nursing microsystem? Are you prepared to develop a small test of change (Institute for Healthcare Improvement [IHI], 2011b) that includes the costs and benefits of implementing quality improvement interventions?

▨ IMPLICATIONS FOR DNPs

DNPs may largely focus on physiologic measures, laboratory values, and other indicators for assessing and monitoring health and disease in their clinical practice. Utilization, staffing, and financial indicators might be considered more relevant for DNPs in executive roles. However, the outcomes of DNP preparation require a greater emphasis on leadership than for master's-level preparation. DNPs in any setting should adopt a macro-level perspective, and are expected to lead clinical practice initiatives (Dreher & Smith Glasgow, 2011). Many clinical DNPs practicing in hospital settings work closely with case managers, discharge planners, and other health team members, and must understand the impact of issues such as patient flow and cost concerns. DNPs must also prepare for change and serve as change agents (Sherrod & Goda, 2016).

Nurses must be prepared to apply business concepts when designing and improving patient care systems (American Association of Colleges of Nursing [AACN], 2006). DNPs must understand the systems and system dynamics in their settings, and be skilled in collecting, analyzing, and presenting relevant data that describe these systems. In hospital settings, utilization and financial indicators are frequently reported and used to monitor and control patient care systems. These data can be used to create an evidence base for systems evaluation and improvement.

This chapter focuses on hospital inpatient and outpatient utilization, staffing, and financial indicators that DNPs should understand as they work to ensure high-quality and cost-effective patient care. Several case scenarios focused on patient flow, staffing, analyzing nursing costs, and planning for outpatient services are presented. These scenarios illustrate the use of indicators in assessing problem situations and in evaluating strategies to resolve those situations.

▨ SCENARIO ONE: THE PROBLEM IS PATIENT FLOW

As the team investigates, problems across the hospital macrosystem emerge. The DNP in the ED reports delays in transferring ED patients to observation beds or admitting units, which pushes the ED to full or excess capacity. This results in ED diversion of patients to other local facilities, which leads to the loss of hospital revenue from potential admissions (Wang, Li, & Howard, 2013). In addition, the state reviews hospital diversion hours and imposes regulatory and financial penalties on hospitals that fail to serve the community when the ED is unavailable.

The ICUs, perioperative care, step-down units, and medical–surgical units all report periodic bottlenecks because transfers are delayed waiting for a bed to become available. This backup in patient flow contributes to the ED capacity and diversion problems. Frequently, transfers ordered on the day shift are delayed until the evening or night, when there are fewer staff available to complete the transfer. Handoff errors on the evening and night shifts have resulted in resistance from evening and night nurses to receive transfers, intensifying the problem. In many instances, patients scheduled for discharge in the morning do not vacate their rooms until the evening shift or the following day, thus delaying admissions for 24 hours or more.

Medical–surgical units report delays in discharges, so that patients often remain in the hospital an additional night, or even longer. Delayed discharge is one of the most frequent reasons for excessive medical–surgical patient length of stay (LOS). Excessive LOS results in fewer available medical–surgical beds, thus delaying transfers from other units such as perioperative services or ICU and increasing the wait time for hospital admissions. Fewer available medical–surgical beds also reduce the availability of observation beds, which increases the likelihood of overcrowding in the ED.

The impact of bottlenecks across the system leads to concerns about the quality of care, as patients are put on hold for hours or even for days to be admitted, discharged, or transferred to the appropriate level of care. In addition, Pacific Hospital incurs substantial costs and loses considerable revenue related to excessive LOS, preventable complications, and diversion to other hospitals in the area.

WHY FOCUS ON INDICATORS?

Up until now, many of these problems with patient flow at Pacific Hospital were reported anecdotally. Nurse managers often blame other nursing units for causing delays and problems with transfers and discharges. Nurses complain that "we just don't have enough staff to admit all these patients," although Pacific Hospital's staffing ratios are consistent with accepted standards of nursing care. The CNO decides to examine the data.

Indicators measure conditions, performance, or results, and can be used to help find the root causes of problems. In this scenario, the CNO asks the team to focus on acute care utilization indicators to better understand the flow of patients through the hospital. One objective is for the team to identify sources of delays and bottlenecks in the system. Inpatient utilization indicators are discussed in the context of patient flow problems at Pacific Hospital.

As these indicators are presented and discussed, it is important to realize that these measures must be collected and analyzed within the same specified time period. In many cases, reporting is on a monthly or annual basis; regardless of the time period, it must be clearly noted and consistent across all the measures in the report. For example, if patient days are reported for a given month, then the number of discharges used to calculate an average length of stay (ALOS) must be reported for the same month. It is important to be aware of factors such as differing days in months that might affect reporting. Institutions may differ in their monthly reporting; some institutions utilize 13 four-week, 28-day "monthly" reports per year. All of the calculations for indicators presented in this chapter assume a specified time period; if monthly, a 30-day month is used; if annual, a 364-day year is used.

Indicators may be measured and reported in absolute amounts, or converted to rates or percentages. For example, hospital readmissions may be reported as the number of readmissions over a specified time period, or as a readmission rate. Converting numbers to rates or percentages makes it possible to compare indicators across time or between settings.

Although the definitions and calculations of these inpatient utilization indicators are taken from accepted sources, indicators may be defined and calculated in various ways across health care settings. For example, the term *available bed* is commonly defined as a bed that is equipped but not staffed for patient admissions. However, many health professionals might use the terms *available bed* and *staffed bed* (a bed both available and staffed for admissions) interchangeably. Be sure to understand the definitions and calculations of indicators in the practice setting, and be consistent with the practice setting's reporting and interpretation of these indicators.

IDENTIFYING PATIENT FLOW PROBLEMS

The CNO and the team review several categories of inpatient utilization indicators. These indicators provide clues for addressing patient flow problems, including bottlenecks, delays, and inefficiencies.

Bed capacity—An inpatient facility may have more beds licensed for operation than are equipped to be available. Licensed and equipped available beds represent the hospital's *fixed* capacity, which remains constant over a fiscal year. However, these licensed or equipped available beds might not all be staffed for patient occupancy, and patients may not occupy all the staffed beds. Staffed bed occupancy is therefore *variable* rather than fixed, as occupancy may change on a daily or hourly basis. Hospital capacity largely depends on the availability of inpatient beds staffed for patient care, so the terms *available beds* and *staffed beds* are often used interchangeably. An implication is that occupied beds are the only beds that are utilized and generate revenue; staffed beds have the immediate potential for utilization and revenue.

Potential patient days—These patient days represent the maximum number of patients who would occupy all staffed beds (Horton, 2010). Comparing potential to actual patient days enables the estimate of potential revenues or costs that would be generated beyond the current, actual occupancy. For example, a medical–surgical unit has 25 licensed beds and 20 staffed beds. The potential patient days per 30-day month are 600; if the unit reports 80% occupancy for the month, there are 480 actual patient days generating costs and revenues for the unit.

Studies show that hospitals at or above 90% occupancy rates for more than 50% of the time may face problems with resource availability and delays in transfer from the ED (Cesta & Keeling, 2009; Forster, Stiell, Wells, Lee, & van Walraven, 2003; IHI, 2003). As a result, inpatient occupancy benchmarks are often set at 65% to 85% to allow for resource needs (Kelleher & Parker, 2007). Pacific Hospital's ICUs frequently operate at 90% or greater occupancy levels, which is likely related to some of the bottleneck problems in Pacific Hospital's ED.

Another problem is *boarding* or "parking" patient admissions in holding locations such as the ED or hallway, waiting to be moved to the destination nursing unit. Parking refers to holding patients temporarily, but parking more than 2% of admitted patients for any length of time, more than 50% of the time, indicates patient flow problems (IHI, 2003). Boarding is a greater concern as patients may be held waiting for appropriate transfer for hours or days. Many experts consider parking a patient for more than 2 hours as boarding (Rabin et al., 2012). The CNO at Pacific Hospital does not have complete or accurate statistics on patient parking, but has data and increasing concerns about boarding problems in the ED.

Monitoring patient days is important for purposes such as capacity planning, measuring utilization, billing, and controlling LOS. Another critical time frame is the nursing care hour. Nursing care directly delivered to patients, staffing, and patient care intensity and acuity are usually measured in hours, not days. This distinction between patient days and nursing care hours is important in managing resources to deliver care as well as control capacity. Reimbursement, which is based on patient days, will remain the same whether the patient is discharged at 10 a.m. or at 6 p.m. However, the patient will require more hours of nursing care, and thus generates higher costs, if the discharge is delayed from 10 a.m. to 6 p.m. More discussion of nursing care hours is found in Scenario Two.

Census—The census or count of patients in a nursing unit is important in understanding hospital utilization and staffing requirements, but census data alone provide limited information. Historically, the census of all hospital patients has been conducted at midnight, assuming this is a time of low activity, when patients can be counted in the beds they occupy. The midnight census is also used for billing purposes in counting a patient day for reimbursement (Green, 2004).

Admissions, discharges, and transfers (ADTs)—Since the 1990s, reductions in LOS and increased patient turnover require more attention to ADT tracking and reporting. A midnight census does not adequately capture the staff workload involved in a high intensity of ADTs, nor does the midnight census adequately account for the care of observation patients who are admitted and discharged within 48 hours. As a result, in the current environment of rapid patient turnover, the actual number of patients cared for on a nursing unit may be far greater than a midnight census indicates (Jacobson, Seltzer, & Dam, 1999). Park, Dunton, and Blegen (2016) point out that the added ADT workload may fragment nursing services and impede patient safety and quality of care.

The usefulness of the daily census is therefore enhanced by incorporating ADT data with the census using an indicator such as the Unit Activity Index (UAI). When the ADT volume (including observation patients admitted for less than 24 hours) is divided by the total number of patients treated (ADT plus the census for the entire 24 hours), the resulting UAI serves as an indicator of the intensity of patient flow through the nursing microsystem. A UAI greater than 50% indicates a likely need for more staffing to manage the patient flow (Jacobson et al., 1999). Institutions may measure ADT intensity using tools and methods other than the UAI. What is important is that patient turnover is monitored, in addition to the census, particularly on units where patient flow efficiency is of the most concern.

A review of Pacific Hospital's UAIs for each of the medical–surgical units shows considerable variance, with two medical–surgical units reporting UAIs of 50% or greater more than 50% of the time. It therefore appears that the volume of patient flow is much more intense for two of the medical–surgical units compared to the others.

Bed turns—These indicators help in understanding how efficiently hospital beds are utilized. Bed turns measure how frequently a given hospital bed changes occupancy over the reporting period. The number of discharges is divided by the number of staffed beds, so that a unit with 20 staffed beds and 105 discharges for a given month would have 5.25 bed turns during that month.

Bed utilization—The actual number of bed turns is then compared to the maximum possible number of bed turns to determine bed utilization, expressed as a percent. The maximum possible number of bed turns (also referred to as theoretical bed turns) is calculated by dividing the reporting time period by the ALOS. The example unit's maximum possible bed turns are 6.3, or 30 days divided by an ALOS of 4.8 days. Bed utilization is calculated by dividing the actual bed turns by the maximum possible bed turns (5.25 divided by 6.3), or 83.3%. When calculated using overall hospital data, bed utilization may also be referred to as *hospital efficiency* (IHI, 2011a).

Bed turnover interval and bed cleaning interval—The bed turnover interval indicates the amount of time beds are unoccupied until the next patient admission following a patient discharge (Tortorella, Ukanowicz, Douglas-Ntagha, Ray, & Triller, 2013). The *bed cleaning interval* is the amount of time required for the unoccupied bed to be cleaned and readied for the next admission, which contributes to the bed turnover interval (IHI, 2011a). Settings such as procedure rooms might require a much longer time for cleaning and preparation for the next patient than other settings, such as medical–surgical units, where the room can be cleaned within a couple of hours. The team is not surprised that the two medical–surgical units with the most intensive patient flow also report the highest bed turns and the lowest bed turnover and bed cleaning intervals.

Wasted capacity to boarders—The excessive amount of time patients occupy a bed while waiting for transfer, admission, or discharge represents wasted capacity for the hospital. This ratio of wasted to total capacity is particularly important to track in the ED, ICUs, and postanesthesia care units (PACUs), because bottlenecks in these microsystems can lead to ambulance diversion as well as patient flow problems throughout the hospital. Patients may be designated as boarded patients if their ED bed occupancy after hospital admission exceeds 2 hours. Boarding not only impedes patient flow, but also leads to patient safety concerns when the transfer of new admissions to the appropriate nursing unit is delayed (Welch, Augustine, Camargo, & Reese, 2006). If wasted capacity is excessive in medical–surgical units, it indicates the need to better control LOS and to improve discharge planning.

As the CNO and team continue to analyze bed turnover indicators, it becomes more apparent that two of the medical–surgical units have been managing more than their share of patient admissions and transfers, whereas other medical–surgical units are lagging behind in bed utilization efficiency. Upon investigation, it is found that nurses in these less productive microsystems may delay notifying the housekeeping staff of discharges for several hours or more, thus impeding the opportunity to admit or transfer patients.

Readmission rates—Measured 7, 15, or 30 days following discharge, the readmission rate is a quality indicator under increasing scrutiny by the Centers for Medicare and Medicaid Services (CMS) and other payers. Not only does the Affordable Care Act of 2010 (ACA) implement financial penalties for hospitals with high readmission rates, but 30-day readmission rates for Medicare heart attack, heart failure, and pneumonia patients are also included in the CMS Hospital Compare website (www.cms.gov) for public review (Medicare.gov, n.d.). The future of the ACA and health reform is currently uncertain, but the cost savings to Medicare from the Hospital Readmission Reduction Program are projected at $10.3 billion from 2018 to 2026 (Dobson, DaVanzo, Haught, & Luu, 2016). Table 3.1 presents selected utilization indicators discussed in this section.

STRATEGIES TO IMPROVE PATIENT FLOW

Based on their analysis of the utilization indicators, the Pacific Hospital's CNO directs the team to develop system-wide strategies to improve patient flow. One of the first priorities is for the clinical DNPs, CNLs, and nurse managers in each clinical area to work together as nurse leaders to improve the efficiency of transfers and discharges. Additional tasks are to better control LOS, increase bed turnover, reduce diversion hours, and reduce wasted capacity to boarders.

The medical–surgical nurse leaders develop a business plan to convert currently available but unstaffed beds to a 10-bed skilled nursing facility (SNF) that will reduce excessive medical–surgical unit LOS. The unit is expected to be cost-effective because many of these patients qualify for skilled nursing care reimbursement. The SNF unit is less expensive to staff compared

TABLE 3.1 Selected Inpatient Utilization Indicators

Indicator	Calculation
Admissions	Admissions + newborns + transfers into the unit + observation patients
Average daily census (ADC)	Patient days ÷ days in time period
Average LOS (ALOS)	Total patient days ÷ discharges
Average Unit Activity Index (UAI)	(Admissions + observation + discharges + transfers in and out)/all patients treated × 100%
Bed turnover interval	(Potential patient days − patient days) ÷ discharges
Bed turnover rate (bed turns)	Discharges ÷ staffed beds
Bed utilization	Actual bed turns/theoretical bed turns
Discharges	Discharges + deaths + transfers off the unit
Diversions	Number of patients diverted to another facility
Occupancy rate	Total patient days ÷ (staffed beds × days) × 100%
Patient days	Sum of census for specified time period
Potential patient days	Staffed beds × days in time period
Readmission rate (7, 15, or 30 day)	Readmissions ÷ total cases
Theoretical bed turns	Time period/ALOS
Total LOS or discharge days	Total days of inpatients discharged during a specific time period

LOS, length of stay.

to medical–surgical units, as the care level is subacute. The community also benefits, as there is a chronic shortage of SNF facilities in the local area.

The nurse leaders in perioperative services work with the admissions department and the chief of surgery to coordinate and more closely control elective surgery admissions and scheduling. Currently, most elective surgeries are scheduled Monday through Wednesday, putting perioperative services at maximum capacity on those days, as well as intensifying nursing unit transfers and patient flow. This intense activity approaches full capacity and increases the risk of delays and cancellations in surgery, the likelihood of bottlenecks in patient transfer, and the probability of errors across all the systems of care. The new scheduling initiative allows a steady, more predictable flow of surgery patients admitted Monday through Friday. This approach allows leeway in the operating room (OR) schedules for emergency surgeries or complications that require extra time (IHI, 2003). Even though only a few surgeons are participating in this initiative, the smoother schedule reduces the high intensity of patient flow through medical–surgical units and the ICUs. Smoothing the schedule helps nurse managers match staffing to actual patient needs, and reduce handoff and other medical errors.

Another initiative is the introduction of an admissions and discharge RN (A-D RN) to one of the medical–surgical units. Evidence indicates that an A-D RN not only improves patient flow by ensuring more timely admissions and discharges in nursing units, but improves nurse satisfaction as well. In addition, improved discharge teaching and medication reconciliation may reduce at least some preventable readmissions (Lane, Jackson, Odom, Cannella, & Hinshaw, 2009).

The ED DNP makes a business case to set up a two-bed, 23-hour observation unit as part of the ED. The plan is to cross-train ED nurses to manage both emergency room and observation room patients. The ED nurses will coordinate with admissions to efficiently transfer these patients if they are admitted, or to discharge the patient within 24 hours. The observation unit will employ a multidisciplinary team, including social workers, discharge planners, and case managers. This enables the unit to better serve patients with multiple chronic conditions at risk for preventable readmissions. Preadmission discharge planning will be initiated for these complex cases, so that LOS and postdischarge needs are addressed as part of the admitting treatment plan.

Another project for the ED DNP is a business plan for embedding nurse practitioners (NPs) or physician assistants in the ED to triage and treat less urgent cases. This approach makes more efficient use of the ED physicians and reduces wait times, ED overcrowding, and ambulance diversion (Cesta & Keeling, 2009).

On the medical–surgical units serving as step-down cardiac care, the DNP explores the strategy of assigning a case manager to conduct telephone follow-up of all recently discharged cardiac patients. This approach would improve continuity of care by making sure that patients are following their treatment plan at home. Telephone follow-up has been shown to reduce preventable ED visits, observation days, and readmissions for patients with congestive heart failure (Inglis et al., 2010).

Additional interventions include educating staff RNs about patient flow concerns and establishing bed turnaround benchmarks in each unit for patient discharge and bed cleaning (Enriquez, Sisson, Kirby, & Gupta, 2009). Nurse managers are encouraged to ask staff RNs for feedback and ideas to help improve patient flow problems, and to engage staff RNs in generating solutions. The Pacific Hospital case scenario shows how inpatient utilization indicators can be applied not only to identify problems, but also to help guide DNPs to improve the productivity and quality of care in nursing microsystems.

▨ SCENARIO TWO: INPATIENT CARE STAFFING INDICATORS

Nurse staffing costs consume the highest percentage of the labor budget in acute care settings and represent the largest segment of the overall institutional budget (Douglas, 2010). The investment in nursing care is among the most critical of all resources managed by nurse executives and nurse managers. Hospitals are called to deliver better health, and their reputation and image in the community is a reflection of the quality of patient care delivered. How much a hospital invests in attracting, developing, and retaining its nursing staff determines the success at achieving that core value. At the same time, the high cost of RN staffing is an important concern.

Pacific Hospital's CNO meets with the nurse manager of the East Wing Medical–Surgical Unit to discuss microsystem productivity. The nurse manager assumed responsibility only 2 months ago, and is new to the management role. East Wing is a very busy unit with 20 beds, an average daily census (ADC) of 16.7 patients (83.3% average occupancy rate), and 17 budgeted staff RN FTEs.

The CNO points out that East Wing is increasingly over its staffing budget. The manager needs to better control the hours per patient day (HPPD) of care provided and the numbers of staff scheduled on the unit. There are several full-time (FT) staff positions that need to be filled, resulting in excessive overtime and agency nurse hours. In addition, most of the activity on the East Wing occurs between the hours of 10 a.m. and 4 p.m., with very high activity Mondays through Wednesdays, leading to overtime and handoff errors. This is one of the units with patient flow problems reported in the first case scenario. Table 3.2 presents selected RN staffing indicators discussed in this section. Table 3.3 presents the East Wing monthly staffing budget report.

KEY INDICATORS FOR NURSE STAFFING

This section presents nurse staffing indicators and their interpretation, followed by examples for using these indicators to plan strategies that lead to staffing success. Note that nurses and staff are RNs unless otherwise specified.

TABLE 3.2 Acute Care RN Staffing Indicators

Indicator	Calculation
Direct care hours per patient day (HPPD)	Productive hours/patient days
HPPD, derived	(N/P) × 24 hours
Indirect hours	Count of hours of indirect activities
Productive hours	Direct hours + indirect hours
Nonproductive hours	Paid days off + paid nonproductive per shift
Overtime hours	Count of hours of overtime
Agency hours	Count of hours of agency nurses
Total paid hours	FTEs × hours recorded in time period
FTE	Annual hours/FTE = 8 hours/week × 52 weeks = 2,080
Daily FTE for one 8-hour shift	1.0 FTE/5 days worked per week = 0.2 FTE
7 days per week coverage factor for 8-hour shifts	7 days a week coverage × 0.2 FTE per day for 8-hour shifts = 1.4
24/7 days per week coverage factor for 8-hour shifts	7 days a week/5 days a week worked by 1.0 FTE × 3 shifts per day = 4.2
Nurse-to-patient ratio (N/P ratio)	Productive nursing hours/(patient days × 24)
Skill mix	% RN FTEs compared to other direct care staff

FTE, full-time equivalent; N/P, nurse-to-patient.

Full-time equivalent (FTE)—An FTE represents a FT employee working 8 hours a day, 5 days a week, for 52 weeks a year, which totals 2,080 hours per year. Because many acute care staff nurses are hired on a part-time (PT) basis, and most staff nurses are paid hourly wages, it is more accurate to think of nurse staffing in terms of FTEs rather than job positions. A unit employing 30 nurses, with 20 of these nurses working FT (1.0 FTE) and the other 10 nurses half time (0.5 FTE), therefore employs 25.0 FTEs. A FT staff nurse working 8-hour shifts would work 10 shifts per 2-week pay period for 1.0 FTE. A staff nurse working 3 days a week would work 6 shifts per pay period or 0.6 FTE.

In many inpatient settings, staff nurses work 12-hour rather than 8-hour shifts. Staff nurses working 12-hour shifts are frequently scheduled for three shifts a week, or 72 hours over a 2-week pay period, which equals 0.9 FTE. In settings such as the OR, nurses may be scheduled to work 10-hour shifts 4 days a week. This chapter focuses on staffing for the standard 8-hour shift. More information is available in the supplemental exercises regarding staffing for 12-hour and 10-hour shifts.

FTEs capture the hours that are to be paid (in 1 year a FT nurse or 1 FTE will be paid for 2,080 hours). These calculations are an important tool for determining the number of positions that will be needed to cover a given workload, but are not to be confused with productive hours (the bedside hours actually worked). We will discuss this important difference after reviewing fixed and flexible FTEs.

Fixed FTEs—Fixed FTEs, also referred to as permanent staffing or indirect staffing, represent staff hours scheduled regardless of patient volume. For example, most nursing units require a nurse manager, a unit clerk, and a minimum level of nursing staff every day to keep the unit open, even if the census is low.

Flexible FTEs—Flexible FTEs represent staff hours scheduled based on actual or projected patient volume (Kirk, 1981). In other words, as the census increases, more staff nurses are required

TABLE 3.3 Pacific Hospital, East Wing Medical–Surgical Unit, Monthly Staffing Report, November 2017

Line Item	November 2017		
	Budget	Actual	Variance
Licensed beds	25	25	0
Days in time period	30	30	0
Utilization and acuity			
Staffed beds	20	20	0
ADC	16.7	16.2	(0.5)
Occupancy rate	83.3%	80.8%	(0.03)
Patient days	500	485	(15.0)
Discharges	105	86	(19.0)
ALOS	4.8	5.6	0.9
HPPD	8	9.2	1.2
RN direct care hours (target)	4,000	3,880	(120.0)
FTEs PPD			
N/P 1 RN to:	3	2.6	(0.4)
N/P ratio	33%	38.3%	0.05
Direct care hours per patient per shift	2.7	3.1	0.4
Total direct care hours	133.3	148.5	15.2
RN FTEs per occupied bed	1.0	0.9	(0.1)
RN staffing per day	17	18.6	1.9
FTEs monthly			
Total RN FTEs	30	26.1	(3.9)
RN productive hours	4,000	4,455	455.0
% RN productive hours/direct care hours	100%	115%	0.15
RN paid nonproductive %	13%	14.3%	0.01
RN adjusted FTEs	33.9	29.9	(4.0)
RN overtime hours	336	543	207
RN agency hours	0.0	145	145
Total paid hours	4,856.0	5,780.1	924.1

ADC, average daily census; ALOS, average length of stay; FTEs, full-time equivalents; HPPD, hours per patient day; N/P, nurse-to-patient ratio; PPD, per patient day.

to manage the patient load than if the census drops. Flexible FTEs depend not only on the number of patients, but also on patient acuity that influences the hours of direct care that patients require each day, on standards for nurse-to-patient ratios, and, in some settings, on the intensity of unit activity (ADTs). If there are unit or institutional policies for staffing for direct care hours, then there may be a staffing standard for flexible FTEs. To comply with demands for high-quality patient care and regulatory requirements, and to manage the costs of RN staffing, executives and managers must closely monitor the budgeted and actual use of flexible FTEs. Table 3.2 focuses solely on RN staffing, not the fixed positions on the East Wing unit.

HPPD—Patient utilization is the fundamental driver of acute care nurse staffing because nursing care is a fundamental reason for hospitalization. In acute care settings, the most relevant unit of service is the patient day. An indicator based on the patient day that is essential in nurse staffing is the HPPD, which represents the amount of time required for nurses to provide direct patient care per inpatient day. HPPD may also be referred to as direct care hours, productive hours, nursing hours per patient day (NHPPD), productive nursing hours per patient day (PNHPPD), or hours per unit of service (HPUOS). This indicator is so important to nursing budgets and performance that it is often reported to the 1/100th of an hour, for example, 4.85 HPPD. Patient acuity is typically the basis for determining standard HPPD, although in some states regulatory requirements may mandate minimum HPPD (California Nurses Association and National Nurses Organizing Committee, 2009). Hospitals or units may establish minimum HPPD policies as well. FTEs are scheduled based on the hours needed for direct patient care.

Nurse-to-patient ratio (N/P ratio)—The nurse-to-patient ratio, also referred to as the nurse–patient ratio or N/P ratio, represents the maximum number of patients allowed per nurse as specified by institutional policy, or, as in California, by regulatory mandate (California Nurses Association and National Nurses Organizing Committee, 2009). The N/P ratio allows the assignment of a patient workload to a nurse related to an estimated required HPPD, rather than simply dividing patients by the number of nurses that happen to be scheduled, which may or may not adequately cover patient care needs. The HPPD may be derived from the N/P ratio by multiplying the N/P ratio by 24 hours. For example, an N/P ratio of three patients per nurse equals 1/3 × 24, or 8 HPPD, so that each patient receives 8 hours of direct RN care per day.

Staffing ratio mandates have financial implications, and are not always optimally efficient. For example, a policy or mandate may require that to ensure an N/P ratio of 1:4, a minimum of five nurses must be assigned to a shift if the census is 17 to 20 patients. As a result, the staffing costs for 17 patients are the same as for 20 patients, whereas the revenue generated by 17 patients is substantially less than for 20 patients. In addition, staffing ratios do not allow for workload differences between shifts. A busier day shift may need more nurses than the ratio requires, whereas the night shift may be overstaffed. However, the N/P ratio mandates at least help ensure that inpatient facilities comply with minimum acceptable staffing levels. The American Nurses Association (ANA) provides online information about staffing laws and initiatives in states across the United States (ANA, 2017).

Nonproductive hours—No employee is expected to actually work a full 40 hours a week for 52 weeks a year. Labor laws and institutional policy allow paid leave for FT employees, including vacation, holiday, and personal time off. In addition, employees are allowed a given amount of paid time for lunch, and can schedule paid or unpaid break time. For example, a staff nurse working an 8-hour shift in California may be allowed 30 minutes paid time for lunch, and two paid 15 minute breaks (California Nurses Association, 2006). Institutions might include activities such as orientation and in-services as nonproductive paid time. On average, 16% of an RN's total time is nonproductive time (The KPMG Health Care and Pharmaceutical Institute, 2011).

24/7 coverage factor—In many industries, FTEs can be assigned based on a 40-hour workweek, but inpatient facilities must remain in operation 24 hours a day, 7 days a week. A 24/7 coverage factor must be calculated to determine the additional FTEs required for acute care staffing. In an inpatient setting staffing 8-hour shifts, scheduling is for a 56-hour week multiplied by three shifts per day, so 168 hours must be scheduled. As a result, 4.2 FTEs are needed to cover all three 8-hour shifts for all 7 days of the week.

Adjusted FTE—In order to determine how many staff persons to assign per day, shift, or other time period, the direct care FTEs must be adjusted for 24/7 coverage and nonproductive time. This indicator is the adjusted FTE, also referred to as the caregiver FTE or staffing FTE. The FTE adjusted for staffing is calculated by multiplying the ADC by HPPD, then by the 1.4 weekend coverage factor and by the adjustment for nonproductive time. This amount is then divided by the hours in a shift. FTEs may be adjusted for other time periods by multiplying the number of patient days in the time period instead of the ADC.

Skill mix—Another important indicator in nurse staffing is skill mix, or the proportion of RNs staffed on an inpatient unit compared to other skill levels such as licensed vocational nurses (LVNs, also referred to as licensed practical nurses or LPNs) and certified nurse assistants (CNAs). There are financial incentives to reduce the proportion of RNs in the skill mix, as LVNs and CNAs cost substantially less than RNs. Although the ideal skill mix has not been conclusively determined (Clarke & Donaldson, 2008; Dunton, Gajewski, Klaus, & Pierson, 2007; Institute of Medicine [IOM], 2004), executives and managers must adhere to nursing scope of practice standards and regulations, and consider patient safety and care needs.

Total paid hours—Total paid hours are the sum of total productive and total nonproductive hours for all the staff in the nursing unit. This is an important indicator for tracking the financial impact of productive and nonproductive hours. The calculation of total paid hours is complex because of the mix of FT nursing staff with benefits and PT staff who do not have benefits, such as paid vacation leave, as well as adjustments for scheduling FTEs and for nonproductive hours during the shift. In addition, there are differential salary increases for weekends, holidays, evening shifts, and night shifts. Overtime hours are costly; they must be closely monitored and are subject to approval to be sure overtime does not become excessive.

The use of agency (travel) nurses when hospital staff nurses are not available also influences the number of paid hours, although the costs of agency nurses may be similar or even somewhat less than for staff nurses (Spencer, 2017). However, excessive use of agency nurses may impact the quality of care, so regardless of cost concerns, agency nurse hours should be monitored (IOM, 2004; Page, 2008). More discussion of agency nurse utilization and costs is presented in Scenario Three.

STAFFING INDICATORS AND STAFFING STRATEGIES

The CNO discusses East Wing's monthly staffing report (see Table 3.3) with the new nurse manager. The direct care hours (flexible target) are calculated by multiplying the unit's standard 8 HPPD by the actual number of patient days for the month (485). In other words, with 485 patient days for the month and 8 HPPD targeted per patient, the direct care hours should be targeted as 3,880 direct care hours for the month. However, nurses actually report 4,455 productive (direct care) hours for the month, 15% above the targeted hours. Comparing the projected direct care hours with the actual productive hours provides helpful insights about the actual extent of excessive staff hours and costs. The CNO points out that the overtime hours are also substantially over budget.

Other indicators reinforce the concerns about staffing. The actual HPPD are more than an hour longer than required by staffing standards (9.2 HPPD rather than the targeted 8.0 HPPD), and the N/P ratio is more intense than targeted (2.6 patients compared to 3 patients per RN). Some of this excess in direct care hours likely stems from the excessive overtime and agency nurse hours, which are approximately twice the budgeted amount (688 overtime and agency hours compared to 336 budgeted overtime hours). Absenteeism (excessive use of sick leave) might be a reason that the nonproductive hours are higher than budgeted. The report indicates that the total paid hours for East Wing are nearly 20% over budget for the month (5,780.1 actual hours compared to 4,856.0 budgeted hours). Staffing reports for prior months (not shown) indicate that staffing and overtime hours have been creeping upward for some time.

The CNO and nurse manager use this information as a starting point for staffing strategies. The new nurse manager has been so focused on learning the manager role and coping with day-to-day crises that she has not attended to filling the vacant nurse staff positions. Filling these positions will likely reduce the need for overtime and agency hours, so the nurse manager makes this task a top priority.

Another strategy is for the nurse manager to more carefully monitor overtime hours, absenteeism, and to coordinate approved leave with anticipated staffing needs. Charge nurses are directed to more closely monitor and report staff overtime hours. The nurse manager will begin to review all reported overtime hours and determine whether these hours are approved or not, counseling employees who request overtime pay for activities that are not approved for overtime, such as catching up on charting. Staff absenteeism, most apparent over weekends in East Wing, is another source of overtime and agency hours that the nurse manager will more closely monitor and attempt to control.

Better control of patient flow helps in managing and controlling staffing hours and costs. An analysis of patient flow indicates that the most intense patient activity is currently focused on Mondays through Wednesdays, resulting in shortages of staff and greater use of overtime and agency hours on those days. The CNO and patient flow team work with the nurse manager, so admissions and occupancy are smoother throughout the week and better fit staff scheduling (Fieldston et al., 2011). As a result, more scheduled patient admissions occur Mondays through Fridays, with more shorter stay patients admitted on Thursdays and Fridays so they may be discharged over the weekend. This strategy not only smooths out demands on staff during the business week, but also makes better use of weekend staff who were previously underutilized.

The manager develops strategies to better distribute nurse workload across all of the shifts. Currently, the most intense care in the East Wing is provided by the day shift, from 10 a.m. to 4 p.m. ADTs are typically scheduled during the day, as are physician rounds and most of the patient procedures. Although many of these patient care activities cannot be rescheduled, the nurse manager works with the nursing staff to find solutions to address the uneven workload. For example, some patient care, such as baths, can be scheduled during the evening shift, rather than the day shift. The night shift staff can review patient charts and prepare checklists for activities such as discharge planning, so the day shift nurses can manage these activities more efficiently. These strategies help the unit better utilize the staff over the entire 24 hours of scheduling.

Another strategy is to allocate the FTEs for daily staffing so that staff are optimally distributed. The report for November 2017 describes typical staffing requirements for East Wing, with 17 nurses budgeted each day, on average. The CNO advises the nurse manager to schedule the RNs so that there are seven nurses on the day shift and five nurses on the evening and night shifts. Even small adjustments that increase staffing and smooth patient flow can considerably ease the stress on nursing staff and help improve patient care. The nurse manager will monitor the impact of these changes, expecting that patient outcomes, nurse satisfaction, and patient flow will improve.

■ SCENARIO THREE: THE TRUE COST OF A PRODUCTIVE NURSING HOUR

Although the CNO sees improvements in patient flow and staff scheduling, reports indicate that Pacific Hospital's staffing costs remain higher than those of other similar hospitals in the area. The CNO investigates the flow of the staffing dollar in more detail. The following case scenario describing the CNO's review of staffing expenses demonstrates how drilling down aggregate data to a greater level of detail can improve understanding about cost or quality problems. This case example focuses on the actual hourly cost of RNs, based on all sources of staff nurse costs. The scenario demonstrates the importance of using data to provide evidence for better informed decisions rather than relying on commonly held assumptions.

When analyzing the cost of nursing staff, executives can make mission-critical decisions based on incomplete data. The cost of a staff nurse is important in budgeting for nursing microsystems. Many nurse budgeting experts estimate the cost of staff nurses as the hourly wage, plus benefits ranging from 25% to 35% of the hourly wage (Finkler & McHugh, 2008; Penner, 2016; Waxman, 2015). The CNO assumes the cost of Pacific Hospital nurses at the hourly wage of 74.95 plus 30% benefits, or $97.45 per hour. The common wisdom at Pacific Hospital is that agency nurses, costing $100.00 per hour, are substantially more expensive than staff nurses.

Cost and quality concerns limit nurse agency use at Pacific Hospital. However, if staff nurse costs actually approach or exceed that of agency nurses, it may affect decisions about using agency nurses versus assigning overtime or double shifts to staff nurses. Overlooking sources of costs also impacts on the budget and makes budget control more difficult.

Table 3.4 presents an example for assessing the true cost of a staff nurse based on paid productive hours, wage-related costs, and other RN costs. This example is based on the hourly and annual costs of a 1.0 FTE "average" staff nurse with 5 years of seniority (Spencer, 2017). It is important to understand that the focus of the analysis is on the staff nurse's *productive* hours and costs. Agency nurses are utilized to provide direct care and are not budgeted for indirect or nonproductive hours. In order to compare staff nurse to agency nurse costs, the CNO views the staff nurse costs based on productive hours.

Therefore, the CNO also must identify all costs associated with staff nurse employment, including some costs that may have previously been overlooked. These costs and wages may vary considerably across institutions, so the estimates presented in Tables 3.4 and 3.5 may differ in other settings. The scenario is a guide for thinking about these costs and their impact on the staffing budget and staffing decisions. Note that the analysis is based on the northern California RN market, where nursing salaries are among the highest in the nation. However, the relationships remain the same regardless of the starting wage.

Nonproductive hours—The staff nurse wage is estimated at $74.95 an hour, or $155,896 annually, which includes all paid nonproductive hours as well as productive hours. Paid vacation leave is estimated at 120 hours per year. There are 10 paid holidays, which total 80 hours. It is assumed that the staff nurse has 120 hours of sick leave, with 75% of the hours utilized, for a total of 90 hours of paid sick leave. Forty hours of educational leave are authorized, with nurses utilizing on average 80%, or 32 hours. Bereavement leave is estimated at 40 hours, with the assumption that on average the staff nurse will use 20% or 8 hours. Jury duty leave is estimated at 4 hours per year. Note a total of 16 hours of training and in-service are paid per year but are treated as overtime cost and not as nonproductive hours. All these sources of nonproductive hours add up to 334 hours per year.

Productive hours and hourly cost—When the 334 paid nonproductive hours are removed from the 2,080 hours in 1.0 FTE, there are 1,746 annual productive staff nurse hours. In order to convert the base wage to an "initial productive hourly wage," the annual salary of $155,896 is divided by the 1,746 productive hours equaling $102.63 (see Table 3.4). This initial productive wage is used as the base for additional nursing costs discussed in the scenario.

Wage-related costs—Federal and state taxes are estimated at 6.94% and vary as wages increase, as there is no limit on the 1.45% Medicare contribution. Workers' compensation and professional liability insurance are estimated at 3% of wages. Institutions that cannot self-insure or that have high experience modification ratings may need to budget workers' compensation at a higher rate. In some settings, an additional amount of workers' compensation funds may need to be set aside as a reserve (GuideStar, 2008a, 2008b). Retirement benefits are estimated as 5% in this example. These wage-related costs add $11.20, increasing the base of $74.95 to $86.15 per productive hour (see Table 3.4).

Other costs: health, disability, and life insurance—The highest and probably most variable cost in this category is health insurance. Disability and life insurance are additional costs. It is difficult to find estimates for health, disability, and life insurance costs for hospitals. The estimate in this example values the cost of health, dental, vision, disability, and life insurance at $9,352.

Other costs: recruitment and orientation—The CNO estimates that a staff nurse works 8 years on average before changing jobs, so 12.5% is Pacific Hospital's turnover rate. If it costs $8,000 to

Table 3.4 Pacific Hospital, Sources of Costs of a Staff Nurse, 2017

Sources of Costs	Percent of Hourly Wage or FTE	Annual Paid or Productive Hours	Annual Wage or Cost	Hourly Wage or Cost
Nonproductive and productive hours (% FTE):				
Vacation	—	120	—	—
Holidays	—	80	—	—
Sick leave	—	90	—	—
Educational leave	—	32	—	—
Bereavement	—	8	—	—
Jury duty	—	4	—	—
Training and in-service	—	16	—	—
Total nonproductive	—	350	—	—
Hours and wages				
Total productive hours and wages	—	1,730	—	$54.10
Total FTE hours and wages	—	2,080	$93,600	$45.00
Wage-related cost (% productive hourly wages):				
Federal and state taxes	7.2%	2,080	$6,749	$3.24
Workers' compensation and professional liability	3.0%	2,080	$2,808	$1.35
Retirement benefits	5.0%	2,080	$4,680	$2.25
Total wage-related costs	15.2%	2,080	$14,237	$6.84
Total productive wages and wage-related costs	—	2,080	$107,837	$60.95
Other RN costs:				
Health, disability, and life insurance	—	1,730	$9,352	$5.41
Recruitment, termination, and hiring	—	1,730	$1,250	$0.72
Orientation	—	1,730	$375	$0.22
Total other RN costs	—	1,730	$10,977	$6.35
Total RN costs based on productive hours	—	1,730	$118,814	$67.29
RN overtime @ 50%	—	2,080	$154,637	$74.34
Including wage-related costs				
Agency nurse hourly rate	—	1,730	$121,100	$70.00

FTE, full-time equivalent.

recruit a nurse, the annual recruitment cost is therefore $1,000. Orientation costs are determined using the same approach, so orientation costs of $3,000 per new hire plus 80 hours at base rate + wage-related costs ($86.15) are annualized at $1,236 a year.

Other costs: in-service training and education reimbursement—The CNO allocates 16 hours per year at overtime (OT) for in-service training and assumes that nurses on average utilize 50% of the $2,300 education reimbursement authorized in the current labor contract. These costs are summarized in Table 3.4.

The productive hourly wage of $111.11 is 48.2% greater than the beginning wage of $74.95. This scenario reinforces the observation that the true cost of a productive nursing hour is likely closer to 50% more than the hourly wage versus prevailing estimates of 25% to 30% (Spencer, 2017). When the productive wage is compared to the $100 hourly expense of agency nurses, the actual cost difference is much less than the CNO had assumed.

Some additional considerations support costing out the true cost of a staff nurse compared to an agency nurse. Overtime pay for a staff nurse at Pacific Hospital is 1.5 times the hourly wage plus wage-related costs, or $129.23 per hour ($86.15 × 1.5), as shown in Table 3.4. The cost per productive hour must also be considered for shift differentials, weekend coverage, and short hour nurses and are summarized in Table 3.4. The CNO realizes that agency nurses are cost-effective compared to staff nurses, particularly when overtime or differential pay is involved.

Although the use of agency nurses must be closely monitored for quality, there are also serious quality concerns when staff nurses work for more than 12 hours (IOM, 2004). Rather than simply assuming that agency nurses are too costly or that they cannot provide quality care, it may be important to instead consider how to best balance costs and quality in staffing and scheduling. In many situations, a careful mix of staff and agency nurses could reduce problems from double-shift fatigue while ensuring that agency nurses supplement rather than replace FT staff.

RN OVERTIME STAFFING STRATEGIES

The CNO shows the nurse leadership team an analysis of costs for FT RN staff and FT RN overtime expenses compared to the costs of using an RN agency (see Table 3.5). For a number of years, the nursing leadership at Pacific Hospital believed that agency fees were much higher than staff RN coverage, and that staff RNs always provide better care than agency nurses. As a result, most RN overtime coverage has been provided by FT staff RNs, with PT RNs utilized to cover unfilled positions, holiday and weekend coverage, vacations, and other leave.

At Pacific Hospital, agency nurse utilization tends to be unplanned and unbudgeted. Recently, exit surveys indicate that the demands to work overtime increasingly contribute to job dissatisfaction and FT RN turnover (IOM, 2004). Hospital reporting and research evidence reinforce that serious medical errors are more likely to occur when RNs work excessive overtime (IOM, 2004). These errors are frequently costly, so better long-term staffing strategies for overtime coverage are needed.

The analysis indicates that the total productive hourly cost of a FT day RN is $111.11 and that overtime is $129.22, comparable to agency fees of "+/–" $100 an hour. A nursing shortage reduces the availability of PT nurses for overtime coverage, requiring some rethinking about policies that limit agency nurse utilization. The CNO proposes a small test of change (IHI, 2011b) directed at improving the quality of staffing decisions, reducing medical errors, and fostering nurse satisfaction and efficiency. In collaboration with Pacific Hospital's nurse managers, the CNO and team develop overtime staffing guidelines that are evidence-based and tailored to the needs of medical–surgical, intensive care, and other nursing units across the institution.

Pacific Hospital's new overtime staffing guidelines specify that, whenever possible, RN staff should not be scheduled for more than 12 hours in a day or more than 48 hours in a week (IOM, 2004). In other words, agency nurses should be considered, rather than asking RN staff to work a double shift. To safeguard quality as well as continuity of care, nurse managers work with staff to develop criteria for the desired mix of FT to agency nurses. As shown in Table 3.5, a target of increasing agency nurse usage to cover 30% of overtime hours is established for the coming fiscal year. Supplementing staff nurses with agency nurses to reduce double-shift fatigue will potentially reduce errors and improve RN performance, without additional cost.

Another concern is that Pacific Hospital's overtime hours and costs are substantially over budget compared to other institutions. FT RNs at Pacific Hospital work an estimated 6.5 hours of overtime per week, compared to the national average of 4.0 hours per week (The KPMG Health Care and Pharmaceutical Institute, 2011). The CNO establishes a performance

TABLE 3.5 Pacific Hospital, RN Overtime Staffing Cost Analysis, 2017

Item	Amount to Basis
Staffed beds	780
Occupancy rate	80.0%
Patient days	227,136
Discharges	61,000
ALOS	3.7
HPPD	7.8
Productive hours RNs	1,771,660.8
Total RN FTEs	851.8
FT RN FTEs	596.2
RN hourly wage	$74.95
FT RN total cost including benefits	$111.11
RN overtime wage (150% hourly wage plus wage-related costs)	$129.22
Agency nurse hourly expense	$100.00
2017 actual RN overtime hours	201,526
2017 RN overtime expense	$14,982,381
2018 budgeted RN overtime hours (70%)	108,514
2018 budgeted overtime RN expense	$8,067,436
2018 budgeted agency hours	46,506
2018 budgeted agency expense	$3,255,427
2018 total budgeted RN and agency overtime hours	155,020
2018 total budgeted RN and agency overtime expense	$11,322,862
Target reduction overtime hours 2011–2018	–46,506
Target reduction overtime expense 2017–2018	–$3,659,518

ALOS, average length of stay; FT, full-time; FTEs, full-time equivalents; HPPD, hours per patient day.

target attempting to reduce RN overtime to 5 hours per week in 2018, thus potentially reducing annual overtime by 46,506 hours and $3,659,518 (Table 3.5). Given the improvements in patient flow and scheduling, greater attention by nurse managers to abuse of overtime, and the judicious use of agency nurses, the CNO believes this goal may be achievable.

SCENARIO FOUR: OUTPATIENT CARE INDICATORS

According to the American Hospital Association (AHA, 2016), inpatient admissions in community hospitals in the United States dropped 5.8% from about 35.1 million admissions in 2004 to about 33.1 million admissions in 2014. Over the same time period, outpatient visits in community hospitals rose 21.3% from about 571.6 million visits in 2004 to about 693.1 million visits in 2014. Improved technologies allow for more tests and procedures in ambulatory care settings. Financial incentives to keep patients out of the hospital also contribute to this ongoing trend from hospital inpatient to outpatient care (Vesely, 2014).

One of the 2012 proposals of the DNP managing Pacific Hospital's cardiac step-down units was telephone follow-up for all discharged cardiac patients (discussed in Scenario One). This

TABLE 3.6 Heart Failure Clinic Outpatient Benchmarks, 2017

Indicator	Benchmark
Annual Statistics:	
Capacity (available appointments)	2,000
Patients (new and established)	180
Encounters	1,800
Urgent care referrals	72
Specialty appointments	250
Current visit rate	10
Readmission rate (30-day)	6%
Daily Statistics:	
Average appointments per day	5
Average NP encounters per day	8
Wait Times:	
Average wait time for clinic appointment (days)	7
Average office visit cycle time (hours)	1
Financials:	
Average revenue per encounter	$150
Average expense per encounter	$115
Net profit or loss	$35

NP, nurse practitioner.

proposal was implemented and demonstrated some improvement in patient outcomes as well as some reduction in preventable readmissions. The proposed nurse-directed heart failure clinic expands this project by offering routine face-to-face patient visits tailored to the needs of persons with heart failure and their caregivers. Heart failure clinics providing specialized services to this patient population provide comprehensive care and provide evidence of improved outcomes (Hauptman et al., 2008).

The DNP managing the cardiac step-down units writes a business plan that includes indicators and benchmarks for outpatient care (Table 3.6). The business plan is submitted in 2017, and it is assumed that if approved, the heart failure clinic will open in January 2018. The indicators and benchmarks are discussed in the following section.

AMBULATORY CARE PERFORMANCE INDICATORS

In this chapter, *ambulatory* refers to care or measures provided in any ambulatory care setting, such as a free-standing clinic. *Outpatient* care or measures refer to ambulatory care provided in a hospital setting, such as the heart failure clinic proposed at Pacific Hospital. These terms are often used interchangeably. Indicators and benchmarks for the heart failure clinic begin with statistics reported on an annual basis.

Capacity—The capacity, or ability of a service to meet consumer demand (Penner, 2016), is measured by the number of appointments available over the fiscal year. The benchmark of 2,000 encounters per year is calculated by estimating that the clinic is staffed by two NPs who each manage four encounters per day. The total 2,080 projected encounters are rounded down to

2,000 because health settings and health care complexity require planning that is somewhat less than maximum capacity (IOM, 2015; Penner, 2016).

Patients—The count of patients served in ambulatory settings includes new patients and established patients (IOM, 2015), and is a measure of demand for ambulatory services. For 2018, the year the heart failure clinic is proposed to open, the DNP anticipates that most of the 180 projected patients are new patients, as the follow-up care of recently discharged heart failure patients has not been monitored systematically in the past. As more patients become established, the DNP anticipates growth in demand and a need for more NPs to increase the clinic's capacity. Patients in ambulatory or outpatient settings might also be classified using categories such as age, disorder, or source of payment.

Encounters—Face-to-face contact between the patient and provider is often referred to as a visit. Patient encounters are defined as visits that are billable or otherwise reimbursed (Penner, 2016). The terms *visits* and *encounters* are often used interchangeably. The DNP estimates 1,800 patient encounters for the start-up year 2018.

Urgent care referrals—A substantial proportion of heart failure patients are at high risk, related to their recent hospital discharge or comorbidities (Hauptman et al., 2008). The DNP therefore benchmarks urgent care referrals at 4% of all patient encounters, or 72 referrals. In this setting, urgent care referrals include referrals of a patient encountered in the clinic to the ED, or advice to patients scheduling appointments to call 911 if their situation appears to be urgent.

Specialty appointments—The DNP assumes that the NPs will refer an estimated 15% (270) of their annual patient encounters to cardiac specialists for nonurgent care. The specialty appointment should be made within 1 week. The actual number of specialty appointments is benchmarked at 250. The DNP will closely monitor this measure to ensure that patients have appropriate access to specialty services.

Current visit rate—The average number of encounters per patient per year represents the current visit rate. The estimated number of patients (180) times the estimated current visit rate (10) results in the estimated demand or number of patient encounters for 2018 (1,800). In other words, the number of patients and the current visit rate help the DNP plan for the capacity required for the heart failure clinic to meet demand (IOM, 2015).

Readmission rate—The readmission rate (also referred to as the *rate*) is defined and discussed in Scenario One. The DNP benchmarks the readmission rate at 6% of the heart failure clinic patients, based on outcomes from research evidence (Walker, Jacobson, & Sumodi, 2012). The current (2017) readmission rate for heart failure patients who are discharged, then readmitted within 30 days is 25% at Pacific Hospital. This measure therefore reinforces the potential value of the heart failure clinic in managing preventable readmissions.

Average appointments per day—Another measure of demand is the number of appointments generated each day, including same-day and future appointments (IOM, 2015). The DNP estimates that five appointments are a reasonable benchmark. This benchmark can be tracked daily and over monthly and annual time periods to monitor changes in demand, such as the anticipated growth as the clinic becomes established and accepts more new patients discharged from Pacific Hospital.

Average NP encounters per day—Another capacity measure is the number of patient encounters with an NP per day. If one or more NPs are unable to maintain the benchmark average of eight encounters per day, there may be performance problems or a higher level of complexity in caring for this patient population. If one or more NPs report more than the benchmark average of eight encounters per day, there may be reason to increase the NP workload or to increase capacity (NP staffing) to manage demand.

Average wait time for clinic appointment—Patient flow is important to monitor in ambulatory settings as well as inpatient settings. The average wait time for a clinic appointment is measured by the amount of time between a patient's request for an appointment and an available opening in a provider's schedule (IOM, 2015). Although wait time is considered to be a nationwide concern in ambulatory care, there are no specific benchmarks. The DNP establishes a benchmark of no more than 7 days for clinic appointment wait times. The DNP will also closely monitor wait time *outliers* (Secretary of Defense, 2014), or excessively long wait times, currently benchmarked as an appointment wait time in excess of 14 days.

Average office visit cycle time—The amount of time required to manage a patient encounter is another measure of patient flow in ambulatory care. Excessive cycle time may indicate concerns such as performance problems, system bottlenecks, or higher than anticipated patient complexity. Office visit cycle time is measured from the time the patient checks in to the clinic to the time the patient checks out for an appointment (IOM, 2015). This measure can be divided into the cycle steps, such as time spent in the waiting room or time required for a procedure. These steps can also be classified as value added or not, such as time spent with the provider (value-added) or time spent waiting for the next step in the appointment (non-value added). The DNP estimates a benchmark of 1 hour for heart failure appointment cycle time. The DNP also plans to monitor outliers in cycle time and cycle time steps to manage heart failure clinic patient flow.

Average revenue per encounter—The DNP includes all sources of revenue such as Medicare, Medicaid, private insurance, and grant funding for clinic services. It is important for the DNP to project anticipated changes in revenue or revenue sources. For example, revenues are expected to increase as the number of heart failure clinic patients increases. The DNP projects the average revenue per encounter at $150 for 2018.

Average expense per encounter—The DNP includes all sources of expense required for a patient appointment. Tracking the expense of selected procedures, such as lab tests or ECGs, also helps the DNP monitor expenses. Budget management responsibilities and skills help inform the DNP's assessment of expenses per encounter (Penner, 2016). The DNP projects the average expense per encounter at $115 for 2018.

Net profit or loss—Profitability is an indicator of financial health (Penner, 2016). The sustainability of health care programs may depend on the maintenance of financial benchmarks. If demand is not reasonably matched to capacity, profitability may be reduced. For example, if the heart failure clinic only serves two patients per day in 2018, the clinic, with a capacity for eight patients per day, is underutilized and is only generating 25% of anticipated revenues. Profitability is also a performance indicator (IOM, 2015). For example, if the heart failure clinic serves only two patients per day in 2018 with a capacity for eight patients per day, it may represent system bottlenecks or staff performance problems. The DNP projects the average net profit per encounter at $35 for 2018.

PROPOSING A NURSE-LED HEART FAILURE CLINIC

The cardiac step-down unit's DNP must make a business case to Pacific Hospital executives for the proposed nurse-led heart failure clinic. The DNP presents convincing evidence supporting substantial financial savings associated with the implementation of heart failure clinics (Henrick, 2001; Paul, 2000). A business plan with detailed budgets of projected revenue sources and revenues as well as sources and amounts of expenses is prepared and presented to make the business case for the heart failure clinic (Penner, 2016). The DNP presents the benchmark indicators shown in Table 3.6 in the business plan. This information is included in a discussion of ongoing performance monitoring and annual performance evaluation of the heart failure clinic.

The IOM endorses expansion of nursing roles to the full scope of practice to help achieve more cost-effective health care outcomes while improving health care quality and access (National Academies of Sciences, Engineering and Medicine, 2015). The CNO supports the step-down unit's DNP's proposal for a nurse-led heart failure clinic at Pacific Hospital.

CONCLUSION

This chapter presents several case scenarios with examples for using indicators to analyze and solve problems in hospital nursing microsystems. The scenarios demonstrate how critical analysis of data can help DNPs lead change and improvement in acute and outpatient care settings.

CRITICAL THINKING EXERCISES

1. *Hospital readmissions.* A 2017 Medicare Payment Advisory Commission (MedPAC) report found that Medicare hospital readmission rates have declined in recent years, but remain a concern. Incentives are needed to further reduce readmission rates and improve care coordination (MedPAC, 2017). Review this report or find another report more current or more specific to your acute care setting. Using the Hospital Compare website (www.medicare.gov/hospitalcompare/search.html) or data from your setting, compare your hospital's 30-day readmission rate with these research findings. Propose at least three reasons for your setting's 30-day readmission rate, as well as at least three ideas for interventions to reduce and control readmissions at your hospital.

2. *24/7 coverage factor.* Calculate and compare the 24/7 coverage factor for RNs working 8-hour and 12-hour shifts. Explain differences and similarities in the results.

3. *RN overtime hours and costs.* As discussed in the third scenario in this chapter, the CNO of Pacific Hospital realizes that overtime hours and costs are excessive. The budget target is to reduce weekly overtime hours per FT RN from 6.5 to 4.0 hours. Strategies may include substitutes for overtime (Berney, Needleman, & Kovner, 2005), interventions such as rapid response teams to quickly address patient complications (Thomas, Force, Rasmussen, Dodd, & Whildin, 2007), or other ideas. Use evidence-based approaches to propose strategies to reduce overtime at Pacific Hospital, and prepare a table showing your analysis of reduction in overtime hours and related cost savings.

4. *Ambulatory care budget.* The fourth scenario in this chapter presents an example of planning an outpatient nurse-led heart failure clinic. Develop a budget that includes performance and financial indicators and benchmarks for another type of outpatient service that might be provided at Pacific Hospital. Adapt and expand on the indicators and benchmarks presented in Table 3.6.

5. *Staffing guidelines for covering last minute shortages.* The third scenario in this chapter presents the methodology for calculating cost per productive hour. Determine the wage variables for your unit/institution and calculate the productive costs per hour, per shift and per overtime shift. Establish the current agency rates for your institution. Develop guidelines for covering a shift when no internal non-overtime resources are available and calculate the true cost of each alternative. *Bonus:* Calculate the annual cost savings if this guideline was 70% effective in eliminating use of staff double shifts.

REFERENCES

American Association of Colleges of Nursing. (2006). *The essentials of doctoral education for advanced nursing practice.* Washington, DC: Author.

American Hospital Association. (2016). *TrendWatch chartbook 2016: Trends affecting hospitals and health systems.* Washington, DC: Author. Retrieved from http://www.aha.org/research/reports/tw/chartbook/2016/2016chartbook.pdf

American Nurses Association. (2017). Nurse staffing. Retrieved from http://nursingworld.org/MainMenu Categories/Policy-Advocacy/State/Legislative-Agenda-Reports/State-StaffingPlansRatios

Berney, B., Needleman, J., & Kovner, C. (2005). Factors influencing the use of registered nurse overtime in hospitals, 1995–2000. *Journal of Nursing Scholarship, 37*(2), 165–172.

California Nurses Association. (2006). Missed break pay starts January 1. Retrieved from http://www.calnurses.org

California Nurses Association and National Nurses Organizing Committee. (2009). The ratio solution. Retrieved from http://www.calnurses.org; http://www.nnoc.net

Cesta, T., & Keeling, B. (2009). Stop inappropriate admissions to improve your hospital's patient flow. *Hospital Case Management, 17*(1), 1–16.

Clarke, S. P., & Donaldson, N. E. (2008). Nurse staffing and patient care quality and safety. In R. G. Hughes (Ed.), *Patient safety and quality: An evidence-based handbook for nurses* (AHRQ Publication No. 08-0043). Rockville, MD: Agency for Healthcare Research and Quality.

Dobson, A., DaVanzo, J., Haught, R., & Luu, P. (2016, December 6). Estimating the impact of repealing the Affordable Care Act on hospitals. *Dobson|DaVanzo*. Retrieved from http://www.aha.org/content/16/impact-repeal-aca-report.pdf

Douglas, K. (2010). Taking action to close the nursing-finance gap: Learning from success. *Nursing Economic$, 28*(4), 270–272.

Dreher, H. M., & Smith Glasgow, M. E. (2011). *Role development for doctoral advanced nursing practice*. New York, NY: Springer Publishing.

Dunton, N., Gajewski, B., Klaus, S., & Pierson, B. (2007, September 30). The relationship of nursing workforce characteristics to patient outcomes. *The Online Journal of Issues in Nursing, 12*(3), manuscript 3. Retrieved from http://nursingworld.org/MainMenuCategories/ANAMarketplace/ANAPeriodicals/OJIN/TableofContents/Volume122007/No3Sept07/NursingWorkforceCharacteristics.html

Enriquez, M., Sisson, M., Kirby, A., & Gupta, N. (2009). Increasing hospital capacity using existing resources to improve patient flow management. *Nurse Leader, 7*(1), 26–31.

Fieldston, E. S., Hall, M., Shah, S. S., Hain, P. D., Sills, M. R., Slonim, A. D., . . . Pati, S. (2011). Addressing inpatient crowding by smoothing occupancy at children's hospitals. *Journal of Hospital Medicine, 6*(8), 462–468. Retrieved from http://www.journalofhospitalmedicine.com

Finkler, S. A., & McHugh, M. L. (2008). *Budgeting concepts for nurse managers* (4th ed.). Philadelphia, PA: Elsevier/Mosby/Saunders.

Forster, A. J., Stiell, I., Wells, G., Lee, A. J., & van Walraven, C. (2003). The effect of hospital occupancy on emergency department length of stay and patient disposition. *Academy of Emergency Medicine, 10*(2), 127–133.

Green, L. V. (2004). Capacity planning and management in hospitals. In M. L. Brandeau, F. Sainfort, & W. Pierskalla (Eds.), *Operations research and health care: A handbook of methods and applications* (pp. 15–42). Norwell, MA: Kluwer Academic.

GuideStar. (2008a). Kaiser Foundation Hospitals Form 990. Retrieved from http://www.guidestar.org/FinDocuments/2008/941/105/2008-941105628-0578411b-9.pdf

GuideStar. (2008b). Marin General Hospital Form 990: 2008. Retrieved from http://www.guidestar.org/FinDocuments//2008/942/823/2008-942823538-056ec0a9-9.pdf

Hauptman, P., Rich, M., Heidenreich, P., Chin, J., Cummings, N., Dunlap, M., . . . Philbin, E. (2008). The heart failure clinic: A consensus statement of the Heart Failure Society of America. *Journal of Cardiac Failure, 14*(10), 801–815.

Henrick, A. (2001). Cost-effective outpatient management of persons with heart failure. *Progress in Cardiovascular Nursing, 16*(2), 50–56.

Horton, L. A. (2010). *Calculating and reporting health care statistics* (3rd ed.). Chicago, IL: American Health Information Management Association.

Inglis, S. C., Clark, R. A., McAlister, F. A., Ball, J., Lewinter, C., Cullington, D., . . . Cleland, J. G. F. (2010). Structured telephone support or telemonitoring programmes for patients with chronic heart failure [Review]. *The Cochrane Collaboration*. Hoboken, NJ: John Wiley. Retrieved from http://www.thecochranelibrary.com

Institute for Healthcare Improvement. (2003). *Optimizing patient flow: Moving patients smoothly through acute care settings* (Innovation Series 2003). Cambridge, MA: Author.

Institute for Healthcare Improvement. (2011a). Patient flow tools. Retrieved from http://www.ihi.org/IHI/Topics/Flow/PatientFlow/EmergingContent

Institute for Healthcare Improvement. (2011b). Science of improvement: Testing changes. Retrieved from http://www.ihi.org/knowledge/Pages/HowtoImprove/ScienceofImprovementTestingChanges.aspx

Institute of Medicine. (2004). *Keeping patients safe: Transforming the work environment of nurses*. Washington, DC: National Academies Press.

Institute of Medicine. 2015. *Transforming health care scheduling and access: Getting to now*. Washington, DC: National Academies Press. Retrieved from http://www.nationalacademies.org/hmd/Reports/2015/Transforming-Health-Care-Scheduling-and-Access.aspx

Jacobson, A. K., Seltzer, J. E., & Dam, E. J. (1999). New methodology for analyzing fluctuating unit activity. *Nursing Economic$, 17*(1), 55–59.

Kelleher, C., & Parker, P. (2007). Medical/surgical bed occupancy rate targets. *APHA Health Planning Today, 29*(2), 7.

Kirk, R. (1981). *Nursing management tools*. Boston, MA: Little, Brown.

The KPMG Healthcare and Pharmaceutical Institute. (2011). KPMG's 2011 U.S. hospital nursing labor costs study. Retrieved from http://www.natho.org/pdfs/KPMG_2011_Nursing_LaborCostStudy.pdf

Lane, B. S., Jackson, J., Odom, S. E., Cannella, K. A. S., & Hinshaw, L. (2009). Nurse satisfaction and creation of an admission, discharge, and teaching nurse position. *Journal of Nursing Care Quality, 24*(2), 148–152.

Medicare Payment Advisory Commission. (2017). *Report to the Congress: Medicare payment policy*. Washington, DC: Author. Retrieved from http://medpac.gov/docs/default-source/reports/mar17_entirereport.pdf

Medicare.gov. (n.d.). Hospital compare hospital returns. Retrieved from https://www.medicare.gov/hospitalcompare/Data/Hospital-returns.html

National Academies of Sciences, Engineering and Medicine. (2015). *Assessing progress on the Institute of Medicine report The Future of Nursing*. Washington, DC: National Academies Press. Retrieved from http://www.nationalacademies.org/hmd/reports/2015/assessing-progress-on-the-iom-report-the-future-of-nursing.aspx

Page, A. E. (2008). Temporary, agency, and other contingent workers. In R. G. Hughes (Ed.), *Patient safety and quality: An evidence-based handbook for nurses* (Chap. 27, Prepared with support from the Robert Wood Johnson Foundation. AHRQ Publication No. 08-0043). Rockville, MD: Agency for Healthcare Research and Quality.

Park, S. H., Dunton, N., & Blegen, M. A. (2016). Comparison of unit-level patient turnover measures in acute care hospital settings. *Research in Nursing and Health, 39*(3), 197–203.

Paul, S. (2000). Impact of a nurse-managed heart failure clinic: A pilot study. *American Journal of Critical Care, 9*(2), 140–146.

Penner, S. J. (2016). *Economics and financial management for nurses and nurse leaders* (3rd ed.). New York, NY: Springer Publishing.

Rabin, E., Kocher, K., McClelland, M., Pines, J., Hwang, U., Rathlev, N., . . . Weber, E. (2012). Solutions to emergency department "boarding" and crowding are underused and may need to be legislated. *Health Affairs, 31*(8), 1757–1766.

Secretary of Defense. (2014, August 29). *Military health system review final report. Appendix 3. Access to care.* Department of Defense. Retrieved from http://www.health.mil/Military-Health-Topics/Access-Cost-Quality-and-Safety/MHS-Review

Sherrod, B., & Goda, T. (2016). Higher learning: DNP-prepared leaders guide healthcare system change. *Nursing Management, 47*(9), 13–16.

Spencer, M. D. (2017). *Assessing the true cost of a productive nursing hour*. Unpublished white paper.

Thomas, K., Force, M., Rasmussen, D., Dodd, D., & Whildin, S. (2007). Rapid response team: Challenges, solutions, benefits. *Critical Care Nurse, 27*(1), 20–28.

Tortorella, F., Ukanowicz, D., Douglas-Ntagha, P., Ray, R., & Triller, M. (2013). Improving bed turnover time with a bed management system. *Journal of Nursing Administration, 43*(1), 37–43.

Vesely, R. (2014). The great migration. *Hospitals and Health Networks, 88*(3), 22–27.

Walker, D., Jacobson, A., & Sumodi, V. (2012). Hospitalization and rehospitalization rates of patients in a network of nurse-led heart failure clinics. *Heart and Lung, 41*(4), 419.

Wang, J., Li, J., & Howard, P. K. (2013). A system model of work flow in the patient room of hospital emergency department. *Health Care Management Science, 16*(4), 341–351.

Waxman, K. T. (2015). *Finance and budgeting made simple: Essential skills for nurses*. Marblehead, MA: HCPro.

Welch, S., Augustine, J., Camargo, C. A., & Reese, C. (2006). Emergency department performance measures and benchmarking summit. *Society for Academic Emergency Medicine, 13*(10), 1074–1080.

Budgeting, Scheduling, and Daily Staffing for Acute Care Nursing Units

Chrys Marie Suby

The focus of this chapter is to provide the doctor of nursing practice (DNP)/nurse leader with knowledge of the financial, scheduling, staffing, and reporting tools, as well as leadership commitment, required to be successful in the management and retention of their workforce and the delivery of care to the patients. The DNP/nurse leader has ultimate accountability for the cost center budget for labor resources, salary and expense dollars, staff satisfaction, and the delivery of care to the patients on the unit. From the perspective of optimized staffing, high retention, and low turnover of less than 10% in nursing and 5% organizationally, the top 10 workforce management characteristics of organizations of performance excellence include the following:

1. Bold, inspiring, agile, adaptable leadership
2. Creative and collaborative partnerships between leaders and staff
3. Financial discipline
4. Respectful and optimized staffing
5. Focused accountability and execution of business goals
6. Proficiency in patient-centric care and operations
7. Clearly defined nursing and/or workforce management model(s) of care
8. Continuous learning with insight and application
9. Technology that realizes the impact of system integrations to provide actionable information for change-forward decision making
10. A human resources (HR) center committed to data-driven staff retention, aggressive recruitment, and leadership support

From the bedside to the executive office, the growing complexity and rapid changes occurring in health care increasingly require that all care providers collaborate and maximize their efficiency. In 2017, it is estimated that three quarters of all people working in a health care system today are nurses or are on the nursing team, touching patients at every level of care and possessing a unique perspective that health care leadership needs. The staff nurses of today are the charge nurses and unit leaders of tomorrow; yet, we continue to have an aging workforce, high turnover, and a projected leadership vacuum.

The shortage of RNs in the United States continues to be well publicized and is being felt by many hospitals. In 2014, the projected shortage was described as a "tsunami of change" based on research studies between 2000 and 2016. According to a 2014 fact sheet from American Nurses Association (ANA), the estimated overall number of new RNs needed (new replacements) is 1.13 million; this value is based on data from the U.S. Department of Labor, Bureau of Labor Statistics. The projected number of current RNs retiring or leaving the labor force between 2012 and 2022 is 555,100. The need for nurses is due to the retirement of one third of the nursing workforce; the pending retirement of an estimated 70 million baby boomers with multiple chronic conditions, health care reform, and the pending physician shortage further contribute to this "tsunami of change" (American Association of Colleges of Nursing [AACN], 2017; ANA, 2014).

Dr. Peter Buerhaus, PhD, RN, FAAN, a health care economist and a professor of nursing at Montana State University, conducts research on nursing workforce economics, forecasts supplies of nurses and physicians, and determines public and provider opinion on care delivery issues. His 2015 study forecasts a shortage of about 130,000 nurses in 2025 (Auerbach, Buerhaus, & Staiger, 2015). Projecting the nursing shortage is contingent on people still entering the nursing profession at the current rate as well as projecting the future demand for RNs. U.S. nursing school enrollment growth has begun to plateau, while 64,067 qualified applicants for baccalaureate and graduate nursing programs were turned away in 2016 due to insufficient number of faculty, clinical sites, classroom space, clinical preceptors, and budget constraints (AACN, 2017).

The increase in RN salary levels and the unprecedented use of bonuses since the credit crisis of 2007–2008 has allowed RNs to reduce shifts and delay retirement.

Adding to the shortage of nurses is the impact of nursing turnover (AACN, 2017). Nurse turnover for both experienced RNs as well as newly licensed hospital-based RNs is an expensive and disruptive trend that threatens the quality of care and patient safety. High vacancy and turnover is associated with overtime or the use of agency nurses to fill vacant positions as well as the cost associated with recruiting qualified nurses. Also, nursing turnover is increasing because of a more robust job market. In addition, nurses nearing retirement age are feeling better about their portfolios and thinking about an exit strategy.

The RN Work Project Study found that 43% of newly licensed hospital-based RNs left their first jobs within 8 years of employment. The 1-year turnover rate among all newly licensed RNs was 17.5% and the 2-year turnover rate was 33.5% (Kovner & Brewer, 2013).

Annually, the Labor Management Institute (LMI) publishes its Perspectives in Staffing and Scheduling (PSS) Annual Survey of Hours Benchmark Report (Suby, 2015). Participation in 2015 included all 50 states from 632 teaching, community, and rural hospitals. The survey asked responding hospitals for their vacancy and turnover rates for their organizations, the nursing departments, and for RNs in the organization. In 2015, LMI reported the following employee turnover and unit erosion statistics from 206 teaching, community, and rural hospitals:

All hospitals: Employees organization-wide:

1. Percent of total employees leaving the organization in the last fiscal year: 7.6%
2. Percent of total employees transferring units within the organization: 3.5%
3. Total organizational turnover with unit erosion: 11.1%

All hospitals: Employees nursing department-wide:

1. Percent of total nursing department employees leaving the organization in the last fiscal year: 12.2%
2. Percent of total nursing department employees transferring units within the nursing department: 6.7%
3. Total nursing department turnover with unit erosion: 18.9%

All hospitals: Organization-wide RNs only:

1. Percent of total RN employees leaving the organization in the last fiscal year: 10.5%
2. Percent of total RN employees transferring units within the nursing department: 6.7%
3. Total RN turnover with unit erosion: 17.2%
4. Average number of RNs per hospital who have left in the last fiscal year: 79.1

In light of the projected shortages, nursing programs must work to produce nurses with skills to be accountable for cost and quality; hospital leaders are challenged on how to engage and retain experienced RNs who have the skills to help organizations transition to a value-based care delivery system to ensure the mission of the organization as well as the survival of the hospitals. It is said that people join companies, but they leave managers. The loss of nurse leaders and strong correlation between staff nurses' positive relationship with their nurse leader and their engagement and tenure to the unit and the organization continues to be of great concern. The nurse leader is the key to staff nurse engagement (Auerbach, Buerhaus, & Staiger, 2007).

The DNP/nurse leader is an essential leadership role in health care, providing the backbone of the organization and setting the culture for their unit. The quality of patient care, success of staff retention, and recruitment rest with the nurse leader. The DNP/nurse leader is pivotal to the success of the organization because that is where the operations happen. Over time, it is the strength of the nurse leader's skills that determines the success or failure of nursing and executive leadership.

It is crucial to the DNP/nurse leader's success, as well as the success of the organization, that they acquire operational, financial, and management skills as well as the skills of balancing the challenges between quality and cost, negotiating with multiple stakeholders, presenting conflicting agendas, and implementing the processes needed to ensure that individualized compassionate care is provided consistently in the most efficient and effective manner possible.

■ NURSING UNIT LEADERSHIP/ACCOUNTABILITY

Although clinical and leadership experience is very important to DNPs'/nurse leaders' success, their understanding and accountability for their unit's financial budget, schedule requirements, schedule development and employee request management, supplemental staffing response to deficit demands, proactive daily staffing, and management reporting will guarantee them their greatest success as they manage their employees and work with their executive leadership. Accountability for the unit's labor and supply expenses, delivery of quality patient care, and management of HR at the cost center level requires the nurse leader to be both the chief executive officer as well as the chief encouragement officer.

With health care reform and the Affordable Care Act (ACA) here to stay and the unknowns of pending changes in continued implementation and reimbursements, the bottom line is that the DNP/nurse leader must have the leadership skills and competencies to figure out how to get things done for less when there is a decrease in revenues from all sources.

Accountability and teamwork are crucial to achieving best practices, as well as engagement by frontline staff to improve patient safety and the quality of care. Health care leaders in all departments are under continued pressure to know their financial numbers with a critical eye toward cutting costs to bare-bone bottom lines, and making their strategic plans for 2017 and beyond. They are working with their staff to creatively and collaboratively improve basic services, look for ways to optimize their efficiency, eliminate redundancy, improve quality, and manage costs to maximize revenue sources. At the same time, leaders are trying to keep their employees motivated and engaged, prevent and avoid turnover, and, where possible, reduce the cost of new employee orientation.

In the economic reality of 2017, there is no more low-hanging fruit to help with budget reductions because hospitals are operating on slim margins. Hospitals are trying to maximize revenues while staying closely aligned with their quality indicators. At the same time as reimbursements are going negative, employees are continuing to look for at least a 1% to 3% cost of living increase in salary and other benefits. Innovative solutions include "flexible scheduling" offering shorter shifts of 4 and 6 hours, and salary increases for all nurses. Some organizations are looking outside of health care to companies such as Google and Apple to consider retention options for on-site fitness centers, free meal service, and financial and retirement planning.

As nursing workforce budgets have been reduced, there is more emphasis on flexing staff to cover fluctuating and erratic changes in volumes, determining ways to cope with the loss of indirect support hours (clerks, monitor techs, case managers, educators), expanding DNP/nurse leader spans of control, and realizing more employees are working second and third jobs, working longer hours at each job, and caring for sicker patients. All these factors challenge patient care delivery; contribute to increasing employee unexpected absences, leave of absence (LOA), and family medical leave of absence (FMLOA) usage; and create an environment that drives nurses from the bedside. To counter these issues, nurse leaders are implementing solutions to improve engagement and retention through "flexible" scheduling, improved communications, and improved orientation programs.

There is no question that nursing care and quality patient care are inseparable. Safe staffing saves lives and a growing body of evidence documents that adequate nurse staffing improves patient outcomes, resulting in shorter lengths of stay and fewer complications and patient deaths. Scheduling and staffing practices must be patient-centric and employee-sensitive to work–life balance while safeguarding against errors, omissions, and accidents due to schedule-related fatigue.

Applying best practices (the techniques and methodologies that, through experience and research, have proved to reliably produce results) to scheduling and staffing is more critical now than it has ever been to ensuring that organizations have the right staff with the right competencies on the right day and shift for the right cost. DNPs/nurse leaders who understand basic financial budgets, scheduling, and daily staffing principles are critical to the success of addressing these challenges.

DNP/NURSE LEADER SPAN OF CONTROL

As organizations have reduced full-time equivalents (FTEs) and blended their unit's patient populations (e.g., oncology/telemetry), DNPs/nurse leaders are being assigned increasing numbers of cost centers and employees to manage. At the same time, the indirect support hours from clerks, case managers, and clinical nurse specialists (CNSs) are being reduced for many types of units. This is creating increasing challenges in communications, as well as controlling overtime, shift bonuses and/or incentives, supplemental staffing to replace deficit demands, and creating and supporting high-performance teams.

For any DNP/nurse leader to perform his or her responsibilities effectively, he or she must have a reasonable "span of control." Span of control is defined as the number of people reporting to one DNP/nurse leader and can be measured by the number of employees (not only FTEs) in the cost center. Span of control defines organizational structure and has financial, HR, and quality of care implications.

Research studies in the 1990s focused on helping hospital leadership better manage labor expenses during a time when cost control and managed care's ever-growing influence in the health care arena was being heavily emphasized, rather than trying to analyze factors such as the variety of services and levels of management in which a manager can be involved. None of the studies examined the effect of span of control on patient safety.

A study done by Dr. Christine Meade published in 2008 revealed that various levels of manager span of control had differing results on quality outcomes. The largest numbers of lower

TABLE 4.1 Labor Management Institute's 2015 Nurse Manager Span of Control Findings

Labor Management Institute's *2015 PSS Annual Survey of Benchmark Hours* Nurse Manager Span of Control Findings	2015 (*n* = 201)
Average cost centers per manager	2.21
Average number of employees to manage per manager per unit	25
Average *total* number of employees to manage per manager	56
Range of employees per manager	1–350
Percent of units with dedicated assistant manager per manager	15.2%
Percent of units with permanent charge nurses for each shift	18.7%

Source: Suby (2015). Reproduced with permission from the Labor Management Institute (LMI).

quality outcomes were associated with spans of control ranging from 46 to 71 employees. The next largest number of lower quality outcomes was associated with employee spans of 1 to 45, and then 72 to 152 employees (Meade, 2008).

The LMI finds that, on average, nursing managers are responsible for 2.1 cost centers, with an average of 25 employees/cost center and mean average of 56 total employees to manage, based on data from 201 of 632 total hospitals that volunteered data for the *2015 PSS Annual Survey of Hours Benchmark Report* (Suby, 2015). This is an increase from an average of 1.5 cost centers per manager and a decrease from 38 employees/cost center in the last 5 years based on the 2012 report. Based on hospital responses in 2015, only 15.2% of unit managers have designated assistant managers and 18.7% have permanent "charge nurses" to help them manage their unit's budget, coordinate staffing, facilitate communications, and monitor care delivery during off-shifts, weekends, and holidays, as displayed in Table 4.1 (Suby, 2015).

DNP/NURSE LEADER HOURS SPENT ON BUDGETING, SCHEDULING, AND STAFFING

DNPs/nurse leaders continue to report that they are more than occasionally taking patient assignments and picking up unfilled shifts when core staff will not work extra hours or overtime. Every DNP/nurse leader has done this on occasion, under unusual circumstances. However, for best practice, DNP/nurse leader's hours should be spent on staff development, enforcing the unit budget, supporting staff, monitoring care delivery, and providing strategic leadership.

Annually, LMI collects data on manager span of control for the *PSS Annual Survey of Hours Benchmark Report*. Responding hospitals provided the following number of hours nurse leaders spent on budgeting, scheduling, and staffing activities in Table 4.2 (Suby, 2015).

LMI finds that where scheduling and staffing is truly autonomous and collaborative, and HR and payroll worked and paid hours policies and practices work in synchrony, nurse leader hours/schedules should average 4 to 6 hours or less/month and daily staffing should average 4 to 6 or less hours/month for an average-size unit of 60 employees.

Schedules driven by shift combinations unmatched to the budget FTEs and schedule requirements; conflicts in worked and paid hour policies and practices; an absence of position control or hiring plan management and employee's working above or below their hired FTEs; unplanned absences; an imbalance of full-time (FT)/part-time (PT)/per-diem staffs; unenforced discipline policies; unclear line and staff functions between the unit leadership, employees, and staffing office; and an underresourced float pool and unclear unit and resource pool goals for the use of supplemental staff for deficit demand replacement will drive up the hours of scheduling

TABLE 4.2 Labor Management Institute's *2015 PSS Annual Survey of Hours Benchmark Report*; Nurse Manager Average Hours/Month/Unit Spent on Budgeting, Scheduling, and Staffing

Survey Year	Manager Hours/Month Scheduling	Manager Hours/Month Staffing	Manager Hours/Month Budgeting	Mean Average Total Manager Hours/Month on Budgeting, Scheduling, and Staffing	Percent of Manager Hours/Month on Budgeting, Scheduling, and Staffing
2015 (n = 159)	19.5	22.8	14.9	57.2	35.8
2012 (n = 151)	18.6	21.3	14.6	54.5	34.1

Source: Suby (2015). Reproduced with permission from the Labor Management Institute (LMI).

and staffing, which, in turn, drives up overtime, use of bonus and incentive pay, and unnecessary hours and costs.

In states such as California and New York that are heavily unionized, leadership challenges are even more complex due to mandated caregiver ratios, meal break and rest period coverage, practices for employee shift cancellation with less than 24-hour notice without penalties, and much more.

As health care providers and DNPs/nurse leaders, our challenge is to find solutions to the logistical problems in maintaining continuity of care. Many of our patients have short-term average lengths of stay (e.g., average length of stay [ALOS] of less than 3 days), increasing acuity levels, increasing pressure from health maintenance organizations (HMOs) and insurers to discharge patients faster, and fractured continuity of care from 4-, 6-, 10-, and 12-hour shifts that result in more scheduled single and split shifts.

■ ESSENTIAL BUDGET COMPONENTS

The DNP/nurse leader needs to understand the essential components of the budget, which identifies the expected workload volume (e.g., patient days, visits, procedures, and so forth) or units of service (UOS), allocates HR in the form of hours and FTEs, and defines the budget key performance indicators (KPIs) including RN, direct, indirect, and total worked hours per unit of service (UOS). Increasingly nursing departments are being asked to include respiratory therapy and pharmacy. Their KPIs need to include their required key skill mix such as registered respiratory therapists (e.g., RRTs) and registered pharmacists (RPHs).

Given proper information and expectations, most DNPs/nurse leaders can perform to the levels expected. However, there is little incentive when information is not available for each DNP/nurse leader. Alternatively, when the information is provided and DNPs/nurse leaders cannot manage their budgets, managerial knowledge should be evaluated for their ability to hold this position. Accountability is the imperative at every level of leadership.

WORKLOAD UNITS OF SERVICE (UOS), VOLUME AND REVENUE PROJECTION

Effective budgets cannot be planned without workload UOS or volume forecasts. A primary workload UOS is defined for every unit. The UOS for inpatient units is patient days, which are the sum of the census at midnight for the survey period; the metric by which we compare care delivery is reported as worked labor hours per patient day (HPPD).

The worked labor hours are grouped into four components comprised of the (a) direct care HPPD, which are reflected in the unit's variable staffing plan (VSP); (b) the indirect care HPPD; (c) total worked or productive HPPD; and (d) total paid HPPD.

The worked hours per UOS will vary by the type of work done in the unit. For example, in perioperative units, the primary workload type is hours/surgical case (H/S case); in obstetric units, the primary workload type is hours/delivery (H/Del).

Secondary workload or UOS may be possible. For example, bedded outpatients in a unit will create hours of work to admit, discharge, and/or transfer patients within a cost center that is not counted in the midnight workload. Finance may agree to a productivity credit formula that gives the unit credit for this work, which is represented as equivalent or adjusted workload. A commonly accepted formula is 24 observation hours = 1 patient day.

Workload variations should be identified according to day of the week or season, as planning for these trends can reduce costs without reducing care. The workload UOS or volumes can be viewed in the following ranges:

Peak volume—Capacity of the unit

Possible volume—Workload between the most frequent and peak UOS or capacity of the unit

Probable volume—Includes the most frequent workload, actual average daily workload, and actual average daily workload by weekday and weekend

Certain or most common—The most common workload that rarely drops below this volume

The "most frequent workload UOS or volume" (e.g., most frequent census or MFC) is one that occurs for 50% or more of the survey period. Defining the most frequent workload UOS or volume helps unit leadership know their "range of staffing elasticity" that direct care staff should be able to flex to accommodate changes in workload volumes due to admissions, discharges, and transfers (ADTs) within the shift that may or may not require additional staff (Suby, 2008b). Refer to the example in Figure 4.1.

The volume forecast is a basic element in estimating workload and unit revenue. It is essential for the patient care services/nursing and finance departments to work together to determine and agree upon the volume forecasts. Revenue forecasts follow forecasted volumes, which are usually provided by the finance department.

The revenue forecast includes both gross and net revenue and will be reviewed in Chapter 7. *Gross revenue* is all charges for projected care for the forecasted patient volume. *Net revenue* is the amount the hospital expects to receive after contractual allowances are made on charges (i.e., diagnosis-related group [DRG] payment, preferred provider organization [PPO], or HMO contracts). *Patient days* are the sum of the census at midnight for the survey period. For example, the midnight census of 22 for two nights is a total of 44 patient days. There is common agreement between nursing and finance that the midnight census does not fully describe the impact of the work on the unit, as it usually excludes the bedded outpatients, unit-based outpatient procedures (e.g., blood transfusions), and outpatient observation hours, visits, and treatments in the obstetric units.

ADMISSION, DISCHARGE, AND TRANSFER (ADT) WORK INTENSITY INDEX

LMI worked to develop a formula to describe how "busy or intense" a unit was during some periods of the day (Suby, 2008a). These periods of work intensity may also be called "churning." Often,

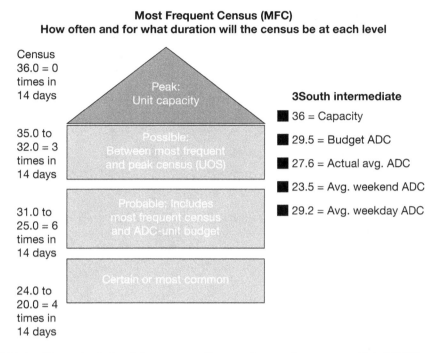

FIGURE 4.1 Example: Labor Management Institute's most frequent workload UOS and range of staffing elasticity.

ADC, average daily census; UOS, units of service.

Source: Suby (2015). Reproduced with permission from the Labor Management Institute (LMI).

the ADT Work Intensity is not captured accurately. One formula developed by LMI to calculate the ADT Work Intensity is:

$$\frac{\text{Total admissions} + \text{Discharges} + \text{Transfers in 24 hours}}{\text{Midnight census}}$$

If hours/UOS (HPPD of H/UOS) is above budget and the workload units are at or below budget, often the reason is that the ADT Work Intensity is very high and turnover in patients is not being captured in the midnight census (refer to Table 4.3).

In 2013, an analysis of 183 units from 32 hospitals in the United States from the LMI Workforce Assessment Two-Week Survey of Hours was used to calculate nurse staffing requirements to meet unit workload using three different metrics (Hughes, Bobay, Jolly, & Suby, 2015). The three metrics were midnight census, the inverse of the length of stay (I/LOS; Unruh & Fottler, 2006) and ADT Work Intensity Index (Suby, 2008a). Respondent units collected unit-level data in 4-hour increments by shift by day of week for 2-week pay periods that excluded holidays. Units collected midnight census, ADTs, RN, and direct, indirect, and total worked hours of care, med errors and patient falls for intensive care, intermediate care, and medical–surgical units to account for expected differences in patient flow and staffing requirement standards.

Most commonly, midnight census is the UOS used to predict nurse staffing, and the unit-level workload increases with the movement of patients into and out of the unit (ADT). The patient turnover method by Unruh adds the I/LOS to the midnight census that considers the turnover

TABLE 4.3 Labor Management Institute's Unit Thresholds for the ADT Work Intensity Index

Unit Type	Range in ADT Index Percent (%)
Critical care	85–90
Intermediate care (telemetry/SD)	70–75
Medical–surgical	50–55
Mother–baby/postpartum NICU/PICU	85–90
Mental health	35–40
Rehab-skilled nursing	25–30

ADT, admission, discharge, and transfer; NICU, neonatal intensive care unit; PICU, pediatric intensive care unit; SD, step down.

Source: Suby (2015). Reproduced with permission from the Labor Management Institute (LMI).

of the same hospital bed within a 24-hour day (Unruh, 2006). This metric adds more staffing to units with shorter LOS and less staff to units with longer LOS and is not usable by shift.

The analysis showed that midnight census and LOS alone did not account for the workload intensity. When ADT is considered, the workload of nurses increases beyond the patient care workload demands based only on the midnight census. Shift-level staffing by unit type was used to evaluate whether ADT increases nurse staffing requirements more than midnight census alone. After differences in staffing were taken into account, about 37% of the variance in staffing over the midnight census requirement was related to ADT.

The ADT Work Intensity Index produced a larger increase in calculated nurse staffing requirements than the patient churn using LOS compared to midnight census by an average of 2.35 RN HPPD in telemetry and medical–surgical units. When the ADT Work Intensity Index was used in determining RN staffing across all hospitals and all three shifts, each type of hospital unit would have needed additional RN staffing in the range of 0.91 to 6.98 additional RNs when patient churn was the highest because of ADT.

The number of RNs assigned per shift within each patient care unit is often based on the budgeted average daily (midnight) census and adjusted for the acuity of the actual patients and the target RN-to-patient ratios. When unit workload is assessed each shift for actual census, ADT activity, and acuity, and staff are deployed to maintain target hours/UOS and RN-to-patient ratios, there is lower stress and greater job satisfaction.

The ADT Work Intensity will reflect the workload when the shift census is at or below the midnight census. For example, when the HPPD is above target and the patient volume is at or below budget, the volume of ADTs will be above target. When unit-level workload fails to address ADT activity by shift, the deployment of nursing staff is considered ineffective, which in turn increases employee feelings of stress and dissatisfaction from working short, which contributes to increased turnover.

ADT activity should be measured by time of day to see when it is the highest and schedule requirements should be adjusted to accommodate this pattern of activity. DNPs/nurse leaders may consider the benefits of an "ADT nurse" during times of peak activity to ensure that the work is being completed in a timely manner. Often nursing negotiates with finance to reduce or elimi-nate nursing assistants (NAs) to maintain or increase RNs in the units. Very often, the "charge nurse" role is negotiated as a direct care position with an expectation that he or she takes a reduced patient assignment while also serving as the shift "resource" and ADT nurse until a patient can be assigned to another staff nurse who has had a discharged patient or until the mutually agreed-upon ratio has been met and the unit receives another RN. It is important that the DNP/nurse leader monitor the workload of the designated charge nurses who become overburdened and too overwhelmed to be a resource to the staff on the shift. This becomes a source of staff dissatisfaction, burnout, and turnover.

COST CENTER

Financial accountability demands that the costs of one area be separated from those of every other. This is done with cost center-specific budgets. Each first-level DNP/nurse leader should have specific reports for her or his unit. With identified costs allocated to each cost center, definitive corrective action can be taken when appropriate.

The cost center or cost unit is a financial unit or code from which wages are paid and costs are identified and controlled by a specific DNP/nurse leader. Accounting practice is to assign all labor costs to the home cost centers and to allocate to all other cost centers the hours worked on those units. Other common names for cost center include cost unit and department number. It is critically important in organizations where scheduling, staffing, and time and attendance have been automated that all employees correctly punch in and out to their shifts using the correct codes. For example, employees in orientation or education activities must correctly document their time in these automated systems.

HOURS PER PATIENT DAY OR UNIT OF SERVICE

The number of HPPD is the usual standard for comparing levels of care between cost centers in the same hospital or facility. Workload UOS or volume comparisons by unit type and their formulas are listed in Table 4.4.

Comparisons, within or among facilities, are valid only when comparable data are available. Departments have often rejected comparisons on the basis that "categories included in the hours at one facility were not necessarily included at another facility." Once legitimate, this argument is no longer valid.

It is essential to determine whether compared hours are total worked (or productive) or total paid (or annual) because the difference between the two may vary significantly in any analysis or comparison. A definition of the essential hours includes the following key terms:

Hours classification—A distinct grouping used to classify hours, correlated with financial industry standards. Standard hour classifications include direct, indirect, total worked (or productive) hours, nonproductive hours (benefit and, at some hospitals, education, meeting, and orientation [EMO]), and total paid (or annual) hours.

Direct care worked hours—The number of hours of direct labor used in providing a service or making a product. In acute care, it is the hours of all staff providing direct, hands-on care to patients. These hours are variable and are adjusted to respond to patient census and/or acuity or other identified unit workload UOS or volumes. *If the hospital does not separate direct and indirect hours, the total worked hours and direct hours will be the same.*

Indirect care (also known as fixed) worked hours—Hours worked by staff (i.e., unit nurse leader, clerical, monitor tech, and others) providing service to the unit, but *not* directly with patients or taking a patient assignment. Indirect (or fixed) hours may also include other personnel not involved in direct care, such as the unit-based educator, CNS, case manager, supply coordinator, and so forth. Most hospitals or facilities include the worked and paid hours for EMO time as indirect hours because the employees are working and getting paid but their time is not directly worked with patients.

TABLE 4.4 Labor Management Institute's Primary Workload Metrics for Nursing Units

Unit Types	Primary Metric	Formula
Inpatient units	Direct hours per patient day (direct HPPD)	Direct care (RN, LPN/LVN, NA) worked hours ÷ total inpatients in the midnight census during the reporting period
	Indirect hours per patient day (indirect HPPD)	Indirect care (nurse leader, clinical nurse specialist or nurse practitioner, clerks, and so forth) worked hours ÷ total inpatients in the midnight census during the reporting period
	Total worked or productive hours per patient day (TW HPPD or productive HPPD)	All hours worked by all personnel in the cost center or unit ÷ total inpatients in the midnight census during the reporting period
Obstetric units	Direct hours per delivery (direct H/Del)	Direct care worked hours ÷ total deliveries during the reporting period
	Indirect hours per delivery (indirect H/Del)	Indirect care worked hours ÷ total deliveries during the reporting period
	Total worked or productive hours per delivery (TW H/Del or productive H/Del)	All hours worked by all personnel in the cost center or unit ÷ total deliveries during the reporting period
Emergency departments	Direct hours per ED visit (direct H/Visit)	Direct care (RN, LPN/LVN, NA, EMT) worked hours ÷ total visits to the ED during the reporting period
	Indirect hours per ED visit (indirect H/Visit)	Indirect care worked hours ÷ total visits to the ED during the reporting period
	Total worked or productive hours per ED visit (TW H/Visit or productive H/Visit)	All hours worked by all personnel in the cost center or unit ÷ total visits to the ED during the reporting period
Procedure units (cath labs, endoscopy, GI labs, infusion, noninvasive labs, observation, special procedures, and so forth)	Direct hours per procedure (direct H/Procedure)	Direct care (RN, LPN/LVN, NA, EMT) worked hours ÷ total visits to the Procedure Units during the reporting period
	Indirect hours per procedure (indirect H/Procedure)	Indirect care worked hours ÷ total visits to the Procedure Units during the reporting period
	Total worked or productive hours per procedure (TW H/Visit or productive H/Procedure)	All hours worked by all personnel in the cost center or unit ÷ total visits to the Procedure Units during the reporting period

(continued)

TABLE 4.4 Labor Management Institute's Primary Workload Metrics for Nursing Units (*continued*)

Unit Types	Primary Metric	Formula
Dialysis units	Direct hours per run (direct H/Run)	Direct care (RN, LPN/LVN, NA, dialysis techs) worked hours ÷ total visits to the total dialysis runs during the reporting period
	Indirect hours per run (indirect H/Run)	Indirect care worked hours ÷ total visits to the total dialysis runs during the reporting period
	Total worked or productive hours per run (TW H/Run or productive H/Run)	All hours worked by all personnel in the cost center or unit ÷ total visits to the total dialysis runs during the reporting period

ED, emergency department; EMT, emergency medical technician; GI, gastrointestinal; LPN, licensed practical nurse; LVN, licensed vocational nurse; NA, nursing assistant.

Source: Suby (2015). Reproduced with permission from the Labor Management Institute (LMI).

TABLE 4.5 2015 LMI Indirect Labor, Education, Orientation Guidelines

Unit Type	Average % Indirect Labor	Average % Education	Average % Orientation	Total % Indirect to Total Worked or Productive Hours
Critical care	13%	2.0–2.4%	2.5–3.6%	17.5–19.0%
Intermediate specialty care	12%	2.0–2.4%	1.2–2.5%	15.2–17.0%
General medical–surgical	12%	2.0–2.4%	2.5–3.6%	16.5–18.0%
Women's and children's	14%	2.0–2.4%	2.5–3.6%	18.5–20.0%
Behavioral health	20%	1.0–2.0%	1.2–2.5%	22.2–24.5%
Rehabilitation and skilled nursing	14%	1.0–2.0%	1.2–2.5%	16.2–18.5%
Perioperative services	14%	2.0–2.4%	2.5–3.6%	18.5–20.0%
Emergency services	21%	2.0–2.4%	2.5–3.6%	25.5–27.0%
Other units/ambulatory care	25%	1.0–2.0%	1.2–2.3%	27.2–29.3%
Outpatient clinics	45%	0.7–1.7%	0.5–1.3%	46.2–48.0%
Dialysis	19%	0.7–1.7%	0.5–1.3%	20.2–21.4%

Source: Suby (2015). Used with permission of the Labor Management Institute (LMI).

Total worked (or productive) hours—Total worked hours. *If the hospital does not separate direct and indirect hours, then direct and total worked will be the same.* Total worked (or productive) hours include actual worked hours by staff that float into the unit from other cost centers or by resource pool, agency, or traveler nurses.

EMO hours—Total worked hours by employees to complete orientation; required education; and meetings for the unit, the department, and shared governance. Most organizations consider the time that employees are absent for these activities as indirect time because employees are working but not directly with patients. However, some organizations classify the EMO hours as nonproductive hours. The time that employees are absent from the unit must be replaced so it requires that the DNP/nurse leader define these hours to create a "backfill replacement plan." The actual time worked by the replacement employees is counted as direct or indirect depending on their skill mix. When EMO time is not correctly recorded in the scheduling, staffing, and time and attendance systems, it will default to direct or indirect worked hours, which will cause the unit to be above the target required hours and viewed as an unnecessary expense. Depending on the unit type and service line, the EMO hours average 1.5% to 4% or more of total worked annual hours and become a driver for unnecessary extra hours and costs in the form of overtime, bonuses, and shift incentives.

Annually the LMI collects the EMO hours in the *PSS Annual Survey of Hours Benchmark Report* and compares them by service line type (refer to Table 4.5; Suby, 2015).

Indirect labor hours—Includes time paid from the cost center that is not included in the VSP (e.g., manager, clerks, charge nurses not counted in the RN-to-patient ratios, educators, case managers, and so forth).

Nonproductive hours—A term used for all hours the hospital defines as "nonproductive." Nonproductive hours always include benefit time or paid time off (e.g., vacation, sick, holiday). Some organizations may also include EMO hours as nonproductive time, although the employee is working and paid. Most time and attendance and payroll systems exclude unpaid absence hours that occur when employees have used up their accrued benefit time or from part-time and per-diem/casual employees that do not accrue benefit time. Replacing unexpected absences, both paid and unpaid, often drives up the hours needed for daily staffing adjustments that are not reflected in the actual nonproductive hours.

Total paid (or annual) hours—All hours paid from the cost center, including total worked (or productive) and nonproductive hours. Total paid hours may also be called total annual hours or total hours.

BASIC FORMULAS

To obtain the average total worked (or productive) hours of care and total paid hours provided to each patient, it is necessary to divide the total worked (or productive) hours and total paid hours on a patient unit for a designated period of time by the UOS during the same period.

For example, 3 South Med–Surg is a blended medical–surgical unit, with the following total worked and total paid hours on the unit for a 2-week period. The total patient days in this sample 2-week period was 348 (total midnight census for the 14-day period). The UOS is HPPD for this unit.

1. *Total worked or productive hours*:   2,096
   1,760 total direct worked hours
   + 336 total indirect hours (nurse leader and clerks)
2. *Total nonproductive hours*:   256
   256 benefit hours for time paid, but not worked
3. *Total paid hours*:   2,352
   2,096 total worked (or productive) hours of work
   + 256 nonproductive benefit hours for time paid, but not worked

4. *Hours per unit of service (hours per patient day or HPPD):*

Total direct (or variable) worked hours per units of service (UOS) or HPPD: $1,760 \div 348 = 5.06$

Total indirect (or fixed) worked hours per UOS or HPPD: $336 \div 348 = 0.97$

Total worked (or productive) hours per UOS or HPPD: $2,096 \div 348 = 6.02$

Total paid hours per UOS or HPPD: $2,096 + 256 = 2,352 \div 348 = 6.76$

5. *Average daily UOS (example average daily census [ADC])* $348 \div 14 = 24.9$

Divide the total UOS (patient days) by days in the survey period

The number of employees required varies with the number of patients or UOS. Many hospitals plan a budgeted number of direct hours for each patient or UOS between the minimum and maximum volume, and hold the DNP/nurse leader accountable for the delivery of care at the budgeted hours per UOS. Total direct hours vary with workload volume. This approach is usually called variable or flex budgeting.

Total paid hours per UOS are usually 12% to 20% higher than total worked (or productive) hours per UOS, depending on what is included in the nonproductive hours. There are two key components in determining this percentage:

1. The amount of benefit time provided by the hospital or facility based on the actual accrued hours of the employees in the unit; or if it is based on the annual average turnover of employees, which is usually the equivalent of an employee who has left after 2 years.
2. Whether the EMO hours are included.
3. Productivity reports do not always make these comparisons available.

FULL-TIME EQUIVALENTS

The concept of FTEs needs to be clearly understood by all DNPs/nurse leaders and other leadership with budget accountability. *FTE* is the term used for comparison of personnel employed by the hospitals. FTE per occupied bed is often used. An *occupied bed* is defined as the number of beds that are licensed and physically available, staffed and occupied by a patient based on standardized definitions developed by the Agency for Healthcare Research and Quality (AHRQ)-supported researchers at Denver Health in Colorado, and vetted by a working group assembled by Denver Health with members from federal and state governments, hospitals around the nation, and the private sector (AHRQ, 2005).

FTEs are often reported in the following ways:

- Direct FTEs
- Indirect FTEs
- Total worked or productive (direct and indirect) FTEs
- Total nonproductive FTEs
- Total paid or annual FTEs

FTE, defined as the number of FT employees needed or worked (hours or shifts) during a specific period (week, pay period, year), is the budgetary term commonly used in comparing cost center budgets. Hospitals are 7-day operations employing a variety of FT, PT, and per-diem/casual or contingent employees. Hospitals offer FT benefits to employees at hours less than 40

TABLE 4.6 Full-Time Equivalents (FTEs) and Formulas

Total Worked or Productive Hours	Formulas
2,096 total worked hours	÷ 80 hours/2 weeks = 26.2 FTEs
2,096 total worked hours	÷ 8 hours/shift = 262 8-hour shifts
2,096 total worked hours	÷ 12 hours/shift = 174.66 12-hour shifts

hours/week or 80 hours/2-week pay period; therefore, computations for FTEs summarize all employees with work agreements less than 40 hours/week or 80 hours/2-week pay period.

The following concepts are important in understanding FTEs:

- When referring to staff required for given time periods, the term *FTE* should be used.
- Because of the number of PT and per-diem/casual or contingent employees, the FTEs of a unit are usually less than the number of required FT and PT employees.
- The same FTE results in different hours or shifts for different time periods (see Table 4.6).

PRODUCTIVE COST OR DOLLAR PER PATIENT DAY

Hospitals are under ever-increasing pressure from insurers to decrease costly inpatient hospital stays. There is also increasing urgency to further reduce Medicare spending growth as that program attempts to deal with declining reserves, the aging baby boom population, the 1997 Balanced Budget Act amendments, and the Patient Protection and Affordable Care Act—ACA (HR 3590, signed March 23, 2010) and the Health Care and Education Reconciliation Act of 2010 (HR 4872, signed March 30, 2010). The health care industry is therefore under tremendous pressure to lower cost while improving quality.

Total worked (or productive) dollars per patient day are a key component in maintaining fiscal accountability. The *cost of care per day or unit of service* is a mathematical calculation of the cost of care in worked hours per day or UOS using average salary costs by category of employee and the primary metric for UOS (e.g., HPPD).

Once hours per UOS and FTEs are determined, average salary information by category of employee is used to calculate dollars or cost per UOS targets by unit. The unit-specific staffing pattern or VSP for each increment of workload is the basis for this calculation.

Department targets for dollars or cost per UOS will vary from unit to unit depending on the tenure of employees, special pay incentives, approved overtime, and use of agency/registry or travelers. Both total worked (or productive) and total paid targets are useful in budget monitoring to evaluate operational decision making. For example, the total worked (or productive) cost or dollars per UOS is budgeted as $18,984.00 for the 2-week period. The budgeted average cost per inpatient day is $1,356.00.

If the total worked (or productive) hours during the 2-week period is 2,096 and the actual total worked (or productive) cost or dollars is $23,730.00, then the actual average cost per inpatient day is $1,695.00. When the actual cost per inpatient day is above budget, and the HPPD is within budget, the DNP/nurse leader staffed the unit with overtime and other premium pay (incentives or agency/registry and travelers). Although the total worked (or productive) hours of care may have stayed constant, LMI finds that there may be an increase in adverse outcomes to the patients by overtime in excess of 5% of total worked hours, a decrease in core staff below 85%, and/or an increase in nonunit supplemental staff greater than 15%.

If the total worked (or productive) hours during the 2-week period is 2,096, the actual total worked (or productive) cost or dollars is $15,187.20, and the HPPD is within budget, then the DNP/nurse leader staffed the unit with fewer RNs and more LPNs/LVNs and NAs. The average salary cost per inpatient day is $1,084.80, which is below the budget of $1,356.00.

If the reduced work hours were due to a reduction in patient acuity during the survey period and safe patient care could be given with reduced hours, then it may be considered good management. However, if the patient acuity was not reduced and the DNP/nurse leader staffed the unit below the target direct and total worked (or productive) hours of care, LMI finds that there may be an increase in adverse outcomes to the patients when direct care RN hours are reduced below 50% of total direct care hours.

In 2015, the national mean average total worked salary cost per inpatient day was $1,338.24 based on data from 164 hospitals in the *PSS Annual Survey of Hours Benchmark Report* (Suby, 2015).

NONPRODUCTIVE BUDGET

Hours paid but not worked are included in the nonproductive portion of a personnel budget. Planned time off usually includes vacation and holidays. Unplanned time off usually includes sick time, emergency absences, funeral, jury duty, and LOA/FMLOA hours. Some hospitals, but not all, include EMO hours in their nonproductive hours.

Deficit demands include all the reasons (paid and unpaid) that scheduled employees are not working and need to be replaced whether they are hired as FT, PT, or per-diem/casual. Paid nonworked hours assume increasing budgetary importance as benefits increase, tenure increases, and PT employees receive improved benefits. Since 1975, average paid time off accruals per employee (FT and PT) has more than doubled in many hospitals. The impact is significant, because increasing costs must be added to the patient's bill for additional employee benefit time. For units that must replace most absences, the nonproductive portion of the budget is used to provide replacement for employees using benefit time. It is important to note that units with high numbers of PT, per-diem, or casual employees may have little or no accrued time off. However, when an individual is absent from a scheduled shift, it represents a deficit demand that must be replaced.

The terms *nonproductive budget* and *benefit replacement* are often used interchangeably. Regardless of the term used, this portion of the budget must be projected and managed separately from the productive (worked) budget.

Some reasons for managing the budget total worked (or productive), direct and indirect, and nonproductive hours separately include:

1. Either portion of the budget, but not necessarily both, may require change.
2. Total worked (or productive) hours reflect UOS. Nonproductive hours correspond to employee paid absences and EMO hours if they are included in the nonproductive hours.
3. The DNP/nurse leader controls total worked (or productive) hours. Organizational policy determines employee benefits as well as EMO amounts.

To budget the appropriate number of nonproductive FTEs, begin by determining the previous year's ratio of nonproductive to productive hours. Then consider any other major changes in EMO time and benefits that could affect this budget figure (Suby, 2009).

In a budget of 30 total paid FTEs, of which 26.5 FTEs are total worked (or productive) FTEs and 3.5 FTEs are nonproductive:

- The ratio of nonproductive-to-total worked (or productive) FTEs is 13% (3.5 ÷ 26.5)
- The ratio of nonproductive-to-total paid FTEs is 12% (3.5 ÷ 30)
- The percentage total worked (or productive)-to-total paid FTEs is 88% (26.5 ÷ 30)

By using such percentages, the DNP/nurse leader can better plan for their employees' nonproductive time and assess actual to budget FTEs to evaluate the source of variations and their acceptability.

ACCRUED VERSUS BUDGETED NONPRODUCTIVE AND CARRYOVER TIME

Most finance departments budget each year's nonproductive time based on the actual hours used in the previous year. Most hospitals do not budget each year's nonproductive time based on the actual accrued nonproductive hours earned by employees in the cost center each year.

Accrued hours are based on the hospital's policy for earned benefit time based on hours worked annually by date of hire or by pay period based on worked hours. Some hospitals' benefit hours plans increase the accrued hours for longevity and sometimes job classification.

It may be possible that employees do not take their accrued time off and "carry it over" to the following year or years based on hospital policy preferring the cash to the time off. Most hospitals limit the total benefit hours that may be "carried over" and held for future payment. The hospital's policy will specify the conditions under which the time can be used for time off or paid or "cashed out" in subsequent years.

The challenge DNPs/nurse leaders encounter when replacing benefit time or dollars in the current year that the employee has accrued from previous years is that the replacement factor or percent in each year is not adjusted to accommodate any unused benefit hours or dollars the employee may be planning to use or cash in for payment.

For example, if the budgeted nonproductive percent this year is 12%, and 5% of the total accrued benefit time earned in the previous year is not taken, the current year's required hours are now increased to 17% to accommodate the total liability while the actual budget is not increased.

Consequently, the actual nonproductive hours may be over budget if employees take their "carryover time" from previous years in the current fiscal year, and the cost of the nonproductive time will be higher than previously budgeted, as it is paid at the current pay rate. If employees elect to be paid for their accrued time from previous years, the nonproductive dollars or costs may be above budget while the hours replaced may be within budget (refer to Table 4.7 and Exhibit 4.1).

■ THE UNIT STAFFING BUDGET–THE LONG-TERM PLAN (1 YEAR)

The focus of this section is to help the DNP/nurse leader interpret the budget FTEs from finance into an annual unit staffing budget that focuses on the distribution of the annual budget FTEs and hours by shift, and the budget hours and FTEs by shift and UOS.

> *Annual budget cost center*—The annual budget is a financial plan for all the financial projected revenues and expenses for the cost centers for the fiscal year that outlines the resources an entity foresees using for a particular time period.

> *Master budget*—The master budget encompasses all the departmental budgets. Based on the organization's strategic goals and vision, the master budget is the actual statement of projected revenues and expenditures for the entire hospital.

> *Unit annual staffing budget*—The unit staffing budget is done for each cost center annually and is the basis for defining the distribution of hours by shift; classification of hours for direct, indirect, and total worked hours; employee category or skill mix (RN, LPN/LVN, NA, and so on); distribution by day and shift; the unit's schedule requirements; and the unit's staffing grid or VSP.

The unit staffing budget focuses on the budget FTEs, daily and annual UOS with any known adjustments for "other workload" (observation hours, ADT Work Intensity, and so forth), distribution of working hours by shift, planned use for the nonproductive (benefit and, at some hospitals, the EMO) hours, and the budget FTEs and hours annually and by shift and UOS. Refer to

TABLE 4.7 Labor Management Institute's Budget Summary Key Points About FTEs and Hours/UOS

Budget Summary Key Points About FTEs and Hours/UOS	
Definitions	
FTE (full-time equivalent) =	The number of employees needed to cover the number of hours or shifts required during a specific period of time, such as a week, pay period, or year. 2,080 hours is the most common definition. Note: Some organizations' finance departments use other definitions such as 2,082 as a blended average to accommodate for leap year. Be sure to use your organization's definition and be sure the definition is the same across all cost centers.
HPPD (total hours divided by patient days) =	The average hours of care provided for each patient during a specific period of time measured in patient days.
H/UOS (total hours divided by the total workload units of service) =	The average hours of care provided for each patient during a specific time period measured in other workload units of service (e.g., visits, procedures, deliveries, etc.).
Categories of hours (direct, indirect, total worked, nonproductive, total paid)	
FTEs and hours/unit of service can both be expressed as:	
Direct (also known as variable) =	FTEs or HPPD for the direct caregivers. Includes RNs, LPN/LVNs, NAs, techs.
Indirect (also known as fixed) =	FTEs or HPPD for the nurse leader, unit clerk, or other fixed personnel. Often includes the education, meeting, and orientation hours.
Total worked (or productive) =	FTEs or HPPD for all worked hours, direct plus indirect.
Nonproductive =	FTEs or HPPD for hours paid out but not worked; vacation, holiday, and sick. At some hospitals this includes the education, meeting, and orientation hours.
Total paid (or annual) =	FTEs or HPPD for worked plus nonproductive hours.
Formulas	
HPPD =	$$\dfrac{\text{Total hours worked or paid for a certain period}}{\text{Patient days for the same period}}$$
H/UOS =	$$\dfrac{\text{Total hours worked or paid for a certain period}}{\text{Other workload units of service for the same period}}$$

FTE formula for a staffing pattern that is the same each day of the week

$$\text{FTE} = \text{shifts per day} \times 1.4$$

FTE formula for a staffing pattern that varies during a week's time

$$\text{FTE} = \frac{\text{Shifts (week's total)} \times 8 \text{ hours}}{40 \text{ hours}}$$

Note: For a week, use 40 hours; for a 2-week pay period, use 80 hours; for a year, use 2,080 hours.

LPN, licensed practical nurse; LVN, licensed vocational nurse; NAs, nurse assistants; UOS, units of service.

Source: Reproduced with permission from the LMI.

Exhibit 4.1 Labor Management Institute's Budget Analysis Worksheet

	Budget	Actual	Analysis
Units of service (UOS)			
Average daily			
Adjustments for other workload (e.g., holding or observation hours)			
Worked hours/patient day or UOS			
Total *direct* hours			
Total *indirect* hours			
Total worked or productive (direct and indirect) hours			
Total paid or annual hours			
FTEs/patient day or UOS			
Total *direct* FTEs			
Total *indirect* FTEs			
Total *worked or productive*			
(Direct and indirect) FTEs			
Total paid or annual hours			
Cost/patient day or UOS			
Direct cost			
Indirect cost			
Total worked or productive cost			
Education, meeting, orientation hours, and FTEs			
Total *paid* cost			
Other labor considerations			
Overtime			
Agency or registry usage			
Travelers			
Other			

FTEs, full-time equivalents.

Source: Suby (2015). Reproduced with permission from the Labor Management Institute (LMI).

the example unit staffing budget for 3M Med–Surg, a medical–surgical unit developed by the LMI, for total worked HPPD of 9.03 HPPD (see Table 4.8.)

The unit staffing budget identifies the budgeted FTEs by employee category or skill mix. The classification of employee worked hours is organized in order of direct caregivers, indirect caregivers, total worked (or productive) caregivers, nonproductive FTEs, and total paid (or annual) FTEs.

The LMI unit annual staffing budget provides the stepping stone from converting the assigned FTE budget by category group or skill mix (RN, LPN/LVN, NA, nurse leader, clerks, and so forth) from finance into a "distribution of hours by shift" across the 24 hours. If the unit is scheduling all employees to 12-hour shifts, the form may be adapted to a day and night 12-hour shift. If the unit is using "flexible scheduling" with 4-, 6-, 8-, 10-, and 12-hour shifts, then the distribution

TABLE 4.8 Example: Current Unit Staffing Budget for 9.03 HPPD for 3M Med–Surg

Unit: 3M Med–Surg   Budget Year: 2011 to 2012   Based on Current Budget of 9.03 Total Worked HPPD

Workload (UOS) type: Census & HPPD   (Bed/UOS) capacity: 21   Budget average daily census (BADC) or UOS: 17.42 with observation

BUDGET DATA AND SUMMARY IN HOURS BY DAY & SHIFT

Budget data	Per day	700	1,500	2,300
Total paid (annual) FTEs	30.20	13.28	8.80	8.12
Total worked (productive) FTEs	27.60	12.13	8.04	7.42
Total hired FTEs	23.01			
Direct hours/census (HPPD) or UOS	8.27	3.21	2.63	2.43
Total worked hours/census (HPPD) or UOS	9.03	3.97	2.63	2.43

Budget summary in hours	Per day	700	1,500	2,300
Average daily census (BADC) or UOS:	17.42	17.42	17.42	17.42
Schedule plan direct hours/census or UOS	8.27	3.21	2.63	2.43
Licensed (RN + LPN) ratio: 1 RN/LPN to 3.76 patients	Skill-mix distribution			
RN ratio: 1 RN to 9.78 patients	29.7%	16	13.4	13.4
LPN ratio: 1 LPN to 6.1 patients	47.5%	24	24	20.44

EMPLOYEE REPLACEMENT AND BACK-FILL PLAN

Nonproductive (NP) data	Value	Hours/day	700	1,500	2,300
Budget NP%	8.6%		44.0%	29.1%	26.9%
Budget NP hours	5,408.0	14.8	6.5	4.3	4.0
Budget NP FTEs	2.6				
Unit replacement NP FTE allocation	2.5	Education/meeting hours/weekday:			0
Resource pool NP FTE allocation	0	Orientation hours/weekday			0

Total per day	Avg.	2015 LMI ASOH™ for community hospitals M/S	Budget Workload UOS or Volume	Amt.
Total per day	52.26	17.42	Direct Low = 8.70 High = 12.6 Avg. = 8.7 Mid-range = 7.2–9.0 Mid-point = 8.11	Annual patient days or UOS	5,728.7
				Total adjusted UOS (*)	629.7
	42.80	14.27	Indirect HPPD Low = 0.1 High = 2.6 Avg. = 1.1 Mid-range = 1.1–1.5 Mid-point = 1.30	Total adjusted or equivalent patient days or UOS	6,358.4
	68.44	22.81		Budgeted-FTEs	Amt.

	Percent of total	Day	Evenings	Nights	Total	Average
NA ratio: 1 NA to 12.4 patients	22.8%	16	8.45	8.45	32.90	10.97
Other direct caregivers:	0.0%				0.00	0.00
Total direct caregiver hours:	100%	56.00	45.85	42.29	144.14	48.05
% Distribution by shift		38.9%	31.8%	29.3%	100.0%	33.3%
Manager/RN charge	Percent indirect of total worked hours:	4.78			4.78	1.59
Clerks		8.38			8.38	2.79
Other indirect caregivers:					0.00	0.00
Total indirect caregiver hours:	8.37%	13.16	0.00	0.00	13.16	4.39
Total worked (productive) hours:		69.16	45.85	42.29	157.30	52.43
% Total worked hours distribution by shift		44.0%	29.1%	26.9%	100.0%	33.3%

Total worked HPPD

Low = 4.0	
High = 13.5	
Avg. = 9.70	
Mid-range = 7.9–9.7	
Mid-point = 8.82	

RN FTEs: (total workload)	7.52
LPN FTEs:	12.01
NA/UAP:	5.68
Other direct FTEs:	
Total direct	25.21
Manager/RN charge FTEs:	0.92
Clerks/other indirect FTEs:	1.47
Total indirect FTEs:	2.39
Total worked (productive) FTEs:	27.60
Budget OT within total worked FTEs:	
Total NP FTEs:	2.60
Total paid (annual) FTEs:	30.20

	Observation hours		Per day	1.7
(*) Other annual UOS:				
Education/meeting hours/year:	0.0	0.0	Orientation hours/year:	0.0

Notes: Annual budget OT is imbedded within the total worked FTEs. It is 2.3 FTEs based on 8 hours/pay period × 23 full-time employees (8 × 23 = 184 hours × 26 pay period = 4,784 hours ÷ 2,080 hours = 2.3 FTEs).

ASOH, Annual Survey of Hours; FTEs, full-time equivalents; HPPD, hours per patient day; LPN, licensed practical nurse; M/S, medical–surgical units; NA/UAP, nursing assistant/unlicensed assistive personnel; OT, overtime; UOS, units of service.

Source: Suby (2015). Reproduced with permission from the Labor Management Institute (LMI).

should be done in traditional 8-hour shift increments across the 24-hour day to synchronize with automated financial systems.

This format helps DNPs/nurse leaders see if they are budgeting the care hours to the shift of need based on where they are estimating the workload will occur. It also provides a budget for the use of the nonproductive hours on a per day basis. It includes a place for the nonproductive time to be budgeted in the same percents as the distribution of care hours by shift.

The unit annual staffing budget also provides for a distribution of the direct and total worked HPPD by shift, so that the charge nurses or shift leaders can compare the hours actually being worked on their shift to the census and see if they are at, over, or under the target HPPD. This helps them be able to negotiate and ask for more staff and/or advise staff why hours are being cancelled and/or floated out of the unit.

Reading the unit annual staffing budget, beginning with the right side of the form shown in Table 4.8, includes the following sections:

The *budgeted FTEs* in the unit annual staffing budget must equal the budget FTEs in the (annual) approved FTEs as agreed upon with finance. If the calculated FTEs in this form are below or above the budgeted FTEs, there is an error in the distribution of hours by shift that must be corrected before proceeding.

The *budget workload* includes the annual patient days for inpatient units or other UOS for noninpatient units (e.g., visits, procedures, deliveries, surgical cases, and so on). It may also include any *adjusted UOS* for which finance is giving the unit credit. This may include "other workload" such as observation or holding hours, ADT Work Intensity hours, and others.

The *equivalent patient days or UOS* is the combination of budget workload and adjusted UOS. This may also be called "adjusted equivalent patient days" or "UOS" in some hospitals.

Employee replacement and back-fill plan: The budgeted nonproductive hours are displayed in FTEs and hours as well as a percent of the budget. The budget nonproductive FTEs are multiplied by the definition of 1 FTE (2,080 hours used in this example) and divided by 365 annualized days in the budget.

The plan identifies what amount of FTE allocation will be made to the resource pool to hire FTEs. This plan should be consistent with the mission and nonproductive replacement goals for the resource plan. If EMO time is included in the hospital's nonproductive budget, then these hours should be identified as a budget per day. If there is no FTE allocation for EMO hours, it means that when the hours occur they will be reported under nonproductive hours even though the employee is working and paid.

All employees require some type of unit-, service line-, and hospital-specific education and meeting time annually and most units have turnover in positions that require orientation. It is critically important that DNPs/nurse leaders identify what these planned hours will be to be sure there is a replacement component within the budget for this time. Unplanned, these hours will drive up the total worked hours of care and are most often the basis for unnecessary extra hours, overtime, bonus, or shift incentive pay.

Good unit management requires that the DNP/nurse leader have an annual plan for the use of education and meeting time. LMI recommends that DNPs/nurse leaders review the average orientation hours over the last 3 years to create a rolling average for their budget. The historical record should reflect the number of hours by each new employee (including new employees who transfer into the unit from another unit) with a reference to whether the employee is experienced or inexperienced. Annually, LMI reports the mean average and range of indirect labor, EMO hours by hospital type (teaching, community, and rural) for eight service lines in the *PSS Annual Survey of Hours Benchmark Report* (Suby, 2015).

Budget summary in hours: The budget summary of hours compares the *average daily census or UOS* by shift as well as per day.

The plan for the worked hours for *direct care* is distributed by shift and per day based on the desired skill mix (RN, LPN/LVN, NAs, or equivalent). The plan includes the target RN-to-patient ratios, licensed caregiver (RN and LPN/LVN if used) to patient ratios, LPN/LVN-to-patient ratios, NA-to-patient ratios, and any other direct caregiver-to-patient ratios. The assignment of direct caregiver hours by shift and day should be the basis for the *skill-mix distribution percent* of total direct care hours.

The direct care RN hours are the basis for calculating the RN-to-patient ratios. If total or all RN hours are used, they will include the nurse leader, educator, CNS, or other advanced practice registered nurse (APRN) and/or case manager. All of these employee types are RNs, but all of these employee types do not usually take patient assignments and are considered "indirect" caregivers. Indirect caregivers support the direct caregivers so that the direct caregivers can stay at the patients' bedside.

The total of the direct worked hours by shift must equal the total budget direct FTEs when multiplied by 365 days and divided by the definition of 1 FTE (2,080 hours).

- If the planned total direct hours divided by the definition of 1 FTE are below the budget total direct FTEs, the hours by shift must be increased or you will be underscheduled and understaffed.
- If the planned total direct hours divided by the definition of 1 FTE are above the budget total direct FTEs, the hours by shift must be decreased or you will be overscheduled and overstaffed. LMI finds that when the total direct hours and FTEs are unmatched, it will often result in a schedule and staffing variance of 2 to 2.5 FTEs over or under the budgeted FTEs.

The plan for the worked hours for indirect care is distributed by shift and per day based on the planned support to the direct caregivers. It is important that a decision is made and standardized across all cost centers to define staff in similar ways. For example, if the shift charge or resource nurses are not expected to take a full patient assignment the same as all other bedside RNs in the unit, then their time should be classified as indirect care. Often the charge or resource nurse will be the "resource" nurse helping the other staff with their assignments and ADTs, or they may take a reduced or limited (one to two patients) assignment so that they are flexible to help all staff on the unit during their shift while being strategic to the DNP/nurse leader for shift-to-shift staffing decisions.

Management productivity reports will be confusing if some units consider the charge or resource nurse as indirect support and some are reporting the hours worked as direct care when the majority of time during the shift is not spent directly with patients.

The *percent indirect of total worked hours* is calculated by dividing the total indirect hours into the total worked hours. All units need some percent of indirect hours to keep direct care nurses at the bedside. LMI annually reports the percent of indirect labor hours by service line in its *PSS Annual Survey of Hours Benchmark Report* and finds that it ranges from 12% to 45% (see Table 4.5; Suby, 2015).

The total of the indirect worked hours by shift must equal the total budget indirect FTEs when multiplied by 365 annualized days and divided by the definition of 1 FTE (2,080 hours).

- If the planned total indirect hours divided by the definition of 1 FTE are below the budget total indirect FTEs, the hours by shift must be increased.
- If the planned total indirect hours divided by the definition of 1 FTE are above the budget total indirect FTEs, the hours by shift must be decreased.

Total worked (or productive) hours include the sum total of the planned direct and indirect worked hours by shift. The total of the total worked (or productive) hours by shift must equal the total worked (or productive) FTEs when multiplied by 365 annualized days and divided by the definition of 1 FTE (2,080 hours).

- If the planned total worked (or productive) hours divided by the definition of 1 FTE are below the budget total worked (or productive) FTEs, the hours by shift must be increased.
- If the planned total worked (or productive) hours divided by the definition of 1 FTE are above the budget total worked (or productive) FTEs, the hours by shift must be decreased.

The *percent total worked hours distribution by shift* is calculated by dividing the total worked hours for each shift into the total worked hours for the 24-hour day.

The annual *budget data and summary in hours by day and shift* identifies the total paid (or annual) FTEs, total worked (or productive) FTEs, and current hired FTEs to determine whether there are any unfilled FTEs or vacancies. It also identifies the direct hours/census (HPPD) or UOS per day and shift and total worked (or productive) hours/census (HPPD) or UOS per day and shift.

Total paid (or annual) FTEs include the sum of total worked (or productive) and nonproductive FTEs based on the planned budget by day and shift. The combined total of the total worked (or productive) and nonproductive FTEs per day must equal the total worked (or productive) and nonproductive FTEs when multiplied by 365 days annualized (refer to the budgeted FTEs in the form).

Total worked (or productive) FTEs include the sum of total worked (or productive) hours based on the planned budget by day and shift. The total of the total worked (or productive) FTEs per day must equal the total worked (or productive) FTEs when multiplied by 365 days annualized (refer to the budgeted FTEs in the form).

Total hired FTEs include the sum total of hired FTEs in the budget. For best practices, the hired FTEs are updated each month from the position control so that DNPs/nurse leaders can see if the actual FTEs are hired above budget in anticipation of turnover, at budget, or below budget. It may be that some FTEs are not authorized to fill if the unit budget volume is below projections or official new programs have not started.

Total direct worked hours/census (HPPD) or UOS include the sum of total direct worked hours based on the planned budget by day and shift divided by the planned workload for each shift. The total of the total direct worked hours per shift must equal the total direct worked hours per day.

The total worked (or productive) hours per day when multiplied by the total annual patient days or UOS and divided by the definition of 1 FTE (2,080 hours) should equal the total direct worked FTEs (refer to the budgeted FTEs in the form; Table 4.8).

Total worked (or productive) hours/census (HPPD) or UOS include the sum of total worked (or productive) hours based on the planned budget by day and shift divided by the planned workload for each shift. The total of the total worked (or productive) hours per shift must equal the total worked (or productive) hours per day.

The total worked (or productive) hours per day when multiplied by the total annual patient days or UOS and divided by the definition of 1 FTE (2,080 hours) should equal the total worked (or productive) FTEs (refer to the budgeted FTEs in the form; Table 4.8).

WORKFORCE MANAGEMENT OPTIONS

Shift scheduling and employee involvement are important to successful schedule development. As the CEO of the unit, the DNP/nurse leader is always accountable for the schedule and allocation of worked hours to ensure the delivery of hours of care and dollars at the budget or target value. To appreciate the art and science of scheduling, DNPs/nurse leaders must begin with some basic scheduling principles that if ignored or violated will result in misaligned resources, increased overtime, and decreased employee satisfaction with their unit.

In workforce planning, it is commonly understood that the employee's schedule and paycheck are very important to them. Errors in the paychecks or perceived unfair scheduling practices are leading factors contributing to staff dissatisfaction and unit turnover.

Creating the schedule is more than putting codes on days to work and be off in a schedule plan sheet. When DNPs/nurse leaders consider the impact of the schedule and its relationship to employee satisfaction and patient outcomes, they must consider the work environment comprised of the unit's culture; policies; practices; and the employee's training, experience, and capacity to handle multiple tasks and patients.

The employee's successful execution of his or her schedule is reflected in his or her health, motivation, and satisfaction. Schedules are just one influence on worker performance and clinical outcomes.

SCHEDULES, WORKER PERFORMANCE, AND THE WORK ENVIRONMENT

The culture of the unit is expressed in the way people treat one another (interpersonal relationships; Suby, 2008b). It is not uncommon to see examples of "great care" in units with limited staffing resources yet very positive staff morale and high patient satisfaction, and, conversely, see examples of poor care (e.g., poor patient satisfaction and staff complaints about "poor staffing" and/or unsafe care) and negative employee morale when the staffing resources were very generous and RN-to-patient ratios were very rich (refer to Figure 4.2).

TRAINING/EXPERIENCE/CAPACITY

Schedules often assume that all nurses are the same, when DNPs/nurse leaders know that nurses have different training, background experience, and, within that, different capacities for numbers of patients and tasks. Medical–surgical units have become the "stepping stone" units for new

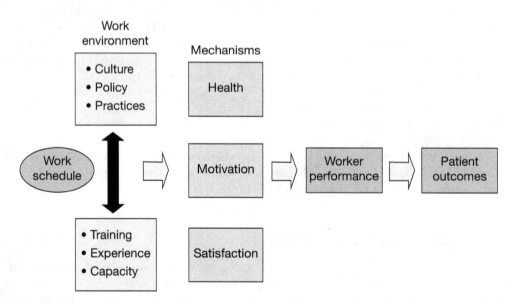

FIGURE 4.2   Labor Management Institute's Model of the Employee Schedule, Work Environment, Worker Performance, and Patient Outcomes.

Source: Suby (2015). Reproduced with permission from the Labor Management Institute (LMI).

employees to enter the organization and then transfer to intermediate and critical care units for higher pay and lower ratios of patients. It is not uncommon to find that medical–surgical units have higher turnover and orientation hours and costs than any other unit type in the organization. If this is your reality, consider establishing minimum tenures of 18 to 24 months before approving unit transfers to help the morale of the unit and reduce the cost of turnover and orientation.

SCHEDULING AND EMPLOYEE HEALTH, MOTIVATION, AND SATISFACTION

Despite the creation of a high-quality schedule, employee performance will be poor and patient care will be negatively impacted if the employee has a chronic illness, lacks motivation to get to work on time or do a good job, and/or is generally dissatisfied in his or her work or personal life.

Employees working hours in excess of 15 hours per 24-hour period or 60 hours per work week will be fatigued. Tired employees make mistakes. Many studies have reported correlations between higher on-the-job injuries, sick-time absences, job dissatisfaction, and turnover when employees are allowed to work fatigued. With many RNs working two or more jobs, it is not uncommon for LMI Schedule Best Practice Audits to identify employees working a 16-hour and a 24-hour shift within a single work week or 40 consecutive hours to satisfy their 40-hour/week commitment, which provides them with 5 days off to work at another hospital.

SCHEDULE ACCOUNTABILITY

The DNP/nurse leader is responsible for the unit budget and the allocation of resources for the delivery of care. Marie Manthey (2004) said it best: "Leaders set the ground rules for interpersonal relationships at the unit level. Management allocates energy; leadership creates energy." We cannot afford to schedule our HR in ways that are misaligned with our patient needs, ignore the unit's budget, and disregard the importance of healthy interpersonal relationships.

Flexible schedules are innovative ways of dealing with variable workload or employee absence due to lifestyle preferences or family demands for child care. Flexible schedules are helpful under the following considerations:

- When the workload requires more than an 8-hour shift but less than a 16-hour shift (e.g., 10- or 12-hour shifts)
- When the workload requires less than an 8-hour shift (e.g., 4, 5, or 6 hours)
- When the workload is variable by day of week (e.g., busier on Mondays than the other days of the week)
- When "call-back" hours occur within 2 hours of the end of a defined shift (e.g., "On Call" begins in the main OR at 3 p.m. and the first "call-back" occurs before 5 p.m.)
- When it meets the needs of the employee, unit, service line, or department and does not cause unplanned overtime or disruption in unit coverage

Many organizations are offering employees "flexible scheduling" in the form of 4-, 6-, 8-, 10-, and 12-hour shifts or "split shifts," meaning they might work 7 a.m. to 11:30 a.m. and 3 to 7:30 p.m. in the same day. Employees who work shifts of less than 4.5 hours in length are not entitled to a lunch break and can have only one 15-minute break. Those who work shifts of 5 or more hours are entitled to a 30- to 60-minute meal break and a mid-shift break of 15 minutes depending on state statutes. DNPs/nurse leaders must be careful to work with human resources and payroll to prevent conflicts between hours worked and hours paid policies and practices. They must also ensure clear and frequent education to both employees and any individuals involved in scheduling so misinformation and misunderstanding are prevented.

SCHEDULING PRINCIPLES

There are basic principles in scheduling that drive the outcome and quality of the schedule. These scheduling principles taught by LMI include the following:

1. Shifts should be developed that deliver resources to the volume of work to assure the consistent delivery of target hours of care at each prescribed UOS and planned cost.
2. Every unit needs FT and PT employees for "staffing elasticity" to cope with fluctuating and erratic changes in workload volumes and planned and unplanned absences. The per-diem/ casual or contingent employees should be a percentage of the PT employees but not comprise all of the PT positions.
3. Weekend requirements determine the total positions needed in position control, total FT staff, and the FT/PT ratios needed (e.g., 70% FT/30% PT).
4. More FT staff will be required when weekday requirements are greater than weekend requirements.
5. More PT staff will be required when the weekend requirements are greater than the weekday requirements.
6. Unequal weekend coverage means greater schedule holes on the weekends and unequal shift distribution during the weekdays.
7. The sum total of the "working" FTEs must be equal to the budgeted total worked FTEs, or the unit hours per UOS will be under or over budget.
8. The defined direct and indirect schedule requirements based on the budget must determine the need for and the required pattern for weekend rotations other than 2 of 4 (or every other weekend), 10- or 12-hour shifts or the mixing of all defined shifts (4-, 6-, 8-, 10-, and 12-hour shifts).
9. Never start 12-hour shifts unless the minimum number of 12-hour shift employees is equal to the minimum weekend requirement for all weekends within the 4-week schedule period and never less than four on the day shift and four on the night shift if the unit is doing all 12-hour shifts.
    If this rule cannot be honored after 12-hour shifts have started, then discontinue them, as it will create unmatched shifts or "schedule holes" that will drive partial shift shortages or produce unnecessary hours or overtime to fill.
10. Always increase or decrease 12-hour shifts in equal increments of two people for each shift. If employees will not commit to working 12-hour shifts and this rule cannot be honored after 12-hour shifts have started, then discontinue them, as it will create unmatched shifts or "schedule holes" that will drive partial shift shortages or produce unnecessary hours or overtime to fill.

SCHEDULING AND STAFFING MODELS

There are three workforce management (scheduling and staffing methods) options for schedule production and daily staffing functionality:

1. *Centralized scheduling and staffing*—All scheduling and daily staffing responsibilities reside in a centralized scheduling and staffing office. The DNP/nurse leader works with a designated scheduler, staffer, and/or timekeeper. The DNP/nurse leader has oversight responsibility and reviews to approve, deny, and/or advise the central staffing office scheduler about employee requests.
2. *Decentralized scheduling and staffing*—The DNP/nurse leader is responsible for all aspects of schedule development and daily staffing. The DNP/nurse leader may delegate tasks to a scheduling/ staffing committee or to permanent charge or resource nurses, but has ultimate accountability for his or her decisions. The DNP/nurse leader approves or denies all employee requests for the scheduling/staffing committee or other designee to implement.

3. *Modified decentralized scheduling and staffing*—Line and job functions are operationally clear for DNPs/nurse leaders versus centralized schedulers and staffers to plan, review, and authorize the publication of schedules every 4 to 6 weeks.

> The DNP/nurse leader approves all "planned absences" within the approved nonproductive budget using PT and per-diem/casual or contingent staff at the regular rates of pay. Within the mutually agreed mission and staffing goals, the central staffing office is most often responsible to find replacement coverage for all "unplanned absences" using resource pool employees, staff from other units or outsourced labor (agency or travelers) inclusive of covering extended absences due to vacant positions or LOA/ FMLOA. Many hospitals include the management of "Sitter or 1 to 1 Observation Hours" as a central staffing office responsibility.

Accountability is jointly held between the DNP/nurse leader and the central staffing office based on the approved workforce management option (e.g., scheduling/staffing method).

Good scheduling requires collaboration, data, and process improvement to control or lower costs and maintain or raise quality. Motivating and retaining employees is always a challenge, and DNPs/nurse leaders must be aware of the relationship between worked hours, fatigue, and performance and patient outcomes.

BUILDING A SCHEDULE: THE 4- TO 6-WEEK BUDGET PLAN

If the annual budget defines the relationship between revenues and expenses for 1 year, the 4- to 6-week schedule is the budget plan for the worked resources for the budget or "most frequent workload UOS or volume" for a portion of the annual plan. The schedule is the short-range plan based on the budget that defines the deliverable clinical resources based on the "5 Rights":

1. Right person
2. Right place
3. Right time
4. Right skills
5. Right cost

Shifts of need:

1. Fill a specific purpose on the unit related to workload or employee competency or skill.
2. Work within the approved budget worked hours of care.
3. Coexist with or complement the other shifts.
4. Provide worked hours at the regular rate of pay.

Shifts of convenience:

1. Focus on meeting the individual employee need versus the patient needs or the needs of the other employees. For example, an ADT shift from 9:00 a.m. to 3:00 p.m. brings an employee on duty after the 7:00 a.m. shift has started, ahead of the most frequent ADT activity, which occurs between 3:00 p.m. and 7:00 p.m., so the ADT nurse misses the peak ADT time.
   a. Often shifts that do not correlate to the intended workload upset the core staff who "rearrange assignments" to accommodate for the late arrival and early departure of the ADT nurse.
   b. Often shifts that do not correlate to the intended workload upset the core staff who feel overworked and frustrated when there is no designated ADT nurse to accommodate the demand.
2. Often incurs overtime to other staff who are waiting for staff to come to the unit when shift start and stop times do not correspond to the other staff.

SCHEDULE TYPES

There are four types of employee schedules. Nurse leaders should choose the best schedule type that reflects their management style and employees' needs.

Self, Autonomous, or Participative Scheduling

Self, autonomous, or participative scheduling is considered the most desirable of all schedule types by DNPs/nurse leaders and employees. Good self-scheduling is dependent on the DNP/nurse leader defining specific schedule requirements or guidelines by shift for direct and indirect caregivers by skill mix or category (e.g., RN, LPN/LVN, NA) and unique experience or skills (e.g., charge nurse or chemo qualified).

Employees will sign up for shifts to work that satisfy their hired work agreement (e.g., FTE commitment every 2 weeks) and meet the DNPs/nurse leader's defined schedule requirements.

Employees feel more autonomy for the unit's schedule and shift coverage. This method requires more shared governance to manage. It preserves the DNP/nurse leader's accountability, but when done correctly, reduces the actual work of schedule development.

Self versus selfish scheduling: The unit's scheduling practices have become more "selfish" than autonomous and collaborative when the following occurs:

1. Employees sign up for their desired shifts and depend on a third party (DNP/nurse leader, unit scheduler, or scheduling committee) to reconcile the employee shifts to the defined schedule requirements.
2. The process of self-scheduling requires the majority of staff to spend many hours working on the schedule without a guaranteed outcome.
3. The shift "sign-up" becomes a "very selfish" approach, whereby adherence to policies is often overlooked because the weekend rotations are unstructured and the schedule requirements are undefined or ignored.
4. Resolution of request conflicts is left to the individual to negotiate with the coworkers, and when it is unsatisfactory to the employee, it often results in a "call-in" for unplanned time off.

Good participative, autonomous, or self- (not selfish) scheduling practices meet the patient care workload demand, comply with budget expectations, enhance staff satisfaction, and minimize the time spent in scheduling.

Good participative or self-scheduling practices require team-driven collaboration, conflict resolution skills, and assertive communication skills to avoid victim behavior.

Self or "selfish" scheduling practices occur when unplanned absences are greater than planned absences, employees expect the DNP/nurse leader and/or schedulers to negotiate all schedule changes, and DNPs/nurse leaders or schedulers are spending more than 6 hours/month (for an average unit of 60 employees) creating a future schedule *and* more than 4 to 6 hours/week making changes in the current and "next" shifts over 24 hours.

Master/Block/Pattern/Core or Cyclical Scheduling

Master/block/pattern/core or cyclical scheduling includes various names for the same type of scheduling practice. These repeating types of schedules include a 21- to 28-day schedule pattern whereby employee requests are superimposed on the "master" schedule plan. This method allows the greatest predictability and stability for employees, DNPs/nurse leaders, scheduling committee members, and central staffing offices. It provides for preplanned weekend and shift balance that corresponds to the budget and position control, and it provides for prebalanced combinations of "experienced" staff to meet unit needs on all shifts.

Master/block/pattern/core or cyclical scheduling can fail the unit when dysfunctional schedule patterns are created that serve some employees while punishing others. This type of scheduling can become unacceptable to the employees if the employee request guidelines are so restrictive that they are punishing to employees. It also can fail the unit when the budget has been changed but the master/block/pattern/core or cyclical schedule is not updated in the scheduling, staffing, and/or time and attendance software systems.

For example, if a pattern needs to have a shift changed permanently and the employee finds another employee willing to make a permanent change in both their patterns but the DNP/nurse leader requires that all the patterns have to be posted and rebid by all employees, then the staff will become frustrated. Staff will come to feel that the change is too cumbersome to support long term, and call-ins for unplanned absences will increase.

Budget and Requirement Driven

The schedule is developed in 28-day or 4-week increments to provide a minimum of 85% of the core staffing needs based on the budget and defined unit schedule requirements as its primary focus. Budget- and requirement-driven schedules require a minimum preassigned weekend pattern for all employees.

Employee requests are superimposed based on the budget nonproductive time. Deficit demands (planned and unplanned absences) are covered from a maximum of the 15% supplemental staffing comprised of unit-based per diem (also called PRN, casual, or contingent) and PT or resource pool staff.

Weekends to work and be off are preplanned and predictable. This method can accommodate up to a maximum of 20% of all the employees having a fixed or repeating schedule pattern.

The budget- and requirement-driven schedule type requires someone to do the scheduling process every 4 to 6 weeks. Employees' weekends may be changed to keep the balance of "experienced" and "inexperienced" staff on each shift. However, employees may be unhappy because of changes in their weekend rotations and unapproved requests often become the responsibility of the employee to trade with other employees for time off. If employees are not collaborative and collegial to trade shifts, then call-ins for unplanned absences will increase.

Employee Request Driven

Employee request-driven scheduling is "selfish" scheduling gone bad. All assigned shifts are secondary to the employees' request to work or not work. It is the most costly, creates the most schedule holes, and is the most dysfunctional of all schedule types. Some of the most common examples of employee request-driven scheduling include:

- Single-shift patterns increase employee "call-ins" or unexpected absences. If the majority of call-ins occur on single shifts, the DNP/nurse leader is dealing with "selfish scheduling." LMI often finds in its Schedule Best Practice Audits between 5% and 25% of all unplanned absence "call-ins" occur on single shifts. Reducing scheduled single shifts by increasing the number of consecutive shifts to two whenever possible will often reduce overall overtime by 1% to 4%.
- Single-shift "call-ins" are usually replaced with overtime and decrease continuity of care for the patient.
- "Unmatched" shifts create "holes" or overlapping shifts, unnecessary hours, and overtime, which is costly to the organization.
- Excessive flexible shifts are disruptive to the delivery of care and ultimately frustrate staff, as it makes it difficult for them to trade shifts.

Scheduling to the Unit Workload Capacity

Creating schedules based on the unit capacity is not a good practice if the unit capacity is not the MFC or UOS for the following reasons:

1. Increases worked hours on the unit if staffing overages are not caught or if staff refuse to float off the unit or take "low workload cancellation" if they are not needed.

2. Increases the use of nonproductive hours when employees want to be paid for their "low workload cancellation" time.
3. Results in hours of care below target thresholds when shift shortages are not caught or if staff refuse to work extra hours or overtime.
4. Increases the risk for greater turnover because of the frequent staffing changes due to shift cancellations, floating out of the home unit, or using benefit time to cover shift cancellations or reductions in hours.

If "shift cancellation" hours are greater than 5% of the total worked hours in the survey period, it is a reflection of scheduling practices that need to be corrected.

TRANSLATING FTEs INTO SCHEDULE REQUIREMENTS

The DNP/nurse leader translates the required clinical resources into the schedule requirements defined as shifts (of need), hours, and FTEs by categories and/or experiences. Defining schedule requirements will determine if you have the budgeted FTEs to accommodate the planned 4-, 6-, 8-, 10-, or 12-hour shifts or reduce the weekend-to-work rotations.

It is critically important that the DNP/nurse leader define the unit's "shifts of need" within the schedule requirements because they serve specific purposes. "Shifts of convenience" usually accommodate employee-specific needs, such as day-care hours.

When "shifts of need" overlap with "shifts of convenience," they create shift overages or shortages, which increase cancellations or floating or increased HPPD if the hours are not floated out of the unit. They increase floating, overtime, and agency usage and ultimately hurt patient care if the shortages are not filled.

DIRECT SCHEDULE REQUIREMENTS

The direct schedule requirements define the number of hours available by shift by day of week in shift lengths (4, 6, 8, 10, 12 hours) that can be scheduled and stay within the budget for the direct caregivers (RNs, LPNs/LVNs, NAs). The default calculation for all finance programs is in 8-hour shifts over a 24-hour day, so doing the calculations in 8-hour shifts helps DNPs/nurse leaders see if they will have enough resources to staff to the target numbers of caregivers they think are necessary.

If schedule needs cannot be met in 8-hour shift increments, the unit's needs will never be met in 12-hour shift increments unless the FTEs are increased by at least 10%. The total shifts and the shifts for the weekends and weekdays are used to calculate the total positions required for the unit in position control as well as the total FT and PT staff needed.

The total required direct FTEs for all shifts must equal the total budget direct FTEs in the unit annual staffing budget. If the calculated direct FTEs in the schedule requirements are below or above the budget direct FTEs in the unit staffing budget, there is an error in the defined direct schedule requirements that must be corrected before proceeding.

The definitions and formulas used to calculate the schedule requirements include the following, grouped by defined shift (refer to Tables 4.9 and 4.10).

Defined shift—Start time, stop time, and paid shift length.

Employee category (skill mix)—The category or skill mix of the employees for each shift.

Day of week requirement (Monday through Sunday)—The number of staff required for each shift by day of week. The number of required staff should reflect patterns for high and low workload.

Total weekday shifts—The sum of all shifts on Monday through Friday.

Total weekend shifts—The sum of all shifts on Saturday and Sunday.

Total shifts—The sum of all shifts on all 7 days of the week.

Total hours—Multiply the total shifts by the paid shift length for the defined shift. For example, total RNs with charge qualification require a total of 14 shifts multiplied by 8 hours/shift = 112 required worked hours.

Targeted FTEs—Divide the total worked hours by 40 hours/FTE. For example, 112 hours divided by 40 hours = 2.8 FTEs.

Repeat these steps for each required employee category or unique skill or experience. For example, RN chemo qualified is a subset of the total RN requirement. The DNP/nurse leader wants a minimum of two employees working each shift, in case one of the chemo-qualified nurses calls in sick. The DNP/nurse leader does not care if all RNs are chemo qualified, as long as it is balanced across all days and avoids days where there are shortages and surpluses.

Totals—Total the required shifts for each day of the week, weekdays, weekends, total shifts, total hours, and target FTEs. The total required FTEs for each unique employee category or skill-mix group must equal the budget FTEs from the unit staffing budget. If the total FTEs are below the budget FTEs, the schedule requirements must be adjusted up or down until they match.

Grand totals—The total of all required shift totals. The total required FTEs in the grand total FTEs for each unique employee category or skill-mix group must equal the sum total budget FTEs from the unit staffing budget for total direct FTEs. If the total FTEs are below the budget FTEs, the schedule requirements must be adjusted up or down until they match.

The best-defined schedule requirements also include a summary of the unit staffing budget, reflecting budget workload UOS or volume and most frequent volumes annually, each 4 weeks, 1 week, and average/day.

It also reflects the budget total worked (or productive), nonproductive, and total paid hours annually, each 4 weeks, 1 week, and average/day. If there is a budget for overtime, education and orientation hours are also displayed. A "Notes" section documents unique variations by unit. For example, do the unit charge or resource nurses take a patient assignment and count as a full staff nurse, impacting the budget FTEs or budget direct, indirect, and total worked hours/UOS (Suby, 2006).

INDIRECT SCHEDULE REQUIREMENTS

The indirect schedule requirements define the number of hours available by shift by day of week in shifts that can be scheduled and stay within the budget for the indirect caregivers (e.g., DNP/nurse leader, clerks, monitor techs, educator, case manager, and any other positions that do not flex to the VSP). Charge nurses that do not take patient assignments would be considered indirect caregivers.

The required indirect FTEs in this exercise must equal the budget indirect FTEs in the unit staffing budget. If the calculated indirect FTEs in the schedule requirements form are below or above the budget indirect FTEs, there is an error in the defined indirect schedule requirements that must be corrected before proceeding (refer to Table 4.11; Suby, 2006).

CALCULATING THE FT/PT RATIOS

An appropriate ratio of FT and PT employees is important when determining the appropriate range of "staffing elasticity" for staffing levels on weekdays and weekends, and defining positions in the position control (Suby, 2007a).

TABLE 4.9 Example: Current Budget Direct Schedule Requirements for 8 Hours

8-Hour Direct Schedule Requirements by Day of Week for 3M-Med/Surg at Somewhere Medical Center Based on Authorized Budget	
2017 Budget direct: 8.27 & 9.03 total worked HPPD Patient days with obs: 6,358.3	Budgeted patient days 6,358/year, 487/8/4 weeks; 243.9/2 weeks 17.42/day Capacity: 21: ADC + obs: 17.42; most frequent census (MFC) range ____ Budget total paid hours: 62,816/year; 4,818.52/4 weeks; 2,409.38/2 weeks; 172.09/day Budget total worked hours: 57,408/year; 4,403.84/4 weeks; 2,201.95/2 weeks; 157.28/day Nonproductive (NP) hours: 5,208/year; 414.4/4 weeks; 207.2/2 weeks; 14.8/day; % NP: 8.3% Overtime (OT) budget 4,784/year; 367.92/4 weeks; 184/2 weeks; 13.14/day %OT: 7.61% Education and orientation are included in nonproductive hours.

Unit 3M-Med/Surg
Manager: ____

Direct Care or Service Personnel   Shift: 7 a.m. to 3 p.m.   Paid Hours: 800

RN-to-Patient Ratio: 1:8.7; LPN-to-Patient Ratio: 1:5.8; Licensed Ratio: 1:3.5	Mon	Tue	Wed	Thu	Fri	Sat	Sun	Weekday Shift Totals (Add Mon–Fri)	Weekend Shift Totals (Add Sat–Sun)	Total Shifts (Add all 7 days)	Total Hours (Multiply Total Shifts by Paid Shift Length)	Targeted FTEs (Divide Total Hours by 40 [1 FTE] in a Week)
RN (w/charge)	2	2	2	2	2	2	2	10	4	14	112	2.8
LPN	3	3	3	3	3	3	3	15	6	21	168	4.2
NA	1	1	1	1	1	1	1	5	2	7	56	1.4
								0	0	0	0	0.0
Totals	**6**	**6**	**6**	**6**	**6**	**6**	**6**	**30**	**12**	**42**	**336**	**8.4**

Direct Care or Service Personnel   Shift: 3 p.m. to 11 p.m.   Paid Hours: 800

RN-to-Patient Ratio: 1:8.7 to 11.6; LPN-to-Patient Ratio: 1:5.8 to 6.9; Licensed Ratio: 1:3.5 to 4.4	Mon	Tue	Wed	Thu	Fri	Sat	Sun	Weekday Shift Totals (Add Mon–Fri)	Weekend Shift Totals (Add Sat–Sun)	Total Shifts (Add all 7 days)	Total Hours (Multiply Total Shifts by Paid Shift Length)	Targeted FTEs (Divide Total Hours by 40 [1 FTE] in a Week)
RN (w/charge)	2	2	2	2	1.5	1.5	1.5	9.5	3	12.5	100	2.5
LPN	3	3	3	3	3	2.5	2.5	15	5	20	160	4.0
NA	1	1	1	1	2.5	2.5	2.5	6.5	5	11.5	92	2.3
								0	0	0	0	0.0
Totals	**6**	**6**	**6**	**6**	**7**	**6.5**	**6.5**	**31**	**13**	**44**	**352**	**8.8**

(continued)

TABLE 4.9 Example: Current Budget Direct Schedule Requirements for 8 Hours (*continued*)

Direct Care or Service Personnel	Shift: 11 p.m. to 7 a.m.						Paid Hours: 800		Weekday Shift Totals (Add Mon–Fri)	Weekend Shift Totals (Add Sat–Sun)	Total Shifts (Add all 7 days)	Total Hours (Multiply Total Shifts by Paid Shift Length)	Targeted FTEs (Divide Total Hours by 40 [1 FTE] in a Week)
RN-to-Patient Ratio: 1:17.4; LPN-to-Patient Ratio: 1:5.8 to 8.7; Licensed Ratio: 1:3.5 to 4.4	Mon	Tue	Wed	Thu	Fri	Sat	Sun						
RN (w/charge)	2	2	2	2	1	1	1	9	2	11	88	2.2
LPN	3	3	3	3	3	2	2	15	4	19	152	3.8
NA	1	1	1	1	2	2	2	6	4	10	80	2.0
								0	0	0	0	0.0
Totals	6	6	6	6	6	5	5	30	10	40	320	8.0
Grand totals	18	18	18	18	19	17.5	17.5	91	35	126	1,008	25.2

Notes: The charge nurse on all shifts takes a patient assignment. Budget total worked RN FTEs: 7.52; total schedule requirement RN FTEs: 7.5.

Budget total worked LPN FTEs: 12.01; total schedule requirement LPN FTEs: 12.0.

Budget total worked NA FTEs: 5.68; total schedule requirement NA FTEs: 5.7.

FTEs, full-time equivalents; HPPD, hours per patient day; LPN, licensed practical nurse; NA, nursing assistant.

Source: Suby (2015). Reproduced with permission from the Labor Management Institute (LMI).

TABLE 4.10 Example: Current Budget Direct Schedule Requirements for 12 Hours

12-Hour Direct Schedule Requirements by Day of Week for 3M-Med/Surg at Somewhere Medical Center Based on Authorized Budget

2017 Budget direct: 8.27 & 9.03 total worked HPPD	Budgeted patient days 6,358/year, 487/8/4 weeks; 243.9/2 weeks 17.42/day
Annual patient days with obs: 6,358.3	Capacity: 21: ADC + obs; 17.42; most frequent census (MFC) range _____; 2,409.38/2 weeks; 172.09/day
	Budget total paid hours: 62,816/year; 4,818.52/4 weeks; 2,409.38/2 weeks; 172.09/day
	Budget total worked hours: 57,408/year; 4,403.84/4 weeks; 2,201.95/2 weeks; 157.28/day
	Nonproductive (NP) hours: 5,208/year; 414.4/4 weeks; 207.2/2 weeks; 14.8/day; % NP: 8.3%
	Overtime (OT) budget 4,784/year; 367.92/4 weeks; 184/2 weeks; 13.14/day %OT: 7.61%
	Education and orientation are included in nonproductive hours.

Unit: 3M-Med/Surg
Manager: _____

Direct Care or Service Personnel   Shift: 7 a.m. to 7 p.m.   Paid Hours: 1,200

RN-to-Patient Ratio: 1:8.7; LPN-to-Patient Ratio: 1:5.8; Licensed Ratio: 1:3.5	Mon	Tue	Wed	Thu	Fri	Sat	Sun	Weekday Shift Totals (Add Mon–Fri)	Weekend Shift Totals (Add Sat–Sun)	Total Shifts (Add all 7 days)	Total Hours (Multiply Total Shifts by Paid Shift Length)	Targeted FTEs (Divide Total Hours by 40 [1 FTE] in a Week)
RN (w/charge)	2	2	2	2	2	1.225	1.225	10	2.45	12.45	149.4	3.7
LPN	3	3	3	3	2	3	3	14	6	20	240	6.0
NA	1.3524	1.3524	1.3524	1.3524	1.3524	1.3524	1.3524	6.8	2.7	9.5	113.6	2.8
								0	0	0	0	0.0
Totals	6.3524	6.3524	6.3524	6.3524	5.3524	5.5774	5.5774	30.8	11.15	41.95	503.0	12.5

(continued)

TABLE 4.10 Example: Current Budget Direct Schedule Requirements for 12 Hours (*continued*)

Direct Care or Service Personnel   Shift: 7 p.m. to 7 a.m.   Paid Hours: 1,200

RN-to-Patient Ratio: 1:8.7; LPN-to-Patient Ratio: 1:5.8; Licensed Ratio: 1:3.5	Mon	Tue	Wed	Thu	Fri	Sat	Sun	Weekday Shift Totals (Add Mon–Fri)	Weekend Shift Totals (Add Sat–Sun)	Total Shifts (Add all 7 days)	Total Hours (Multiply Total Shifts by Paid Shift Length)	Targeted FTEs (Divide Total Hours by 40 [1 FTE] in a Week)
RN (w/charge)	2	2	2	2	2	1.225	1.225	10	2.45	12.45	149.4	3.7
LPN	3	3	3	3	2	3	3	14	6	20	240	6.0
NA	1.3524	1.3524	1.3524	1.3524	1.3524	1.3524	1.3524	6.8	2.7	9.5	113.6	2.8
								0	0	0	0	0.0
Totals	6.3524	6.3524	6.3524	6.3524	5.3524	5.5774	5.5774	30.8	11.15	41.95	503.0	12.5

Direct Care or Service Personnel   Shift: 7 p.m. to 7 a.m.   Paid Hours: 1,200

	Mon	Tue	Wed	Thu	Fri	Sat	Sun	Weekday Shift Totals (Add Mon–Fri)	Weekend Shift Totals (Add Sat–Sun)	Total Shifts (Add all 7 days)	Total Hours (Multiply Total Shifts by Paid Shift Length)	Targeted FTEs (Divide Total Hours by 40 [1 FTE] in a Week)
RN (w/charge)								0	0	0	0	0.0
LPN								0	0	0	0	0.0
NA								0	0	0	0	0.0
								0	0	0	0	0.0
Totals	0	0	0	0	0	0	0	0	0	0	0	0.0
Grand totals	12.7048	12.7048	12.7048	12.7048	10.7048	11.1548	11.1548	61.6	23.30	83.9	1006.0	25.1

Notes: The current budget is for 8.27 direct HPPD and 9.03 total worked HPPD. The charge nurse on all shifts takes a patient assignment. Budget total worked RN FTEs: 7.52; total schedule requirement RN FTEs: 7.52.

Budget total worked LPN FTEs: 12.01; total schedule requirement LPN FTEs: 12.0.

Budget total worked NA FTEs: 5.68; total schedule requirement NA FTEs: 5.7.

FTEs, full-time equivalents; HPPD, hours per patient day; LPN, licensed practical nurse; NA, nursing assistant.

TABLE 4.11 Example: Current Budget Indirect Schedule Requirements

8-Hour Indirect Schedule Requirements by Day of Week for 3M-Med/Surg at Somewhere Medical Center Based on Authorized Budget

Unit name: 3M-Med/Surg   Based on budget of 8.27 direct & 9.03 total worked HPPD

Cost center#:

Indirect Care or Service Personnel   Shift: 7 a.m. to 3 p.m.   Paid Hours:

	Mon	Tue	Wed	Thu	Fri	Sat	Sun	Weekday Shift Totals (Add Mon–Fri)	Weekend Shift Totals (Add Sat–Sun)	Total Shifts (Add all 7 days)	Total Hours (Multiply Total Shifts by Pd. Shift Length)	Targeted FTEs (Divide Total Hours by 40 [1 FTE] in a Week)
Manager	1	1	1	1	1	0	0	5	0	5	40	1.0
Unit secretary	1	1	1	1	1	1	1	5	2	7	56	1.4
								0	0	0	0	0.0
Totals	**2**	**2**	**2**	**2**	**2**	**1**	**1**	**10**	**2**	**12**	**96**	**2.4**

Indirect Care or Service Personnel   Shift: 3 p.m. to 11 p.m.   Paid Hours:

	Mon	Tue	Wed	Thu	Fri	Sat	Sun	Weekday Shift Totals	Weekend Shift Totals	Total Shifts	Total Hours	Targeted FTEs
Unit secretary	0	0	0	0	0	0	0	0	0	0	0	0.0
								0	0	0	0	0.0
Totals	**0**	**0**	**0**	**0**	**0**	**0**	**0**	**0**	**0**	**0**	**0**	**0.0**

Indirect Care or Service Personnel   Shift: 11 p.m. to 7 a.m.   Paid Hours:

	Mon	Tue	Wed	Thu	Fri	Sat	Sun	Weekday Shift Totals	Weekend Shift Totals	Total Shifts	Total Hours	Targeted FTEs
Unit secretary	0	0	0	0	0	0	0	0	0	0	0	0.0
								0	0	0	0	0.0
								0	0	0	0	0.0
Totals	**0**	**0**	**0**	**0**	**0**	**0**	**0**	**0**	**0**	**0**	**0**	**0.0**
Grand totals	**2**	**2**	**2**	**2**	**2**	**1**	**1**	**10**	**2**	**12**	**96**	**2.4**

Notes: The charge nurse is included in the direct RN caregivers.

NAs and unit secretaries are cross-trained. An NA is used as a secretary on the p.m. shift.

The indirect percent of total worked hours is 8.37% and the indirect HPPD is 0.75.

FTEs, full-time equivalents; HPPD, hours per patient day; LPN, licensed practical nurse; NA, nursing assistant.

Source: Reproduced with permission from the Labor Management Institute (LMI).

For units requiring nearly the same weekend and weekday coverage, the following principles apply:

1. Weekend needs determine the total number of employees required.
2. Weekday needs determine the maximum number of FT employees.
3. More FT employees can be used if weekend needs are reduced from weekday.
4. Consistent weekday and weekend staffing requires the highest ratio of PT employees.

Part-time and per-diem/casual or contingent employees are necessary, both for providing alternative weekends of work and for flexibility in dealing with a varying census. A mixture of PT and per-diem/casual or contingent employees is desirable. All PT positions hired at 32 hours/pay period or all per-diem/casual or contingent positions are not best practice and will result in scheduling employees when they are not needed to satisfy their hired work agreement, increased single shifts and decreased continuity of care, and increased call-ins for single shifts.

The ratio of FT to PT, per-diem employees is determined by the weekend and weekday requirements. A ratio of 40% PT provides maximum flexibility. However, availability and management are the key issues in PT staffing.

Many hospitals experience difficulty managing a PT workforce. In today's market and economy, availability of part-timers is an even greater issue. Even good benefit packages are not enough to obtain an adequate supply of workers. Each hospital has to continue to recruit and retain PT employees with benefits and adequate pay.

DNPs/nurse leaders must be careful to not fill PT or per-diem/casual or contingent positions with employees working second jobs. Although it may not be against HR policy, employees working second jobs often exceed 60 total worked hours per work week, and 15 hours per 24-hour period, resulting in significant fatigue. Employees working second jobs often have higher "call-ins" for unexpected absences than other employees, and their performance and interpersonal relationships suffer from the consequences of fatigue.

ROTATING OR PERMANENT SHIFTS

A *permanent shift* is when employees work one shift only. A *rotating shift* is when employees desiring to work the day shift are required to work a designated number of evening or night shifts. Both of these options are used in hospitals. Both have advantages and some disadvantages. Permanent shifts sound good, in theory, because they appear to give employees the opportunity to work the shifts of their choice. In actuality, they often drive the newest, least-experienced employees to work the evening and night shifts—the shifts that are most sparsely staffed.

Greater turnover occurs on these shifts, since employees move to day shifts as soon as positions open. Units with permanent shifts usually find the day shift will have the highest percentage of tenured staff. Vacancies on evening and night shifts are difficult to fill, with no assurance of keeping an experienced group of staff on these shifts. Increasing ADT occurring on the night shifts, combined with charge or resource nurses who are often taking full patient assignments, makes it essential to require even more experienced staff on these shifts.

Rotating shifts have the best potential for providing experienced staff on all shifts when there is not enough permanent shift staff to meet all the unit's needs. However, expectations for employees working rotating shifts have often been unrealistic. This excessive and erratic rotation between shifts can be very difficult for employees to manage. Since rotation is dependent on the number of permanent evening or night staff available, clear guidelines must govern rotation practices. The more shifts an employee is expected to rotate to, the more unhappy he or she becomes. Turnover will increase dramatically when the employee is expected to rotate to four or more shifts. For example, a day, evening, and night 8-hour shift along with a day and night 12-hour shift represents five shifts. This becomes particularly troublesome under "flexible" scheduling that combines 4-, 6-, 8-, 10-, and 12-hour shifts; this has the potential to represent 17 different shifts in 24 hours.

The need to develop and implement plans to provide experienced staff on all shifts is a top priority for DNPs/nurse leaders. Making the least desirable shifts more desirable must be an agreed-upon and sought-after scheduling and staffing goal.

The required shifts from the scheduled requirements form are used to determine the total number of positions needed in the position control if all positions are based on 8- or 12-hour shifts while keeping the weekend rotation equitable to 2 of 4 (or every other) weekends.

POSITION CONTROL OR HIRING PLAN

Position control is also called the unit's hiring plan (Suby, 2007c). It contains the defined and approved positions for each category of employees from FT to PT at the planned FTE work agreement/pay period. Best practice requires that the DNP/nurse leader work with HR and recruiters to keep the position control/hiring plan updated every pay period so that projections can be accurately made of total budgeted positions, total filled positions, and vacant positions compared to positions hired but in orientation or not yet started. Best practice is for the DNP/unit leader to maintain the accuracy of the position control/hiring plan, understanding that HR and finance will also depend on its accuracy. Changes to the planned FTE work agreements and composition of FT and PT positions must be considered against the unit's annual or quarterly budget. Employees who desire to change their hired FTE work agreement should request their FTE change in writing, allowing a minimum of 6 months or more to be approved. Many organizations are limiting employees' change in their hired FTE work agreement to one time per year.

When defining the total employees needed for position control, the FT/PT calculations should address the EMO replacement if it is budgeted as indirect replacement coverage and the nonproductive replacement coverage the unit is responsible for in each schedule.

The PT and per-diem/casual staff should be the first sources used for deficit demand response, and their hired FTE work agreement should reflect an expectation to work weekends (even if they are not needed to work weekends) as well as the minimum number of shifts necessary for them to maintain their individual skills and unit-based competencies in the unit.

LMI recommends that the per-diem/casual staff work no fewer than 8 to 16 hours/2-week pay period or 0.1 to 0.15 FTE, or they are an expense to the unit to maintain their credentials, skills, and competencies.

Defining the total employees and total FT and PT positions is best done for each skill mix individually (RN, LPN/LVN, and NA).

The required FTEs in the LMI Full-Time/Part-Time Form must equal the budget FTEs in the unit staffing budget. If the calculated FTEs in this form are below or above the budget FTEs in the unit staffing budget, there is an error in the direct or indirect defined schedule requirements that must be corrected before proceeding. The position control based on the budget should have the following positions:

8-hour total:	Direct care: 36	Full-time direct: 22	Part-time/PRN: 14
	Indirect care: 3	Full-time indirect: 2	Part-time/PRN: 1
Total:	39	24 or 61.5%	15 or 38.4%
Or combined			
8- and 12-hour total:	Direct care: 30	Full-time direct: 24	Part-time/PRN direct: 6
	Indirect care: 3	Full-time indirect: 2	Part-time/PRN indirect: 1
Total:	33	26 or 78.8%	7 or 21.2%

The calculations will vary depending on the shift length (8, 10, or 12 hours) and the weekend rotation (2 of 4 weekends or 1 of 3 weekends; see Tables 4.12 and 4.13.

TABLE 4.12 Example: Budget Total Employees FT-PT for 8-Hour Shifts for 2 of 4 Weekends

Defining Total Direct Employees (FT/PT) for 8-Hour Shifts and 2 of 4 Weekends for 3M-Med/Surg at Somewhere Medical Center Based on Authorized Budget		
Example Unit: 3M-Med/Surg Current Budget: Direct Care: 8.27 & 9.03 Total Worked HPPD		

Shift			Weekday	Weekend
D:			7 (56 hours)	7 (56 hours)
E:			5.7 (45.9 hours)	5.7 (45.9 hours)
N:			5.3 (42.3 hours)	5.3 (42.3 hours)

	Instructions	Result	Rationale
A	Weekdays: 1 day × 20	360	Multiply 1 day times 20, since there are 20 weekdays in a 28-day scheduling period.
B	Weekends: 1 day × 8	144	Multiply 1 day times 8, since there are 8 weekend days in a 28-day scheduling period.
C	Total: A + B	504	The sum of weekday and weekend shifts equals the total staffing requirements needed to achieve the staffing pattern.
D	FTE: C ÷ 20	25.2	The total required shifts are divided by 20 to calculate the total FTE shifts. The total is divided by 20 since an 80-hour person (1 FTE) would work 20 shifts in a 28-day scheduling period.
E	Total employees: B ÷ 4	36	The number of employees needed to cover weekend requirements is calculated by dividing the total weekend shifts by four, since each employee works half of the 8 weekend shifts.
F	Maximum FT: A ÷ 16	(Use 22) 22.5	Divide the weekday requirements by 16 to calculate the number of weekday shifts a FT person would work in a 28-day scheduling period, since a FT employee must work at least four of the 20 shifts on the weekend.
G	Minimum PT: E − F	(Use 14) 13.5	The remaining number of employees necessary to achieve the staffing pattern.
H	Weekday shifts FT: F × 16	352	Calculate the total weekday shifts for FT employees by multiplying the maximum number of FT employees by 16, since there are 16 weekday shifts available to be worked in a 28-day schedule period.
I	Weekend shifts FT: F × 4	88	Calculate the total weekend shifts for FT employees by multiplying the maximum number of FT employees by 4, since each employee will be working 4 weekend shifts.
J	Weekday shifts PT: A − H	8	Calculate the total weekday shifts for PT employees by subtracting the total number of weekday shifts FT employees will work from the total number of weekday shifts available in a 28-day period.
K	Weekend shifts PT: G × 4	56	Calculate the total weekend shifts for PT employees by multiplying the minimum number of PT employees by 4, since each employee will be working 4 weekend shifts.
L	Total shifts: H + I + J + K	504	The total number of shifts available equals the sum of all FT and PT weekday and weekend shifts to be covered in a 28-day schedule period.

Notes: Whenever the weekend rotation is based on 2 of 4 weekends, the formula is always based on a 28-day scheduling period comprised of 20 weekday shifts and 8 weekend shifts.

This unit needs 36 total employee positions in the position control of which 22 are FT and 14 are PT. The FT to PT ratio is 61% FT and 39% PT.

Recommend hiring four PT employees at 0.4 FTE to work 2 weekday shifts and 2 weekend shifts every pay period and 10 positions hired to work 0.2 FTE and 2 weekend shifts every pay period.

D, day shift; E, evening shift; FT, full-time; FTE, FT equivalent; N, night shift; HPPD, hours per patient day; PT, part-time.

Source: Suby (2015). Reproduced with permission from the Labor Management Institute (LMI).

TABLE 4.13 Example: Budget Total Employees FT-PT for 12-Hour Shifts for 2 of 4 Weekends

Defining Total Employees (FT/PT) for 12-Hour Shifts and 2 of 4 Weekends Based on Authorized Budget for 3M-Med/Surg of Somewhere Medical Center		
Example Unit: 3M-Med/Surg Current Budget: Direct Care: 8.27 HPPD & 9.03 Total Worked HPPD		
Shift	**Weekday**	**Weekend**
D:	6 (72 hours)	6 (72 hours)
E:	NA	NA
N:	6 (72 hours)	6 (72 hours)
Total:	12 (144 hours)	12 (144 hours)

	Instructions	**Result**	**Rationale**
A	Weekdays: 1 day × 20	240	Multiply 1 day times 20, since there are 20 weekdays in a 28-day scheduling period.
B	Weekends: 1 day × 8	96	Multiply 1 day times 8, since there are 8 weekend days in a 28-day scheduling period.
C	Total: A + B	336	The sum of weekday and weekend shifts equals the total staffing requirements needed to achieve the staffing pattern.
D	FTE: C × 12 hours ÷ 160 hours/4 weeks	(336 × 12 = 4,032 hours/160) 25.2	The total required shifts are multiplied by 12 hours to calculate the total worked hours and then divided by 160 hours to get the FTEs. The FTEs are based on the 40-hour/week definition. (A FTE will average 13 shifts/4 weeks.)
E	Maximum employees: A ÷ 8	30	Divide the weekday requirements by 8 to calculate the number of weekday shifts a FT person would work in a 28-day scheduling period, since a FT employee must work at least four of the 12 shifts on the weekend.
F	Maximum FT: B ÷ 4	24	The number of employees needed to cover weekend requirements is calculated by dividing the total weekend shifts by 4, since each employee works half of the 8 weekend shifts.
G	Minimum PT: –E –F	6	The remaining number of employees necessary to achieve the staffing pattern.
H	Weekday shifts FT: F × 8	192	Calculate the total weekday shifts for FT employees by multiplying the maximum number of FT employees by 8, since there are 8 weekday shifts available to be worked in a 28-day schedule period.
I	Weekend shifts FT: F × 4	96	Calculate the total weekend shifts for FT employees by multiplying the maximum number of FT employees by 4, since each employee will be working 4 weekend shifts.
J	Weekday shifts PT: A – H	48	Calculate the total weekday shifts for PT employees by subtracting the total number of weekday shifts FT employees will work from the total number of weekday shifts available in a 28-day period.

(continued)

TABLE 4.13 Example: Budget Total Employees FT-PT for 12-Hour Shifts for 2 of 4 Weekends (*continued*)

	Instructions	Result	Rationale
K	Weekend shifts PT: $G \times 4$	0	Subtract the total weekend shifts by FT employees from the total required weekend shifts. If the balance is 0, then the minimum PT employees in Step G must be PRN/casual employees. If there is a remaining balance, calculate the total weekend shifts for PT employees by multiplying the minimum number of PT employees by 4, since each employee will be working 4 weekend shifts.
L	Total shifts: $H + I + J + K$	336	The total number of shifts available equals the sum of all FT and PT weekday and weekend shifts to be covered in a 28-day schedule period.

Notes: Whenever the weekend rotation is based on 2 of 4 weekends, the formula is always based on a 28-day scheduling period comprised of 20 weekday shifts and 8 weekend shifts.

This unit needs 30 total employee positions in the position control of which 24 are FT and six are PRN/casual. The FT to PT ratio is 80% FT and 20% PRN/casual.

Recommend hiring six PT positions at 0.6 FTE to week 4 weekday shifts and 0 weekend shifts every pay period or 12 positions hired to work 0.3 FTE and 2 weekday shifts every pay period.

D, day shift; E, evening shift; FT, full-time; FTEs, FT equivalents; HPPD, hours per patient day; N, night shift; NA, nursing assistant; PT, part-time.

Source: Suby (2015). Reproduced with permission from the Labor Management Instutute (LMI).

POSITION CONTROL AND NURSE STAFFING

Position control comes in all kinds of formats and is best used as the translation of the budget into the defined total positions FT, PT, and per diem/casual or contingent based on the defined "scheduling requirements" for the unit. The use of CORE FTEs versus supplemental staffing to replace deficit demands is described in the following text.

The direct, indirect, and total worked FTEs defined in the unit annual staffing budget at the budget UOS are considered *core* staff and defined in the unit's position control or hiring plan. The number of FTEs needed to replace the CORE EMO and nonproductive planned and unplanned, paid and unpaid absences are calculated in the unit annual staffing budget, and the sources for replacing those staff must be identified. The staff that replace the CORE staff work supplemental replacement hours and FTEs, and they come from the following sources in order of least to most expensive:

1. Unit-based per-diem or casual staff
2. PT staff willing to pick up extra hours
3. Employees willing to float from other units within and outside of the service line if they are not needed
4. Employees in the float or resource pool
5. Agency RNs
6. Traveler RNs

It is critically important that the DNP/unit leader define the amount and sources of supplemental staffing with the annual budget from the unit-based per-diem or casual and PT employees and incorporate into the position control. It is also important for the nursing department to have a mutually agreed-upon mission and goals for staff replacement by unit and service line for the central staffing or resource office. Once defined and agreed to, DNPs/unit leaders and their service line directors must work collaboratively to flex staff to the mutually agreed-upon goals before any staff are given additional time off. Employees become increasingly angry watching staff on another unit go home early using vacation or paid time off (PTO) time while employees on another unit are working short of staff or incurring more overtime, bonus, and incentive hours.

An example of a central staffing or resource office mission statement is: "Design and maintain a fair and equitable workforce system that ensures stability and appropriate distribution of clinical labor resources 24/7 hours/day."

An example of the total unit and/or service line commitment goals for supplemental staffing replacement includes the following:

1. Unplanned absence FTEs equal to 1/day
2. Vacation/PTO or holiday off FTEs
3. EMO FTEs
4. Unplanned workload fluctuation or acuity greater than 1 up or down of the target VSP

An example of the total central float or resource pool commitment goals for supplemental staffing replacement includes the following:

1. Unplanned absence greater than 5% of total worked hours in the unit(s) or the second or additional call-ins per day
2. LOA/FMLOA FTEs
3. Vacant position FTEs for orientation factoring in any known "overhired" FTEs
4. Unplanned workload fluctuation or acuity greater than 2 up of the target VSP

LMI best practices for cost center position control are based on the following:

1. It is managed by the DNP/nurse leader and used as the unit's hiring plan to guide the approval of employee requests to change from FT to PT to per-diem/casual or contingent status.
2. It is shared with human resources as the unit's hiring plan.
3. It is shared with finance for FTE management.
4. It is shared with the central staffing office as the plan for workload fluctuation greater than the defined "range of staffing elasticity" at the budget or "most frequent workload UOS or volume" as well as the unit-based nonproductive replacement time.
5. Positions are based on the budgeted FTEs and defined weekday and weekend schedule requirements.
6. Identifies filled and unfilled or vacant FTEs.
7. Position control reports identify:
   a. Filled and open or vacant positions compared to the hired and actual FTE positions.
   b. Job category or classes for staff (e.g., RN, LPN/LVN, NA, nurse leaders, clerks, and so forth), or skill-mix caregiver groups (e.g., direct and indirect).
   c. Job codes to track budgeted dollars for the FTE positions.
   d. Hire dates for the employees in the filled positions to track seniority.
   e. Designation for FT or PT or per-diem/casual or contingent status as a check for the optimum or budgeted FT/PT rotation plan.
   f. Tracking positions by shift as a check against the budgeted "care distribution hours" in the unit staffing budget.
   g. Tracking positions for weekday and weekend distribution to:
      i. Compare budgeted positions to the schedule at posting to visually see that resources have been distributed to the shifts for which they were budgeted.

ii. Compare the budgeted positions to the schedule after the schedule period is completed, to see if employees worked to their expected shifts, especially if self- (or selfish, depending on the unit-based guidelines and employee requests) scheduling is the designated scheduling method for the unit.

h. Comparison of actual to budget "paid FTEs with variance" will reflect employees working more hours than they were hired for versus employees working less hours than they were hired for. This comparison often explains unnecessary overtime or the loss of planned experience and competencies when employees trade their shifts away.

i. Comparison of actual "worked" FTEs to the "target" or VSP FTEs with variance.

j. Comparison of actual and budget workload for productivity reference (e.g., how busy was the unit for the time period being evaluated).

DNPs/nurse leaders should aggressively investigate these variances as the root sources for unnecessary hours and overtime, and excessive use of nonproductive hours.

Research conducted by the LMI shows that overtime in excess of 5% is associated with adverse patient outcomes (medical errors and patient falls), so position control reports that can determine how efficiently and effectively employee scheduling and staffing is being done should help in promoting safe staffing for our patients (Suby, 2008b).

CONSTRUCTING THE SCHEDULE

The required steps to constructing the schedule use the unit staffing budget as the foundation for defining the patient care needs and target hours of care. The schedule relies on the defined unit-specific schedule requirements by shift for direct and indirect caregivers, recognizing unique skills and experience to translate whole FTEs into worked hours over the 24-hour day.

Schedule development best practices are based on official policies developed from sound principles and are regularly audited for quality by HR, Payroll, Finance, and, most importantly, by DNPs/nurse leaders and the scheduling/staffing committee members.

Sound scheduling principles define the weekend, weekday, and day-off options:

1. The workweek is seven consecutive 24-hour periods.
2. The weekend is two consecutive 24-hour periods.
   a. Saturday/Sunday is the most common weekend definition for permanent day and evening shift employees or day/evening shift rotators.
   b. Friday/Saturday is the most common weekend definition for permanent night shift employees or day/night shift rotators. However, if this definition is used, then Sunday night is a weekday shift and employees who have been off for a weekend must return to work on Sunday night.
   c. Weekend shifts determine the total employees or positions to hire in the position control.
   d. Weekend needs will determine the total FT positions and total FT/PT ratios.
   e. Weekends drive the weekday shift patterns.
   f. Every other weekend to work and be off (2 of 4) means that one half (1/2) or 50% of the unit's staff will be unavailable every weekend.
   g. Every third weekend to work and be off (1 of 3) means that two thirds (2/3) or 66% of the unit's staff will be unavailable every weekend.
   h. More FT employees can be used if weekend needs are less than weekday needs.
3. The weekdays include five consecutive 24-hour periods.
   a. Day/evening shift rotators may have to work an off-shift prior to their weekend off if the off-shift rotation is 30% or higher of total shifts to work.

   b. Weekday shifts determine the total PT and per-diem/casual or contingent positions in the FT/PT ratios.
   c. Consecutive worked shifts should be limited to:
      i. Five shifts or 40 hours for 8-hour employees.
      ii. Three shifts or 36 hours for 12-hour employees.
   d. Single shifts should be avoided as much as possible. Call-ins for unexpected absence are higher with single shifts. Productivity is 25% higher when employees care for the same patient twice because of continuity of care.
4. Day-off options include the following:
   a. Monday and/or Friday are best if the employee is scheduled to work a weekend.
   b. Tuesday and/or Thursday are the second best option if the employee is scheduled to work a weekend.
   c. Wednesdays are the "hump" or pivot day for employees to work if they are going to have a weekend or Monday/Friday or Tuesday/Thursday off and limit consecutively worked shifts to three or four. Therefore, it is best to plan unit-specific education and meetings on these days to reduce the amount of time an employee must come in on scheduled days off.
5. Equal needs for weekends and weekdays will require the highest ratio of PT employees:
   a. All PT and per-diem/casual or contingent employees should be planned to work the same weekend rotation to keep schedules equitable.
   b. All per-diem/casual or contingent employees should be planned to work at least 8 hours and, ideally, 16 hours/2-week pay period, or an FTE equivalent of 0.2 FTE.
   c. Increases of 0.2 FTE should be based on the required additional weekday shifts to cover the planned nonproductive replacement time and/or EMO.
6. Unequal weekend coverage means greater schedule holes on the weekends and unequal shift distribution during the weekdays.

SCHEDULING ORDER

Scheduling FT employees around the committed PT and the per-diem/casual or contingent employees disincentivizes employees from committing to FT. It is important that employees are scheduled with FT employees first, committed PT employees second, and unit-based per-diem/casual employees third.

1. Permanent shifts:
   All permanent shift FT and committed PT employees should have their default weekend rotation assigned to predict their weekends to work and be off.
2. Rotating shifts:
   All rotating shift FT and committed PT employees should have their default weekend rotation assigned that predicts their weekends to work and be off. The working weekends should identify which weekend shifts are on the day shift and which weekends are on the evening or night shift.
3. Per-diem/casual or contingent employees.
   a. Assign all per-diem/casual or contingent employees a default weekend to work to preplan weekend coverage when workload volumes increase on the weekends, as well as to plan replacement coverage for unexpected absences and vacation coverage when employees take time off on the weekends. This allows the per-diem/casual or contingent employee the ability to make advance plans for his or her weekends to work and be off consistent with the departmental or hospital policy expectation that all employees will work a minimum of 26 of 52 weekends in the year.

b. If the per-diem/casual or contingent employees are not needed on their default weekend to work, they should be expected to be assigned to other shifts and/or float to other units to fulfill their work agreements and maintain their competencies.

c. Per-diem/casual or contingent employees may sign up for additional shifts based on the published "needs list" or identified schedule holes.

d. Per-diem/casual or contingent employees should not "shop their shifts" to other staff to take nonproductive hours above the budget daily allowance while working their minimum work agreement so they are no longer available to meet the strategic staff replacement plan for the unit.

It is important to remember the 20–80 Rule when scheduling! When 20% or more of the employees in a unit have fixed patterns, or more than the equivalent of four requests to work or not to work in 2 or more weeks of the 4-week schedule, the patterns or employee requests will so limit the schedule availability for favorable patterns that the other 80% of the employees will work around this 20% of employees with fixed patterns or excessive requests. DNPs/nurse leaders who encounter this pattern of employee requesting to work and be off will provide better schedules to all employees and save themselves and their schedulers and staff hundreds of hours of frustration by developing repeating core patterns or master schedule blocks for all employees in the unit.

ALTERNATIVE SHIFTS

Alternative shifts are any shifts shorter or longer than the standard 8-hour shifts. Implement alternative shifts to achieve the following needs:

1. Increase the number of FT staff when volumes decrease.
2. When required additional work is less than an additional 8-hour shift (e.g., a 12-hour shift).
3. When evening and night shift requirements must be reduced.
4. Increase days off *but* only if the budget will afford it.

The budget will require approximately 10% more FTEs if all shifts are converted from 8-hour to 12-hour, because FTEs are calculated based on 40 hours while employees are hired for 36 hours per week work agreements.

12-Hour Shift Cardinal Absolute Rules

1. Never start 12-hour shifts unless the minimum number of employees is equal to the minimum weekend requirement for all weekends within the 4-week schedule period.
2. A minimum of four employees based on two working on each shift every other weekend is required. If you cannot find this minimum commitment of staff to work these shifts, then do not start 12-hour shifts!
3. If you are scheduling one of three weekend rotations, then the minimum employees needed to start scheduling 12-hour shifts is six, based on two on each shift working every third weekend. If you cannot find this minimum commitment of staff to work these shifts, then do not start 12-hour shifts!

MANAGING EMPLOYEE REQUESTS

Employees need flexible schedules that help them achieve balanced lifestyles, predictability, and career experience. Best budget practices include providing DNPs/nurse leaders with a budget for the employees to use their accrued vacation and holiday or planned time off (Suby, 2009). The most common budget practice used by hospitals is to budget a percent of the total worked hours for benefit time (e.g., 10%) based on the hours used in the previous year or the annual average turnover of the hospital. It is important to calculate this value into actual paid absence hours, as it is often equivalent to employees who have been employed less than 2 years. Although this may work well for a unit with a lot of turnover, it is often insufficient for units with tenured employees using the maximum benefit package or in units where employees have high "carryover" balances.

For the greatest accuracy, LMI recommends that each DNP/nurse leader calculate the hours that should be planned for all employees to use within the budget year.

Employee request guidelines: LMI recommends the following definitions for scheduling and staffing:

Planned absences—Any employee request(s) made in advance of the schedule posting, so the DNP/nurse leader and/or unit scheduler knows about it in advance and appropriate staff coverage has been secured.

Unplanned absence—Any employee request(s) made after the schedule is published or posted that is left unfilled or is filled at overtime or premium pay.

Schedule request—Any request to work or to be off of work for a specific date and shift.

1. Staff should request time off, *not* days and shifts to work.
2. All employees must work to their hired hours FTE commitment. Schedules must be based on the budget.
3. Determine which two nights define the weekend work in order to define the weekend off for night shift and day/night shift rotators. If the weekend off is Friday–Saturday, then Sunday through Thursday are the weekdays.
4. Ensure equitable weekend rotations by defining the employee's weekends to work and be off as a guide for balancing experience and skills. DNPs/nurse leaders should address this by defining the available shift(s) and expected weekend rotations or master/core pattern when hiring new staff or accepting staff transferring into the unit from other units.
5. Distribute 3- and 4-day weekends off equitably. Mondays and Fridays are the most popular weekdays to have off, followed by Tuesdays and Thursdays.
6. Budget for nonproductive replacement based on the budget and absenteeism history of the unit. Overapproving benefit time may feel like the kindly thing to do, but it creates unreasonable workloads for the remaining employees and engenders disrespect for leadership for all employees.

DNPs/nurse leaders must be operationally clear about who will address employee call-ins for unexpected absences, LOA/FMLOA, and vacant positions at the unit level and at the central staffing office, if they exist.

Employees often want 3- and 4-day weekends off, which means taking a Thursday or Friday prior to the weekend off or a Monday or Tuesday following the weekend off. To best accommodate these requests, the DNP/nurse leader must know (as a historical trend) what is the average workload UOS for each day of the week. Once this is known, the DNP/nurse leader can advise the employees that more requests can be accommodated if the least busy days of the week are selected with the weekend to be off.

Most 4-week schedule patterns can accommodate most FT and committed PT employees to have at least one 3-day weekend every schedule. Most 4-week schedule patterns will not accommodate most FT and committed PT employees having at least one 4-day weekend every schedule. If all FT and committed PT employees cannot have a 4-day weekend every schedule as part of their repeating patterns or master schedules, then DNPs/nurse leaders need to decide what will be the basis by which the 4-day weekends will be awarded. Considerations could include perfect attendance, amount of mentoring/coaching provided, most volunteered committee or project work, and so on.

DNPs/nurse leaders should enter the following information into the schedules for future schedule preparation as soon as it is available:

1. Anticipated dates for LOA/FMLOAs to start. This includes the estimated due dates for maternity LOAs to start.
2. Known educational sabbaticals, reassignment to administrative cost centers for EMR, other informatics software training, and so on.
3. Estimated LOA/FMLOA return dates as soon as they know of a pending absence.
4. Planned resignations/termination dates to identify vacant positions as soon as the resignation or unit transfer is turned in.

CALCULATING THE BUDGET BENEFIT HOURS/DAY PLAN

DNPs/nurse leaders must know the budget hours per year and per day for their benefit time to give staff the option to request time off with planned notification and to decrease the unplanned time off. Too often, the DNP/nurse leader inherits a schedule process that assumes how many staff can be absent per day and it is unclear if the total benefit hours/day can accommodate both the planned and unplanned or call-in absences.

When the actual planned and unplanned absences exceed the budget benefit time, the DNP/nurse leader will find he or she is replacing the hours above the nonproductive replacement budget with extra hours and overtime from unit-based staff, hours from hospital staff floated into the unit from other units or the resource pool, or outside agency or traveler hours.

When the DNP/nurse leader has no plan or an undefined plan for the replacement of planned and unplanned absences, the staff will create their own plan with ever increasing "call-ins" for unplanned absences. The employee's planned time off becomes the DNP/nurse leader's unplanned time off to replace.

The greater number of unplanned absences to planned absences occurring in each schedule is the staff's way of telling the DNP/nurse leader that they do not understand or accept the existing unit-specific employee request guidelines.

To create a budget for your nonproductive replacement hours (Suby, 2009), consider the following steps:

1. Convert the budget nonproductive replacement benefit FTEs into hours by multiplying by the definition of 1 FTE (2,080 hours) and dividing by 365 days in an annualized year.
2. Divide the nonproductive replacement benefit hours/day by 8 hours to determine the number of 8-hour shifts available to assign to employees.
3. Alternatively, if the unit is using 12-hour shifts, divide the nonproductive benefit hours/day by 12 hours to determine the number of 12-hour shifts to assign to employees. For example:

Nonproductive replacement benefit FTEs = 4.46 FTEs

$$\times 2,080 \text{ hours/FTE}$$
$$= 9,280 \text{ hours/year}$$
$$\div 365 \text{ days}$$
$$= 25.42 \text{ hours/day}$$
$$\div 8 \text{ hours/shift}$$
$$= 3.18 \text{ shifts/day}$$

CONSEQUENCES OF NOT BUDGETING THE NONPRODUCTIVE REPLACEMENT BENEFIT TIME

Additional dollars should not be needed to respond to deficit demands from your nonproductive replacement benefit time because the budget includes dollars in the form of FTE allocations for these needs. The consequence of not budgeting the nonproductive replacement benefit time includes the following:

1. Replacement is usually done with overtime and agency, which is more expensive than the "regular rate of pay."
2. Employees may have unused "carryover" time to take back or "cash out," which pays them but does not give them a restful break so they can avoid job burnout and low morale. It also creates an increasing financial liability for the organization.
3. Carryover time is usually not budgeted for use in the following year if the employee chooses to take it as time off. However, the DNP/nurse leader has a responsibility to provide the accrued time off if it meets all other employee request criteria. Remember that replacing absence time due to carryover hours will drive the nonproductive hours above budget.
4. Carryover benefit time is more expensive to use in years other than when it is accrued as the cost of living continues to increase. Paying out the carryover hours will cause the total dollars paid to be over budget while the nonproductive benefit hours may be at budget.

IMPACT OF PLANNED AND UNPLANNED ABSENCES AND EMPLOYEE REQUESTS TO THE NONPRODUCTIVE BUDGET

Once DNPs/nurse leaders know the number of hours and shifts/day budgeted for use, they should consider the average number of unexpected absences or call-ins and FMLOA/LOAs occurring per day. For example, if the unit averages one call-in or FMLOA/LOA per day, it should be subtracted from the budgeted shifts or hours. The remaining balance is what the DNP/nurse leader can afford to approve for planned vacation and holiday absences per day at the regular rate of pay.

$$\frac{3.18 \text{ nonproductive replacement benefit shifts budgeted/day}}{-1 \text{ shift/day call-in or FMLOA/LOA}}$$
$$= 2.18 \text{ shifts/day for planned absence (e.g., vacation)}$$

PLANNING VACATION TIME USAGE

LMI recommended the best practice for managing planned absences for vacation time is to create a "vacation sign-up form" based on the pay period dates for the schedule year, allowing space for staff to sign up for their desired time off as far into the future as they desire (Suby, 2009).

The number of staff allowed to request time off each week should be equal to the number of allowed shifts based on the nonproductive replacement budget calculations. The time should be approved based on defined guidelines.

The DNP/nurse leader should develop a set of guidelines to govern vacation requests, changes, and cancellations and publish them on the unit. Most often, it is based on "first come-first approved" and/or seniority followed by any other (e.g., union) considerations.

1. Create a vacation plan by identifying the target number of staff that can be gone on vacation each week and pay period for the entire year so that all employees have an equal opportunity to use their accrued time.
2. List the number of people that can sign up for each week based on the budget nonproductive replacement benefit hours or shifts/day that can be approved.
3. Request all employees to sign up in 1-week increments no less than 8 to 12 weeks in advance, and work to have employees commit to 6 months to 1 year in advance.
4. Identify a list of employees who would be willing to take vacation time if someone has to cancel by allowing space for one or two additional people to request time off. Do not approve these additional requests unless someone with approved time off wants to trade with them or

something has changed in the unit whereby you need to reduce staff right away. For example, the majority of the orthopedic surgeons go to a ski resort for a conference so patient admissions will be low during their absence.

These additional unplanned absences occurring per day in excess of the budget will most often be paid from extra hours and overtime or premium pay from agency staff or travelers unless the PT and/or the per-diem/casual or contingent employees are used to cover these absences at the regular rate of pay.

A significant complaint from staff when they are dissatisfied with their schedules is the "fairness" of the schedule. Employees watch for equitability in weekends to work and be off, distributions of 3- and 4-day weekends off, numbers of off-shifts they must work prior to a weekend off, numbers of shifts they must rotate to from day to night shifts or day to evening shifts, and consecutive work stretches.

To effectively manage employee requests and develop employee request guidelines, LMI recommends that DNPs/nurse leaders evaluate their existing guidelines against the following:

1. Do the "employee request guidelines" reflect clear policies to help employees request time off and *not* days and shifts to work?
2. Is there a clear definition for which two nights determine the weekend for night and day–night shift rotators?
3. Are all employees scheduled to work to their hired work agreement or committed hours every schedule? Trading away scheduled hours to work below the hired work agreement allows most employees to continue to earn accrued hours based on their hired work agreement. This practice prohibits the DNP/nurse leader from hiring another position as long as the employee is holding that position in position control.
4. Replacing all nonworked time with accrued benefit time so the employee's FTE honors its hired work agreement of hours each work week pay period.
5. Fair and equitable distribution of shift rotations and weekends to work and be off.
6. Fair and equitable work assignments built for employee experience and skills. Assignments should avoid geographic assignment because it is easier or self-serving.
7. The number and type of employee requests is impacted by the culture and morale of the unit.

LMI-RECOMMENDED DNP/NURSE LEADER LINE AND STAFF FUNCTIONS IN SCHEDULING AND STAFFING

It is essential for DNPs/nurse leaders to be responsible for the following line functions:

1. Establishment and control of the unit staffing budget.
2. Development of a master staffing plan based on the patient needs and the method of work assignments.
3. Development of procedures to adjust the staff on a daily and, if needed, shift-to-shift basis.
   a. Units with workload changes greater than the target RN-to-patient ratios are considered to have "erratic" workloads and will need daily staffing adjustments every 2 to 4 hours.
   b. Units with workload changes less than the target RN-to-patient ratios are considered to have "fluctuating" workloads and will need daily staffing adjustments every 6 to 8 hours.
4. Establishment of the defined schedule requirements for each staff position by shift (e.g., all RNs, charge RNs, and so on).
5. Staff development with ongoing evaluations to meet the defined schedule requirements for their positions.
6. Hiring, promotion, discipline, and discharge of employees.

LMI SCHEDULING BEST PRACTICES AND MEASURING FOR QUALITY

LMI scheduling best practices reflect the following:

- Weekend rotations are defined and preassigned; the master/block/core schedules are maintained.
- Core schedule patterns are consistently achieved 85% of the time by *regular CORE-unit* employees.
- Unfilled schedule holes are less than 5% of total worked hours.
- Supplemental staffing from all sources (resource pool, staff floated from other units, agency or travelers) is less than 15% of total worked hours.
- Limited single shifts, shift switches, and/or double-back shifts.
- Single shifts are defined as nonconsecutively worked shifts (e.g., work a day, off a day).
- Shift switches are defined as different shifts scheduled together. For example, a day shift followed by an evening shift followed by a day off.
- Double-back shifts are defined as different shifts scheduled together that result in less than 8 hours off between shifts or 15 or more hours being worked in a 24-hour period (e.g., a day shift followed by a night shift or an evening shift followed by a day shift resulting in 16 hours of work in a 24-hour period).
- Unexpected absences or call-ins less than 5% of total worked hours.
- Work stretches limited to less than 40 hours/work stretch (e.g., 3, 4, 5 consecutive shifts). No consecutive work stretches greater than 5 days for 8-hour employees or 3 days for 12-hour employees.
- Defined employee request guidelines consistent to HR, payroll/time and attendance (T&A) policies.
- Policies and practices are consistent among units.
- Practices match policies unless exceptions are valid.
- Position complement is developed and known for each unit, resulting in achievement of the defined schedule requirements when positions in the position control are filled.
- Shift lengths and shift rotation combinations are appropriate to staff and patient needs.
- Schedules reflect organizational philosophy and standards regarding continuity in patient care and staff retention.

DAILY STAFFING: THE SHORT-TERM 24-HOUR BUDGET

The VSP is also called the staffing grid, matrix, or the daily staffing plan. It is the short-term budget designed to flex the caregivers to the volume of patients or UOS for the concurrent shift (next 2 to 8 hours and 12 to 24 hours), and proactively at 48 and 72 hours, 5 and 7 days.

The VSP is planned for fluctuating and erratic changes in census or other workload UOS or volumes while maintaining the consistency of the target HPPD or H/UOS and the RN percent, which is the underlying driver for the RN-to-patient care ratios. It is designed to reflect the flexing of only those direct caregivers that correlate to a ratio of patients or workload UOS or volumes (e.g., RN, LPN/LVN, NA, and so forth).

The Institute of Medicine (IOM, 2004) gave criteria for adequate staffing in its 2004 report on *Keeping Patients Safe: Transforming the Work Environment of Nurses*, which included the following:

1. Adequate staffing is established by sound methodologies as determined by nursing staff.
2. Mechanisms are in place to accommodate unplanned variations in patient care workload.
3. Enables nursing staff to regulate nursing unit workflow.
4. Is consistent with best available evidence on safe staffing thresholds.

VSPs may be created to guide decisions to flex staff by shift and day of week, by skill mix and experience (e.g., charge), and usually identifies the budget workload and response uniquely from the target staffing response at each workload UOS or volumes between the lowest allowed workload and the unit capacity.

Good VSPs keep the target RN, direct, indirect, and total worked HPPD or H/UOS and the direct care RN percent constant for each number of patients the unit can accommodate. This ensures that patients receive the same target HPPD or H/UOS and direct RN-to-patient ratio regardless of how many patients are on the unit. Most often, direct caregivers have been planned by skill mix in fractions to allow room for the DNP/nurse leader or charge or resource nurse to apply clinical judgment and decide if the acuity of the patient warrants more RNs, for a lower RN-to-patient ratio and/or fewer LPN/LVNs or NAs.

RN-to-patient ratios greater than 1 to 6, even if augmented by LPN/LVNs, will stress experienced nurses, and the higher ratios are allowed to rise to become factors for staff dissatisfaction and turnover as well as contributing factors in adverse patient outcomes.

Refer to Table 4.14; this is designed to deliver 8.27 direct HPPD and a target RN percent of 29.7% at each census level. This unit has all 12-hour shifts. The VSP is designed for 1.84 RNs/shift, 2.95 LPN/LVNs/shift, and 1.41 NAs/shift.

The DNP/nurse leader and charge or resource nurse are empowered to consider patient acuity and professional judgment to decide if they want to go with two RNs (for an RN-to-patient ratio of 1 to 9), three LPN/LVNs (for an LPN/LVN-to-patient ratio of 1 to 6), a licensed (RN and LPN/LVN) ratio of 1 to 3.6 patients, and one NA each shift (for an NA-to-patient ratio of 1 to 18). Alternatively, they could choose to go with two RNs (for an RN-to-patient ratio of 1 to 9), two LPN/LVNs (for an LPN/LVN-to-patient ratio of 1 to 9), a licensed (RN and LPN/LVN) ratio of 1 to 4.5 patients, and two NAs each shift (for an NA-to-patient ratio of 1 to 9). However, if the RN skill mix is increased, be sure that the annual unit budget is revised or the dollars/UOS will be above budget while the H/UOS will be on target.

LMI-RECOMMENDED DAILY STAFFING BEST PRACTICES AND MEASURING FOR QUALITY

It is best practice for the DNP/nurse leader, charge, or resource nurses to know the VSP and how to flex to meet the target hours of care and RN-, LPN/LVN-, and licensed direct caregiver-to-patient ratios.

Daily staffing shift management reports identify the scheduled direct and indirect caregivers and the patients assigned to each caregiver. LMI-recommended best practices for daily staffing by the designated charge or resource nurse include the following:

1. The designated charge or resource nurse for each shift should review the current staffing coverage with the shift charge or resource nurse who is leaving the shift.
2. The designated charge or resource nurse should forecast ahead in 2- to 4-hour increments if the census or UOS is erratic and changing by more than the target direct RN-to-patient ratio within the shift. Alternatively, if the UOS is fluctuating within the target direct RN-to-patient ratio within the shift, the daily staffing decisions can be made in 6- to 8-hour increments for the next shift.
3. The designated charge or resource nurse should forecast proactively to the next 12-, 24-, and 48-hour periods to anticipate the workload volumes and current staff to see if shift exchanges or extra hours need to be made to anticipate the workload and staffing response. As the designated charge or resource nurse forecasts proactively, they need to communicate with the central staffing office to give as much notice as possible to look for additional staff or to make adjustments to downsize staff if volumes decrease.

Refer to the following sample Daily Staffing Shift Management Report as an example of the shift-to-shift proactive staffing plans for the rolling 24 hours (see Figure 4.3).

TABLE 4.14 Example: Variable Staffing Plan Based on Current Practice

		Target	Total 12			LPN	NA	Day Shift			Night Shift		
Census Volume ×	Budget Direct HPPD =	Direct Hours/ Day ÷	Hour Shifts/24 Hours ×	Target RN % =	RN Shifts/24 Hours	Shifts/ 24 Hours (47.5%)	Shifts/24 Hours (22.8%)	RN	LPN	NA	RN	LPN	NA
21	8.27	173.67	14.47	29.7%	4.30	6.87	3.30	2.15	3.44	1.65	2.15	3.44	1.65
20	8.27	165.4	13.78	29.7%	4.09	6.55	3.14	2.05	3.27	1.57	2.05	3.27	1.57
19	8.27	157.13	13.09	29.7%	3.89	6.22	2.99	1.94	3.11	1.49	1.94	3.11	1.49
18	8.27	148.86	12.41	29.7%	3.68	5.89	2.83	1.84	2.95	1.41	1.84	2.95	1.41
17	8.27	140.59	11.72	29.7%	3.48	5.57	2.67	1.74	2.78	1.34	1.74	2.78	1.34
16	8.27	132.32	11.03	29.7%	3.27	5.24	2.51	1.64	2.62	1.26	1.64	2.62	1.26
15	8.27	124.05	10.34	29.7%	3.07	4.91	2.36	1.54	2.46	1.18	1.54	2.46	1.18
14	8.27	115.78	9.65	29.7%	2.87	4.58	2.20	1.43	2.29	1.10	1.43	2.29	1.10
13	8.27	107.51	8.96	29.7%	2.66	4.26	2.04	1.33	2.13	1.02	1.33	2.13	1.02
12	8.27	99.24	8.27	29.7%	2.46	3.93	1.89	1.23	1.96	0.94	1.23	1.96	0.94
11	8.27	90.97	7.58	29.7%	2.25	3.60	1.73	1.13	1.80	0.86	1.13	1.80	0.86
10	8.27	82.7	6.89	29.7%	2.05	3.27	1.57	1.02	1.64	0.79	1.02	1.64	0.79
9	8.27	74.43	6.20	29.7%	1.84	2.95	1.41	0.92	1.47	0.71	0.92	1.47	0.71
8	8.27	66.16	5.51	29.7%	1.64	2.62	1.26	0.82	1.31	0.63	0.82	1.31	0.63
7	8.27	57.89	4.82	29.7%	1.43	2.29	1.10	0.72	1.15	0.55	0.72	1.15	0.55
6	8.27	49.62	4.14	29.7%	1.23	1.96	0.94	0.61	0.98	0.47	0.61	0.98	0.47
5	8.27	41.35	3.45	29.7%	1.02	1.64	0.79	0.51	0.82	0.39	0.51	0.82	0.39
4	8.27	33.08	2.76	29.7%	0.82	1.31	0.63	0.41	0.65	0.31	0.41	0.65	0.31
3	8.27	24.81	2.07	29.7%	0.61	0.98	0.47	0.31	0.49	0.24	0.31	0.49	0.24
2	8.27	16.54	1.38	29.7%	0.41	0.65	0.31	0.20	0.33	0.16	0.20	0.33	0.16
1	8.27	8.27	0.69	29.7%	0.20	0.33	0.16	0.10	0.16	0.08	0.10	0.16	0.08

The top of the table reads: "Direct Care Variable Staffing Plan for 3M-Med/Surg at Somewhere Medical Center Based on Authorized Budget 8.27 Direct Care and 9.03 Total Worked HPPD"

Notes: **Budget workload is 17.42 ADC; budget direct care HPPD is 8.27, and total worked HPPD is 9.03.**

Charge nurses included in the direct care RNs taking a patient assignment.

Target RN-to-patient ratio is 1 RN to 9.45 patients (17.42/1.84).

Target licensed caregiver (RN/LPN)-to-patient ratio is 1 RN/LPN to 3.64 patients (17.42/4.79 licensed caregivers) 1.84 RN + 2.95.

Target LPN-to-patient ratio is 1 LPN to 5.95 patients.

Target NA ratio is 1 NA to 12.35 patients.

ADC, average daily census; HPPD, hours per patient day; LPN, licensed practical nurse; NA, nursing assistant.

Source: Suby (2015). Reproduced with permission from the Labor Management Institute (LMI).

LMI-recommended daily staffing best practices include the following:

1. A 24-hour staffing plan exists for each unit, which includes contingency plans to staff at the target HPPD or H/UOS.
2. There is evidence for collaboration among the units with a merge of numbers for clinical clusters.
3. There is concurrent planning for the next 2 to 8, 12 to 24 hours.
4. There is proactive planning for the next 3 to 7 days.

SAMPLE					
MEDICAL CENTER					
Shift Management Report					
Unit:					
Day:		Day:		Day:	
7 a.m.–3 p.m. Shift		**3 p.m.–11 p.m. Shift**		**11 p.m.–7 a.m. Shift**	
Charge nurse:		Charge nurse:		Charge nurse:	
Ward secretary:		Ward secretary:		Ward secretary:	
Pod A		Pod A		Pod A	
Pod B		Pod B		Pod B	
Pod C		Pod C		Pod C	
Beginning census	**Hours used**	Beginning census	**Hours used**	Beginning census	**Hours used**
Ending census ____	CN ____	Ending census ____	CN ____	Ending census ____	CN ____
Admits/transfer in ____	ADT ____	Admits/transfer in ____	ADT ____	Admits/transfer in ____	ADT ____
Transfers out ____	RN ____	Transfers out ____	RN ____	Transfers out ____	RN ____
Discharges/ deaths ____	LPN ____	Discharges/ deaths ____	LPN ____	Discharges/ deaths ____	LPN ____
Anticipated 11 a.m.–3 p.m. census ____	NA ____	Anticipated 3–7 p.m. census ____	NA ____	Anticipated 11 p.m.–7 a.m. census ____	NA ____
Anticipated 11 a.m.–3 p.m. direct staff ____	UC ____	Anticipated 7–3 p.m. direct staff ____	UC ____	Anticipated 11 p.m.–7 a.m. direct staff ____	UC ____
Anticipated 3–7 p.m. census ____	WS ____	Anticipated 7–11 p.m. census ____	WS ____	Anticipated 7–11 a.m. census ____	WS ____
Anticipated 3–7 p.m. direct staff ____	Total ____	Anticipated 7–11 p.m. direct staff ____	Total ____	Anticipated 7–11 a.m. direct staff ____	Total ____
Target direct HPPD:		Target direct HPPD:		Target direct HPPD:	
Direct staff × 8 hours ÷ census= ____	HPPD	Direct staff × 8 hours ÷ census= ____	HPPD	Direct staff × 8 hours ÷ census= ____	HPPD
RN: patient ratio: ____		RN: patient ratio: ____		RN: patient ratio: ____	
License staff: patient ratio: ____		License staff: patient ratio: ____		License staff: patient ratio: ____	

FIGURE 4.3 Example: Daily shift management report.

ADT, admission, discharge, and transfer; CN, charge nurse; HPPD, hours per patient day; LPN, licensed practical nurse; NA, nursing assistant; UC, unit clerk or secretary; WS, ward secretary.

Source: Suby (2015). Reproduced with permission from the Labor Management Institute (LMI).

5. Criteria have been defined to evaluate staffing responses:
   a. The source of the adjusted staffing (e.g., extra hours or overtime from core staff, per-diem/ casual or contingent employees, staff from the resource pool or other units, and agency or travelers)
   b. Supplemental hours floated into or out of the unit by shift and day
   c. Direct RN-to-patient ratios
   d. Unmet needs or schedule "holes"
6. The process used regarding staffing decisions after the DNP/nurse leader is gone for the day.
7. Identified resources or possible sources to help meet last-minute changes.
8. Evidence of clinical cluster considerations in allocation and organization of central resources. For example, did the central staffing office have staff to send from the medical–surgical float pool, the critical care float pool, or did the service line find resources within the cluster units?

Issues and Concerns									
7 a.m.–3 p.m. Shift				3 p.m.–11 p.m. Shift				11 p.m.–7 a.m. Shift	
JC Requirements	Time		Name	JC Requirements	Time		Name	JC Requirements	Time		Name
Narcotic/misc.				Narcotic/misc.				Narcotic/misc.			
Crash cart check				Crash cart check				Crash cart check			
Refrigerator check				Refrigerator check				Refrigerator check			
Restraint log				Restraint log				Restraint log			

Quality Issues						
	Patient/physician/ family complaints		Patient/physician/ family complaints		Patient/physician/ family complaints
	Medication errors		Medication errors		Medication errors
	Order entry		Order entry		Order entry
	Missed orders		Missed orders		Missed orders
	Security ancillary departments		Security ancillary departments		Security ancillary departments

COMMENTS	COMMENTS	COMMENTS

EXAMPLES OF EXCELLENCE	EXAMPLES OF EXCELLENCE	EXAMPLES OF EXCELLENCE

FIGURE 4.3 *(continued)*

JC, Joint Commission.

IDENTIFYING ROOT SOURCES OF OVERTIME

The Fair Labor Standards Act (FLSA) was passed in 1937 to govern record keeping, minimum wage payment, overtime payment, and child labor standards. Employees are generally aware of its protection. DNPs/nurse leaders as well as anyone else designated to create and publish schedules and make daily staffing decisions must understand overtime rules and comply with them. Enforcement mechanisms are well established through the U.S. Department of Labor and federal courts. Refer to www.dol.gov.

FLSA does not require:

- Vacation, holiday, sick, or severance pay
- Meal or rest periods
- Premium pay for weekend or holiday hours worked
- Pay raises
- Health and welfare or retirement benefits
- Immediate payment of final wages to a terminated employee

All of these factors are governed by state, health care systems, or unions, and not FLSA. Each hospital will define its policies governing these factors and it is important that DNPs/nurse leaders read and understand the policies.

Overtime is paid to nonexempt or hourly employees in all job categories for all hours worked in excess of 40 hours/week unless there is an alternate rule that pays overtime for lower worked hours per week. For example, some unions have negotiated contracts whereby overtime is paid after 30 hours/week, 35 hours/week, or 37.5 hours/week. There are two types of overtime:

Regular overtime is any overtime occurrence 30 minutes or greater per event.

End of shift (EOS) overtime is any overtime occurrence less than 30 minutes per event.

DNPs/nurse leaders should never rely on "hearsay" information passed on from one well-intentioned person to another. DNPs/nurse leaders should always work with HR to know the answers to the questions affecting their approval of payroll hours and dollars. If there are questions, the DNPs/nurse leaders should always contact the payroll supervisor and HR for the correct information.

All unit leadership must care about the overtime occurring on their units because it directly impacts the unit by increasing the cost center's operational costs while reducing the available funds for hiring more staff, obtaining more equipment, or acquiring new or expanded programs.

Indirectly, overtime increases employee job dissatisfaction, burnout, and turnover. It increases employee fatigue, contributing to "failure to rescue," on-the-job employee injuries, and unplanned absences. Overtime also increases the risk of adverse patient outcomes (medical errors and patient falls; Suby, 2007a).

The most frequently identified sources for regular overtime (overtime occurrences greater than 30 minutes/event) range from 0.1% to 10% of total worked hours based on unclear budget, definitions and undefined schedule requirements, position control that is disconnected from the budget, the scheduling method used (e.g., self vs. selfish), the workload and ALOS, availability of supplemental staffing resources to cover deficit demands to the unit's core staff, planned versus unplanned deficit demands, and demand for sitter hours.

Through the application of good budgeting and best practices, the DNP/nurse leader can reduce overtime to a range of 0.5% to 5% for these same root sources. A financial "rule of thumb" in organizational overtime savings says that a 1% decrease in organization-wide overtime is equal to saving $1,000,000.00 (see Table 4.15).

Health care organizations of all types struggle to manage their overtime and identify its root sources or "drivers" (Suby, 2007a). It is important for all DNPs/nurse leaders to have a plan that uniquely identifies the budgeted overtime from the plan.

LMI has developed recommended overtime usage guidelines based on our research for root sources or drivers for overtime and the increase in med errors and patient falls. LMI finds that overtime below 4.9% is reasonable for units with fluctuating workload volumes and normal deficit demand replacement.

LMI finds that overtime between 5% and 7.9% is symptomatic of "financial bleeding." It is most often the result of schedule imbalances, overauthorizing employee requests causing staffing shortages, and excessive tardy/late occurrences.

LMI finds that overtime that is 8% or higher is symptomatic of "financial hemorrhaging" and requires immediate investigation and intervention. It is most often due to excessive vacancies, excessive LOA/FMLOA absences, excessively high ADT Work Intensity causing drastic workload fluctuations, and mismatched 8- and 12-hour shift combinations, in addition to overauthorizing employee requests for time off and excessive tardy/late occurrences.

LMI finds that medical errors and patient falls increase when overtime is above 5% of total worked hours, and the most dangerous overtime is 8% or higher (see Table 4.16).

TABLE 4.15 Labor Management Institute's Source of Regular Overtime and Estimated Savings

Sources of Regular Overtime (Occurrences 30 + Minutes/Event)	OT Savings if Changed (Estimated)	
	% Range	% Avg.
Unclear budget, definitions, and schedule requirements Position control disconnected from the budget Scheduling methods (self vs. selfish)	1.0–3.0	1.5
ADT Work Intensity and average length of stay (ALOS)	0.1–1.0	0.5
Inadequate supplemental staffing resources (unit floating, float pool, unit-based per-diem/PRN/casual/contingent staff, agency, travelers)	0.1–2.0	1.0
Planned deficit demands (vacation/PTO)	0.1–1.0	0.5
Sitter and/or 1 to 1 observation hours Unplanned deficit demands (call-ins, emergency absences, funeral, LOA, FMLOA/intermittent FMLOA)	1.0–3.0	1.5
Total	2.3–10.0%	5.0%

ADT, admission, discharge, and transfer; FMLOA, family medical leave of absence; LOA, leave of absence; OT, overtime; PTO, paid time off.

Source: Suby (2015). Reproduced with permission from the Labor Management Institute (LMI).

TABLE 4.16 Labor Management Institute's Overtime Usage Guidelines

OT%	LMI Overtime Finding/Implication
0% to 4.9%	Reasonable response to fluctuating workload volumes or deficit demands.
5% to 7.9%	*Sign of financial bleeding:* Consider schedule imbalances (e.g., too many on the day shift and inadequate coverage on the off shifts) or overauthorizing employee requests causing staffing shortages.
8% or above	*Sign of financial hemorrhaging:* Consider excessive vacancies, excessive ADT activity within the unit that creates excessive workload intensity and drastic workload fluctuations, and mismatched 8- and 12-hour shift combinations in addition to the previous suggestions.

ADT, admission, discharge, and transfer; OT, overtime.

Source: Suby (2015). Reproduced with permission from the Labor Management Institute (LMI).

Goal comparisons were based on overtime greater than 5% compared to vacation greater than 10%, call-in/unexpected absence greater than 5%, and LOA/vacancy hours greater than 10%. Units that experience an increase from these sources in both levels and occurrences typically show a dramatic increase in overtime.

Overtime root sources—As you consider your overtime levels, it is important to consider the sources for it. Sources of overtime include the following:

- EOS (overtime less than 30 minutes per occurrence) versus regular overtime (occurrences greater than 30 minutes)
- Unexpected absences/call-ins (sick calls) greater than 5% of total worked hours
- Vacancies, LOA/FMLOA absences greater than 10% of total worked hours
- Excessive observation/sitter hours greater than 3% of total worked hours
- Scheduling/staffing practices

TABLE 4.17 Labor Management Institute's Comparison of Overtime to Possible Overtime Drivers

Unit	Total Worked Hours	Total OT Hours	% of Total	Total Vacation	% of Total	Call-in Unex. Absence (Sick)	% of Total	Total 1:1 Obs-Sitter	% of Total	Total LOA or Vacancy Hours	% of Total
Medicine/MED	3,631.0	735.5	20.3	391.5	10.8	202.0	5.6	810.0	22.3	0.0	0.0
Neurosurgery/SURG	2,767.7	418.5	15.1	329.0	11.9	153.0	5.5	330.0	11.9	222.0	8.0
Chest step down/SD	3,127.8	273.0	8.7	285.2	9.1	148.0	4.7	0.0	0.0	543.0	17.3
Surg Oncology/ONCOL	2,738.2	291.5	10.6	556.5	20.3	130.0	4.7	201.0	7.3	455.5	16.6
CT step-down unit/SD	2,841.0	366.0	12.9	468.0	16.5	356.0	12.5	115.5	—	120.0	4.2
Med-telemetry/TELE	3,605.5	693.2	19.2	371.5	10.3	164.0	4.5	358.5	9.9	480.0	13.3
Cardiac ICU-Med/CCU	3,128.5	180.5	5.8	370.0	11.8	202.0	6.5	22.5	0.7	365.5	11.6
Total	**21,839.7**	**2,958.2**	**13.5**	**2,771.7**	**12.7**	**1,355.0**	**6.2**	**1,837.5**	**8.4**	**2,186.0**	**10.0**
LMI-recommended thresholds			**Less than 5%**		**Less than 10%**		**Less than 5%**		**Less than 3%**		**Less than 10%**

LOA, leave of absence; OT, overtime.

Source: Suby (2015). Reproduced with permission from the Labor Management Institute (LMI).

TABLE 4.18 Labor Management Institute's Essential Financial Management Information Key Performance Indicators (KPIs)

| | KEY PERFORMANCE INDICATORS | | | |
Hours	Direct	Indirect	Total Worked (or Productive)	Total Paid (or Annual)
FTEs	Direct	Indirect	Total worked	Total paid
$/UOS	Direct	Indirect	Total worked	Total paid
Workload volumes	Inpatient and adjustments for observation, holding hours, ADT, or other workload			
Other	RN H/UOS RN, LPN/LVN, licensed and nursing assistant skill-mix ratios Overtime (%) Turnover/vacancy rates with unit erosion			

ADT, admission, discharge, and transfer; FTEs, full-time equivalents; LPN, licensed practical nurse; LVN, licensed vocational nurse; UOS, units of service.

Source: Suby (2015). Reproduced with permission from the Labor Management Institute (LMI).

DOCUMENTING OVERTIME DRIVERS OR ROOT SOURCES

To find the overtime drivers, the DNP/nurse leader must be able to clearly document and trend the unit's overtime usage. In the following example, overtime usage at a teaching hospital was compared to vacation, call-in, or unexpected absence (sick), 1:1 observation/sitter, LOA/FMLOA, and vacancy hours (Table 4.17).

MANAGEMENT REPORTS: THE REFLECTION OF THE DNP/NURSE LEADER OPERATIONAL DECISION MAKING

You can't manage what you can't measure. You can't change what you can't document.
—Author Unknown

Measuring the right data and having real-time access to that information is essential to controlling labor costs. Management reports are the reflection of the DNP/nurse leader's operational decision making. Management reports provide the information loop between the budget, the schedule, and our daily staffing decisions.

Reviewing labor and productivity targets on a daily basis is the most optimal method to allow for daily trending of volume and labor hours. Daily monitoring encourages the unit to respond to changes in the volume/work units on a real-time basis to ensure appropriate use of staff 24 hours/day. DNPs/nurse leaders should remember that "What gets measured gets done," (author unknown).

Management information from different sources should be interactive. Together it should answer the question and tell the story. The KPIs are the foundation for our financial management (see Table 4.18).

The DNP/nurse leader is the most knowledgeable source of information about the business of the unit. Biweekly reporting helps to ensure that interventions are on target. If we do not like the numbers, we must change something operationally. Our choices must consider:

- What is the reason the numbers are doing what they are doing?
- Are we satisfied with the reason?

- Does the reason represent best practice?
- Are we satisfied that this reason cannot be improved?

Potential causes for increased labor standards above target:

1. Additional FTEs above budget from overstaffing or overhiring
2. New programs that require additional worked hours
3. High overtime
4. Contract labor that cannot be cancelled or floated out of the unit
5. Changes in patient acuity or ALOS. Often this is due to not having the patient in the appropriate unit type (e.g., a step-down patient in med–surg)
6. Working inefficiently

Potential causes for decreasing labor standards below target:

1. Reduction in FTEs below budget from understaffing or high vacancies
2. Elimination of programs requiring a reduction in worked hours
3. Unfilled vacant positions
4. Elimination of extra hours, overtime, or contract labor
5. Changes in patient acuity or LOS
6. Working efficiently

In Gapenski, Vogel, and Langland-Orban's study, "The Determinants of Hospital Profitability" (1993), it was found that "a decrease in labor intensity by 1/100th FTE per adjusted inpatient day would increase the after-tax operating margin by approximately 3.5%." This suggests that relatively large gains in profit margins are available from even very small increases in workforce efficiencies (p. 72).

It should be noted that not-for-profit and public hospitals' median operating margins declined slightly in fiscal year (FY) 2016 from 3.4 % in FY 2015 to 2.7% in FY 2016. Moody's Investors Service Report found that hospitals' annual operating expenses outpaced operating revenues with expenses growing by 7.5% in 2016 compared to a 6.6% increase in hospitals' annual operating revenues. The increase in the hospitals' expenses were largely driven by growth in spending on prescription drugs and labor expenses (Wexler & Smith, 2017).

PEER REVIEW MANAGEMENT MEETINGS

Peer reporting is a process in which DNPs/nursing leaders meet with their service line directors to report to each other on their unit(s)' labor resource outcomes for the most recent 2-week pay period. Peer reporting is information sharing, collaborative, and focused on problem solving.

- It requires 1 hour every other week.
- No "secret culture."
- Open book/open door.
- Quality outcomes are reviewed.
- Financial outcomes are shared ("Am I on target, over budget, under budget? Do I know the reasons why my numbers look the way they do? Am I satisfied with the reasons? Do the reasons represent best practice? Am I satisfied that this reason(s) cannot be improved?").

Peer review ground rules:

- All DNPs/nurse leaders come prepared.
- Limit reporting to 1 to 3 minutes/cost center.
- Report successes.

LABOR MANAGEMENT INSTITUTE PEER REVIEW MANAGEMENT REPORT-NURSING UNITS

Unit leader name: _____ Unit name: _____; Time period: _____ to _____

Units of Service and Workload:

1. Unit capacity: _____ Budgeted: _____ Average: _____

2. Range: High: _____ Low: _____   3. *Explanations*:

Impact of Workload Using ADT:

4. Total ADT averaged ____/PP

5. Ranging from a high of: ____ to a low of: ____

6. Unit-based ADT average % [*Average ADT for the 2 weeks divided by the average MN census × 100 = ADT%*]

7. Compared to the LMI national threshold of ____%, we were ____ [e.g., *busy, reasonable, light*]

8. "Other workload" impacting our unit that contributes to higher direct care hours

was ____ due to [*state reasons, not excuses, why: examples include sitters, ECMO, RRTs, OBS hours, etc.*]

9. Target sitter hours/day: ____

10. Actual avg. sitter hours/day: ____

11. Actual avg. sitter hours % of total worked hours (TWH): ____ [*LMI-recommended threshold less than 3%*]

Planned Absences/Nonproductive (NP) Time to TWH:

12. Budget total NP hours/day: ____ (all reasons)

13. Actual avg. NP hours/day: ____ (all reasons)

14. Budget total NP% of TWH: ____%

15. Actual avg. NP% of TWH: ____% [*LMI-recommended threshold less than 10% TWH*]

16. Target planned PTO NP hours/day: ____

17. Actual avg. planned PTO NP hours/day: ____

Unplanned Absences/Nonproductive (NP) Time to TWH:

18. Target unplanned PTO (call-in) hours/day: ____

19. Actual avg. unplanned PTO call-in hours/day: ____ [*LMI-recommended threshold less than 5% TWH*]

20. Actual avg. unplanned call-in hours% of TWH: ____% [*LMI-recommended threshold less than 5%*]

21. Actual avg. LOAs/FMLOA hours/day: ____

22. Actual avg. LOA/FMLOA hours% of TWH: ____% [*LMI-recommended threshold less than 10%*]

23. Actual avg. vacant hours/day: ____

24. Actual avg. vacancy% of TWH: ____ % [*LMI-recommended threshold less than 10%*]

25. *Explanations*:

Key Performance Indicators (KPI) and RN: Patient Ratios:

26. Target RN H/UOS: ____

27. Avg. RN H/UOS: ____

28. Target RN: patient ratio: ____

29. Avg. RN: patient ratio: ____

30. Target direct H/UOS: ____

31. Avg. direct H/UOS: ____

32. Budget total worked H/UOS: ____

33. Avg. total worked H/UOS: ____

34. Avg. productivity%: ____% [*Recommended range: 95%–105%*]

35. Budget total worked FTEs: ____

36. Avg. total worked FTEs: ____

37. *Explanations*:

FIGURE 4.4 Labor Management Institute's peer review report for nursing units.

ADT, admission, discharge, and transfer; ECMO, extracorporeal membrane oxygenation; FMLOA, family medical leave of absence; FTEs, full-time equivalents; H/UOS, hours/UOS; LOA, leave of absence; OBS, observation hours; OT, overtime; PP, pay period; PTO, paid time off; RRTs, registered respiratory therapists.

Source: Suby (2015). Provided with permission of the Labor Management Institute (LMI).

OT, on-call/call-back, incentive/bonus hours:

38. Avg. total OT hours/day: _____

39. Avg. OT% TWH: _____ % *[LMI-recommended threshold: less than 4.9%]*

40. Avg. incidental OT hours/day: _____

41. *Explanations*:

42. Avg. on-call hours/day: _____

43. Avg. on-call% of TWH: _____ % *[LMI-recommended threshold: less than 3% for inpatient units and less than 60% perioperative units]*

44. Avg. call-back hours/day: _____

45. Avg. call-back% of total on-call hours: _____% *[LMI-recommended threshold: less than 10% inpatient units and less than 60% perioperative units]*

46. Avg. incentive/bonus hours/day: _____

47. Avg. incentive/bonus% of TWH: _____ %

Other Hours:

48. Target education hours/day: _____

49. Avg. education hours/day: _____

50. Avg. education hours% TWH: _____%

51. Target meeting hours/day: _____

52. Avg. meeting hours/day: _____

53. Avg. meeting hours% TWH: _____%

54. Target orientation hours/day: _____

55. Avg. orientation hours/day: _____

56. Avg. orientation hours% TWH: _____% *[LMI-recommended threshold% by service line. Refer to the PSS Annual Survey of Hours Benchmark Report]*

Supplemental Staffing Response to Deficit Demands:

57. Avg. core staff% of TWH: _____%

58. Avg. supplemental staff% of TWH: _____% (all sources) *[LMI-recommended threshold %: Core = 85% or higher TWH; supplemental: less than 15% TWH]*

59. Target indirect H/UOS (e.g., charge nurse without patient assignments): _____

60. Avg. indirect H/UOS: _____

61. Avg. unit-based per diem% of TWH: _____%

62. Avg. float-into unit% of TWH: _____%

63. Avg. central resource pool% of TWH: _____%

64. Agency/travelers% of TWH: _____%

Response to Lower Volumes With Flex Down (Down-Staffing—if applicable):

65. Avg. daily census (ADC) was below budget ADC _____ days of the 14 days during the reporting period.

66. Avg. low workload cancel hours/day: _____

67. Avg. low workload cancel% of TWH: _____% *[LMI-recommended threshold%: less than 5%]*

68. Avg. float-out% of TWH: _____%

69. Avg. float-out to float-in%: _____% *[LMI-recommended threshold%: less than 40%]*

Staffing Effectiveness Indictors and Summary:

70. Total med errors: _____

71. Total falls: _____

72. Total employee on-the-job injuries: _____

73. Total worker comp claims filed: _____

Other:

I would like your suggestions to help me address _____ _____ [Provide a list of no more than three items]:

FIGURE 4.4 (*continued*)

- Focus on areas of opportunity.
- Elicit questions and comments.

    The benefits of peer reporting include:

- Disciplined review of the unit
- Open-book sharing
- Collaboration

- Continuous learning
- Problem solving
- Positioning and telling your story

Refer to the following LMI peer review report for NURSING UNITS as an example of the KPIs to share from the previous week or pay period. The peer review format should be adjusted for noninpatient units such as the ED, and nonnursing units such as respiratory therapy and pharmacy. The DNP/nurse leader should be able to obtain the data for this report from the daily shift management reports over the last week or pay period. Teaching the shift charge nurses to assist in the collection and updating of this report is a great opportunity for them to learn and for the DNP/nurse leader to ask them questions to prepare for the service line or department meeting (see Figure 4.4).

DNPs/nurse leaders learn the skills necessary to present their requests for additional staff to their executive leadership, finance representatives, FTE committees, and HR. When DNPs/nurse leaders feel comfortable telling their stories and answering the questions raised by their colleagues, they will feel comfortable with the members of their service line and departmental leadership.

■ CONCLUSION

Balancing available labor resources and workload for optimal workforce management and cost-effectiveness can only be achieved when the DNP/nurse leader truly understands financial principles, formulas, and the interrelatedness of the 1-year annual budget in hours and FTEs to the 1-month budget expressed in the employee schedule to the 1-day or 24-hour budget expressed in the VSP. Employee schedules must be produced and daily staffing decisions must be made that meet both financial constraints and employee needs that address workload volumes, patient acuity, and employee limitations in skills and competencies.

DNPs/nurse leaders who develop their understanding of these financial management, scheduling, and staffing interdependencies and work to strengthen their financial skills will be able to identify the sources for their FTE deficits and monitor scheduling and staffing practices to ensure safe and cost-effective care delivery.

DNPs/nurse leaders with a sound foundation in workforce management theory and evidence-based best practices and tools in financial management, scheduling, and staffing will be more successful in helping their organizations operate efficiently and effectively by having the right employees in the right place at the right time for the right cost and in ways that engage both employees and patients.

CRITICAL THINKING EXERCISES

1. Assume you need two RNs 24/7 (all three shifts) and the rotation would be every other weekend. How many worked FTEs would it require?
   a. 2.0 FTEs
   b. 4.2 FTEs
   c. 8.4 FTEs
   d. 10.6 FTEs

2. A medical–surgical unit with a standard of 8.0 total worked HPPD and a budgeted ADC of 20 patients will need a minimum of _____ FTEs (exclude the nonproductive replacement factor):

    a. 35
    b. 22
    c. 28
    d. 32

3. This 20-bed medical–surgical unit with a standard of 8.0 HPPD has a budget of 14% nonproductive replacement (benefit only) factor. It needs _____ total paid FTEs.
    a. 34
    b. 32
    c. 30
    d. 36

4. Which of the following statements is true when the unit patient volume is below budget?
    a. Total worked FTEs will be below budget.
    b. Direct HPPD is at budget.
    c. Dollars per UOS is above budget.
    d. Total annual dollars per unit are at budget.
        a. 2 only
        b. 3 only
        c. 1 and 2
        d. All of the above

REFERENCES

Agency for Healthcare Research and Quality. (2005). *AHRQ releases standardized hospital bed definitions to aid Katrina responders.* Rockville, MD: Author. Retrieved from http://www.ahrq.gov/research/havbed/definitions.htm

American Association of Colleges of Nursing. (2017). Nursing faculty shortage fact sheet. Retrieved from http://www.aacnnursing.org/Portals/42/News/Factsheets/Faculty-Shortage-Factsheet-2017.pdf

American Nurses Association. (2014). The nursing workforce 2014: Growth, salaries, education, demographics and trends. Retrieved from http://www.nursingworld.org/MainMenuCategories/ThePracticeofProfessionalNursing/workforce/Fast-Facts-2014-Nursing-Workforce.pdf

Auerbach, D. I., Buerhaus, P. I., & Staiger, D. O. (2007). Better late than never: Workforce supply implications of later entry into nursing. *Health Affairs, 26*(1), 178–185.

Auerbach, D. I., Buerhaus, P. I., & Staiger, D. O. (2015). Will the RN workforce weather the retirement of the baby boomers? *Medical Care, 53*(10), 850–856.

Gapenski, L. C., Vogel, W. B., & Langland-Orban, B. (1993). The determinants of hospital profitability. *Hospital and Health Services Administration, 38*(1), 63–80.

Hughes, R. G., Bobay, K. L., Jolly, N. A., & Suby, C. (2015). Comparison of nurse staffing based on changes in unit-level workload associated with patient churn. *Journal of Nursing Management, 23*(3), 390–400.

Institute of Medicine. (2004). *Keeping patients safe: Transforming the work environment of nurses.* Washington, DC: National Academies Press.

Kovner, C., & Brewer, C. (2013). *The RN Work Project: A national study to track career changes among newly licensed registered nurses.* Robert Wood Johnson Foundation. Retrieved from www.rnworkproject.org/resource-library.

Manthey, M. (2004, October). Leadership for Relationship-Based Care. ANCC 8th Annual National Magnet Conference, Sacramento, CA.

Meade, C. (2008). *Nurse manager span of control and effectiveness study.* Charlottesville, VA: Studer Group.

Suby, C. (2006). Staffing implications for increasing c-section rates, Oregon updates nurse staffing law, DOL issues regulations protecting reemployment rights of veterans, defining your schedule requirements. *PSS™ Newsletter, 25*(1), 3–4.

Suby, C. (2007a). Identifying root sources of overtime; managing your overtime plan; taking your overtime pulse; non-productive replacement FTE plan. *PSS™ Newsletter, 26*(2), 1–4.

Suby, C. (2007b). Full-time/part-time employee ratios and percentages. *PSS™ Newsletter, 26*(5), 1–4.

Suby, C. (2007c). LMI workforce management findings regarding overtime & position control, minimum, good & best position control management, what makes a good position control report, position control best practices. *PSS™ Newsletter, 26*(6), 1–4.

Suby, C. (2008a). Impact of admissions, discharges, transfers (ADT) on average length of stay (ALOS), decreasing length of stay impacts admissions, ADT, ALOS. *PSS™ Newsletter, 27*(1), 1–4.

Suby, C. (2008b). Schedulers, worker performance and work environment scheduling principles, defining employee requests, measuring quality with schedule report cards, 10 indicators that your unit's schedule is not working, scheduling best practices. *PSS™ Newsletter, 27*(3), 1–4.

Suby, C. (2009). Managing your non-productive budget. Formulas for calculating your non-productive benefit time. Self vs. selfish scheduling, employee request guidelines, impact of planned vs. unplanned absences. Developing a vacation plan form. *PSS™ Newsletter, 28*(2), 1–4.

Suby, C. (2015). *Labor Management Institute's 2015 PSS™ Annual Survey of Hours Benchmark Report©*. Labor Management Institute Bloomington, MN: Labor Management Institute. Retrieved from http://www.LMInstitute.com

Unruh, L. Y., & Fottler, M. D. (2006). Patient turnover and nursing staff adequacy. *Health Services Research, 41*(2), 599–612.

Wexler, B. I., & Smith, K. M. (2017, May 16). *Moody's: Preliminary FY 2016 US NFP hospital medians edge lower on revenue, expense pressures*. New York, NY: Moody's Investors Service. Retrieved from https://www.moodys.com/researchdocumentcontentpage.aspx?docid=PBM_1064975

5 Nurse Practitioner Strategies for Financial Success

Karen Van Leuven

Advanced practice registered nurses (APRNs) are registered nurses who have completed graduate education that expands their scope of practice via didactic and clinical education. Nurses practicing in APRN roles include nurse practitioners (NPs), clinical nurse specialists (CNSs), certified nurse midwives (CNMs), and certified registered nurse anesthetists (CRNAs). Initially, APRNs were educated at the certificate level; however, as the roles evolved, education transitioned to the master of science in nursing (MSN) degree. With the introduction of the doctor of nursing practice (DNP) degree, the American Association of Colleges of Nursing (AACN) advocated for the transition of these graduate programs to the DNP level.

The DNP degree is based on core knowledge that is best described by the essential components of the degree. These essential components are (a) scientific underpinnings for practice, (b) organizational and systems leadership for quality improvement and systems thinking, (c) clinical scholarship and analytical methods for evidence-based practice, (d) information systems/technology and patient care technology for the improvement and transformation of health care, (e) health care policy for advocacy in health care, (f) interprofessional collaboration for improving patient and population health outcomes, (g) clinical prevention and population health for improving the nation's health, and (h) advanced nursing practice.

Understanding financial aspects of APRN practice addresses *The Essentials of Doctoral Education for Advanced Nursing Practice (DNP) Essential II* as it provides APRNs with the skill set to monitor the cost-effectiveness of individual practice, APRN practice at large, and practice innovations. In addition, financial skills are also needed to accomplish *DNP Essential V*, because it is important to unveil the key role that APRNs play in health care delivery. Unfortunately, this role is often hidden due to billing practices employed by providers and organizations. *DNP Essentials VI and VII* are also addressed, because financial skills are needed to analyze complex practice and organizational issues and evaluate the socioeconomic aspects of care delivery models. Furthermore, financial skills are needed to ensure the viability of APRN roles and practice in an evolving health care system (*Essential VIII*; AACN, 2006).

■ BACKGROUND

APRNs evolved over a lengthy period of time and have become increasingly more important in the delivery of health care in the United States. Nurse anesthetists were the first APRNs, beginning practice in the late 1800s by administering anesthesia, thereby freeing surgeons to concentrate on the surgical procedure (Diers, 1991; Savrin, 2009). Nurse midwives were next to emerge. Although midwives have existed since antiquity, this role, which combined nursing knowledge with advanced skills, is relatively current. Early professional midwifery services in the United States were supplied by nurse midwives from England, who came to the United States to provide perinatal and delivery services to rural and underserved areas that did not have their own physicians. However, in 1925 in rural Kentucky, the Frontier Nursing Service began the first program in the United States to educate nurses to serve as midwives and public health nurses (Frontier Nursing Service, 2000). The third APRN role to appear was that of the CNS. This role evolved as the complexity of health care increased after World War II. The goal of the CNS was to provide clinical expertise to improve patient care. This role placed the CNS in contact with staff nurses, physicians, and patients predominantly in acute care settings (LaSala, Connors, Pedro, & Phipps, 2007). The final APRN role to develop was the NP. In 1963, the Surgeon General recommended, in response to a shortage of primary care providers, the development of the NP role to address this concern (LaSala et al., 2007). In 1965, Loretta Ford, a public health nurse working in rural Colorado, together with Henry Silver, a pediatrician, launched the first NP program. The program was a 3-month continuing education curriculum focused on health promotion, disease prevention, and the health care needs of children and families (O'Brien, 2003). Currently, all NP programs are delivered at the graduate level. Curricula focus on management of health and illness, the NP–patient relationship, teaching and coaching of patients, managing and negotiating health care delivery systems, cultural sensitivity, and quality of care (American Academy of Nurse Practitioners [AANP], 2013). Although NPs are the most recent addition to the APRN group, they represent the largest and most visible group of APRNs (Savrin, 2009).

Since their beginnings, APRNs have been contributing to the delivery of essential care services. However, many remain hidden providers; that is, their financial contribution to health care is difficult to assess. This chapter discusses the myriad of reasons for this problem, using the NP role as the exemplar. Later discussion focuses on essential financial skills for advanced practice.

HIDDEN PROVIDER STATUS

Although NPs have been delivering primary care services since 1965, direct reimbursement for NP services did not commence until 1990 when Medicare offered reimbursement to NPs—but only in rural areas and skilled nursing facilities (SNFs). In 1997, Medicare amended its reimbursements of APRNs to include all geographical regions and included reimbursement for CNS, CNM, and CRNA services. Reimbursement by commercial insurers followed suit (Wound, Ostomy, & Continence Nurses Society [WOCN], 2012).

Although NPs can bill directly for services, the value of their services is often hidden due to the frequent practice of NP care being billed under physician provider numbers. This situation occurs when the NP works as an employee or as contracted labor for a physician or group of physicians. Under Medicare guidelines, when physicians bill for services, reimbursement occurs at 100% of the negotiated physician fee reimbursement. However, when an NP delivers the *same* care, but bills under his or her own provider number, he or she is reimbursed at 85% of the physician fee schedule (Centers for Medicare and Medicaid Services [CMS], 2016). A work-around solution found in many settings is for the NP to deliver care but to bill services under the physician provider number (Buppert, 2015). This allows 100% reimbursement, but because NP salaries are typically below physician salaries, this results in increased profit to the practice.

This custom is an interesting strategy that allows practices to use the work of NPs to deliver care and reap financial benefits by employing lower paid providers. Yet, on the grand scale, it makes it difficult to track the contribution of NPs in care delivery. Without this knowledge, lawmakers and regulators have no real incentive to create laws or positions that are favorable to APRNs.

The legality behind this practice, commonly known as "incident-to" billing, lies in the language of Medicare rules (Balen, 2014). Criteria that must be met to legally bill under the physician provider number are quite detailed. Following is a summary of the criteria:

1. The physician must perform an initial evaluation of the patient.
2. No new patients can be billed as "incident-to"; the patient must be established at the practice.
3. The physician must be physically present in the suite where the care is delivered so that immediate face-to-face consultation is available.
4. The problem treated must be an ongoing problem, and no new problem can be addressed during the visit.
5. The physician must see the patient intermittently in order to oversee continuing management.

All criteria must be met for billing to be appropriately done at the physician fee schedule. Although this practice originated with Medicare, many commercial insurers have their own criteria. Some are identical to Medicare, whereas others have their own specific criteria and protocols. More importantly, some commercial insurers will not "credential" NPs (Yee, Boukus, Cross, & Samuel, 2013). Credentialing is a verification of the qualifications of a provider, which, when successfully completed, allows the provider to conduct business, including billing for that business, at a site or with members of a group. Refusal to credential NP providers is a denial of their legitimacy as health care providers. Furthermore, reimbursement can only be obtained by billing under the credentialed physician.

It is easy to see how the contribution that NPs make to the health care system can be hidden with this billing practice. Furthermore, this system is rife with problems. For example, if a patient is initially seen by the NP in the office, and the NP establishes a plan of care, incident-to billing criteria have not been met. Even if the physician has initially seen the patient to establish a plan of care, if the patient has a new problem when being seen by the NP, incident-to billing criteria have not been met. In fact, incident-to billing criteria are not met if the physician is at lunch outside of the office (Balen, 2014).

As an NP working in an office, if care is billed under a physician's name, the patient is aware of who delivered the care, but insurance companies and regulators may not be aware. Yet, the problem is more complex than that. NP scope of practice is dictated by each state. At the time of this writing, only 22 states and the District of Columbia allow completely autonomous practice for NPs; most require some form of collaboration or supervision by a physician. An annual update is published in the January issue of *The Nurse Practitioner*. However, this is a situation in flux because of numerous pending pieces of legislation. Up-to-the-minute information is available through the AANP and state NP organizations. State laws also dictate a ratio of NPs per supervising or collaborating physician. The most restrictive state is Oklahoma, which allows one MD to supervise two full-time (FT) NPs, or four part-time (PT) NPs. When a ratio is specified, the most permissive state is Texas, which dictates a 7:1 ratio. However, 21 states do not limit the number of NPs a physician can supervise or collaborate with (National Nursing Centers Consortium [NNCC], 2014). As you can see, it is possible for a massive amount of NP work to be hidden under this system.

Fortunately, the practice environment is rapidly changing. In 2016, seven states amended laws favorably affecting NP reimbursement and 16 states enacted legislation that improved the NP practice environment and scope of practice. Countless pieces of legislation are in proposal to grant unrestricted practice to NPs. Much of this momentum has been fueled by shortages of primary care providers nationwide (Phillips, 2017).

The contribution of NPs is also well hidden in inpatient settings. Historically, hospitals were reimbursed based on the fees charged for services, whether inpatient or outpatient. However, soaring fees led Medicare to develop the prospective payment system. This system involves receiving a set amount per patient discharge or outpatient procedure based on the patient's diagnosis, without regard to actual costs. The reimbursement amount is tied to the patient's diagnoses and is set by Medicare based on average regional cost charges as well as knowledge of typical care associated with a disorder. Reimbursement is set before care is delivered, rather than in response to actual costs (Bodenheimer & Grumbach, 2016).

Medicare is the principal insurance company for the most likely users of the health system (older than 65 or disabled). As a result, Medicare rules are quickly adopted by other payers. Many commercial insurance companies and Medicaid have followed Medicare's lead and reimburse similarly. Hospitals must still submit cost reports to Medicare. In these cost reports, the expense of salaries and benefits of hospital employees is delineated. Medicare uses this information to reassess fee structures on a regular basis. However, the costs of direct and indirect care providers listed on the cost report are assumed to be covered under the lump sum payment through Medicare Part A, which covers hospitalization, SNF services, and some home health services. In contrast, physician services are reimbursed under Medicare Part B (CMS, 2016).

Medicare allows NPs to bill under Part B for physician services, defined as diagnosis, therapy, surgery consultation, and care plan oversight (Buppert, 2015). However, if NPs are employees who are included in the cost report to Medicare, their services are not reimbursable under Part B. Instead, the cost of NPs would be considered subsumed under the diagnosis-related fee reimbursement. Because NPs are frequently employees of the hospital, many have been hired under nursing contracts and therefore the cost of their salaries and benefits is included in the cost report to Medicare. Therefore, NP services are not eligible for Part B reimbursement. In addition, because maternity care and surgery services are usually bundled into a global fee, acute care-based NPs who provide service to admitted patients in lieu of the obstetrician or surgeon, such as pain management, removal of a drain, or management of complications, cannot bill for their services because it is assumed that the cost of this care is under the global fee (WOCN, 2012). The physician may indeed reap tremendous benefit from the presence of acute care-based NPs, as he or she is able to engage in other services that are fee generating, yet the NP cannot generate revenue from these activities. In addition, the fact that the NP alters the productivity of the physician is hidden because of the inability of the NP to bill for services. Furthermore, if the NP is employed by the hospital, the hospital is responsible for the cost of the NP, whereas the physician is reimbursed for care.

The services of acute care-based NPs are advantageous to hospitals. As on-site providers, NPs are available to promptly respond to changes in patient conditions, thereby limiting length of stay, which results in improved reimbursement patterns under the prospective payment model (Hoffman & Guttendorf, 2014). In addition, careful monitoring of patients improves quality and safety, reduces use of material and personnel resources, and results in higher patient satisfaction. However, without thorough understanding of reimbursement rules, inpatient-based NPs can appear to be cost centers, rather than enhancements to patient care and potential revenue generators.

As length of hospital stay has diminished, use of SNFs has escalated. SNFs now provide services that have historically been delivered to hospitalized patients. Skilled services include wound care; intravenous therapy; enteral feeding; and speech, occupational, and physical therapy. Yet NPs are hidden providers here as well.

The previously stated incident-to billing rules apply to care delivered in SNFs as well. A physician must have an office for which he or she pays fair market value within the SNF and the physician must be on-site for the NP to bill at the 100% rate. Otherwise, billing must occur under the NP's provider number at the 85% reimbursement rate (CMS, 2016). Although this is the rule, personal experience in a number of offices has proved otherwise. This occurs as an extension of faulty use of incident-to billing practices in offices. For example, take the case of a patient who is normally seen in the office who undergoes hospitalization and requires rehabilitation services posthospitalization. The office practice physician agrees to be the admitting physician to the SNF; however, the physician sends the NP to see the patient in the SNF. Care is billed under the physician name, as the billing manager is accustomed to this practice in the office. However, incident-to billing criteria of maintaining an office in the SNF, being present at the site, and initiating and monitoring care have not been met. In addition, the contribution of the NP to care delivery is hidden from insurers and regulators.

Similar to hospital regulations, all patients must be admitted to an SNF under a physician's care, and the physician must perform the history and physical within 72 hours of admission and see the patient at least every 60 days. However, the initial evaluation, which would include a complete examination and ordering of medications, labs, and treatments, as well as subsequent evaluation of progress, can be conducted by an NP and billed under an NP's provider number.

It is clear from this pervasive hidden provider status that NPs have opportunities to bill that are being missed. Understanding billing codes and acquiring business skills are essential to move away from hidden provider status.

UNDERSTANDING BILLING CODES

In order for NPs to assume a greater role in health care, billing in all settings must consistently be done under NP provider numbers so that the contribution of NPs can be fully appreciated. Billing for care is based on use of a series of accepted codes identified in the *Current Procedural Terminology* (CPT) code set (2017), which is maintained and updated by the American Medical Association (2017). The code set provides a uniform method to describe medical, surgical, and diagnostic services. The CPT code is used in conjunction with the *International Statistical Classification of Diseases and Related Health Problems* (ICD) code for billing purposes. The ICD code identifies the disease, sign, symptom, or complaint that generated the visit. The first step to correctly bill for patient care is to gain an understanding of the CPT evaluation and management (E&M) codes.

CPT CODING

CPT E&M codes evaluate the complexity of care delivered and are associated with reimbursement based on documentation of patient care encounters. E&M codes transform a patient encounter into a five-digit code. The care setting (office, home, hospital, SNF, or domiciliary setting) determines the unique series of codes that may be considered for use. Patient encounters that occur via phone or online also have unique codes. Within settings, codes are divided into those appropriate for patients who are new to the site versus established patients. This distinction acknowledges the fact that when a patient is unknown to the provider, additional data must be gathered in order to deliver care safely. A new patient is defined as an individual who has not received services from a provider in the practice group in the past 3 years. An established patient is someone who has had care delivered by a provider at the practice within the last 3 years (Department of Health and Human Services [DHHS], 2016). Lapses in care of more than 3 years would therefore generate a new visit code, even though the patient may have an old file on record.

Within each series of setting-based codes, the NP must select the billing code that is associated with the level of care provided at the patient encounter. Four levels of care are present for new and established patients. The levels in increasing order of complexity are problem focused, expanded problem focused, detailed, and comprehensive (DHHS, 2016). For example, the code associated with a detailed visit in an office setting with a new patient is 99204, whereas the code for a detailed visit with an established patient is 99214. This differentiation is important, because the new patient encounter is reimbursed at a higher level than the established patient encounter. The history, examination, and medical decision-making components of the visit determine the level of care that should be coded. As complexity increases, documentation requirements increase, as does reimbursement (DHHS, 2016).

The history is the first component that must be evaluated to determine the level of care. Certainly, patient care is crucial, but E&M guidelines follow the old adage, "if it wasn't charted, it wasn't done," so not only must the visit include the required elements, but these elements must also be recorded (K. J. Moore, 2010). Consider the case of a historically healthy patient established at a practice seeking care to determine whether a minor abrasion needs further evaluation. Salient questions the NP should pursue center around the timing and circumstances of the abrasion as well as the patient's current treatment. This would be consistent with a problem-focused visit. However, additional history would be needed if the patient sustained a laceration. A detailed history would be necessary if the patient sustained a laceration from a fall after newly starting medications to treat hypertension. Still, a more complex or comprehensive history is appropriate if you are initiating care for a new patient, or caring for a patient with multiple acute and chronic conditions. Table 5.1 details the history requirements for each billing code.

Physical examination requirements follow a similar pattern, with each progressively higher level of examination requiring more elements. Table 5.2 summarizes the physical examination requirements. Documentation requirements specify the number of organ systems or body areas examined as well as the detail of the examination. Provision is also made for high-level examination of a single-organ system. For example, an NP conducting a women's health examination would correctly code a visit as comprehensive if it included assessment and documentation of vital signs, commentary on the nutritional status or body habitus (e.g., well developed, well nourished), observation, and palpation of the abdomen, as well as at least seven bulleted comments focused on the examination of the breast and external and internal pelvis (DHHS, 2016).

The final aspect of E&M coding focuses on the complexity of medical decision making. Medical decision making is evaluated based on the number of diagnoses or treatment options, the number of tests or consults that must be ordered or evaluated, and the risk associated with care management (DHHS, 2016). A patient with multiple health problems who has had lab or diagnostic testing that must be evaluated, and as a result has medications adjusted, is a high-complexity visit. In contrast, a patient with iron deficiency anemia who is taking iron supplementation and

TABLE 5.1 History Requirements for E&M Codes

Type of History	Chief Complaint	History of Present Illness	Review of Systems	Past, Family, and/or Social History
Problem focused	Required	Brief (one to three elements)	Not required	Not required
Expanded problem focused	Required	Brief (one to three elements)	Problem focused only	Not required
Detailed	Required	Extended (four or more elements or status of three or more chronic or inactive conditions)	Extended (positive and pertinent negative findings for two to nine systems)	Pertinent (at least one specific item documented)
Comprehensive	Required	Extended (four or more elements or status of three or more chronic or inactive conditions)	Complete (positive and pertinent negative findings for at least 10 systems, including the system involved in the present illness)	Complete (at least one item from two of three areas: past history, family history, social history for established patients, and three of three for new patients)

E&M, evaluation and management.

Source: Adapted from DHHS (2016) and Clack, Freeman, and Lewis (2017).

TABLE 5.2 Physical Examination Requirements for E&M Codes

Type of Exam	Requirements
Problem focused	Examination of one to five elements identified by bullet in one or more organ systems or body areas
Expanded problem focused	Examination of six or more elements identified by bullet in one or more organ systems or body areas
Detailed	Examination of at least six organ systems or body areas documented by at least two bullet items per system, or exam and documentation of at least 12 bulleted elements in one or more organ systems or body area
Comprehensive	Examination of at least nine organ systems or body areas documented by at least two bullet items per system; provisions are also made for comprehensive examination of a single-organ system accompanied by review of constitutional elements and related systems

E&M, evaluation and management.

Source: Adapted from DHHS (2016).

TABLE 5.3 Decision-Making Requirements for E&M Codes

Type of Decision Making	Number of Diagnoses or Treatment Options	Amount or Complexity of Data	Risk of Complications, Morbidity, or Mortality
Straightforward	Minimal	Minimal or none	Minimal
Low complexity	Limited	Limited	Low
Moderate complexity	Multiple	Moderate	Moderate
High complexity	Extensive	Extensive	High

E&M, evaluation and management.

Source: Adapted from DHHS (2016).

being seen for follow-up of lab work would qualify as a low-complexity visit. Table 5.3 details the requirements for medical decision making.

To determine the billing code for a visit, the NP needs to examine his or her documentation regarding the history, examination, and medical decision-making components of the visit. For an established patient, two of three of the components must meet criteria for the level, whereas all three components must be at the level for a new patient (DHHS, 2016). Although this may seem quite complex, in reality the levels reflect the degree of investigation and thought that are required when assessing and diagnosing patients in the clinical setting. As the complexity of care increases, the appropriate level code rises. Higher level codes are reimbursed at a higher rate, so the NP is being reimbursed more as the evaluation and management of the patient become more complex.

Visits that are focused on counseling or coordination of care are billed entirely differently. Time is the key billing consideration. Documentation should include time spent in face-to-face counseling or on the unit coordinating care, along with a thorough description of the counseling and coordination activities. Time increments associated with visit levels are 10 minutes for a problem-focused encounter, 15 minutes for an expanded problem-focused visit, 25 minutes for a detailed visit, and 40 minutes for a comprehensive visit.

It is important for NPs to become proficient in coding care so that reimbursement reflects services delivered. In a study involving randomized chart reviews of outpatient visits conducted by NPs in a clinic setting, four coding problems were identified:

1. Failure to recognize that new patients require more documentation than established patients. Recall that all three components must be at the designated level in order to use the corresponding code for new patients, whereas only two areas must be at the level for established patients. This can result in coding too high for new patients and overpayment for services.
2. Failure to select the new versus established patient code, which can lead to underpayment for the visit.
3. Failure to thoroughly code all aspects of the visit, resulting in underpayment for the visit. For example, a patient was seen for a general prevention-oriented exam, but the NP also needed to address a health problem. Correct coding for this visit would include one code for the prevention visit and an additional-level code for the problem that was addressed.
4. Failure to detail the elements of an examination by using catch-all phrases such as "within normal limits." The result is a need to code lower due to lack of documentation even though the work was done (Allen, Reinke, Pohl, Martyn, & McIntosh, 2003). The concerns raised by this study are likely; however, a more recent follow-up study has not been conducted.

ICD CODING

ICD coding complements E&M coding by defining the patient situation that warranted the services rendered. Prior to 1851, diseases were not uniformly categorized. Descriptions varied widely between providers and locales. However, the Great Exhibition in Paris of 1851 fostered an interest in statistical tracking of health problems. Two years later, at a follow-up conference in Brussels, several learned attendees set off on the task of tracking causes of death. There was no standard nomenclature for disease, so attempts to devise a classification system ensued. After many attempts to define and classify illness, the first globally accepted system was launched in 1893, entitled the *International List of Causes of Death* (Moriyama, Loy, & Robb-Smith, 2011).

Since these early attempts, the *ICD* has undergone significant change. The World Health Organization, in cooperation with the National Center for Health Statistics in the United States, oversees all changes to the classification. The first revision of the list in 1909 was known as *International Statistical Classification of Diseases and Related Health Problems–First Edition (ICD-1)*. The most recent revision, *International Statistical Classification of Diseases and Related Health Problems–Tenth Edition (ICD-10)*, was endorsed for acceptance in 1990 and launched into use in 1994. Globally, the *ICD-10* classification is widely used. However, its adoption in the United States was not mandated until October 2015. Delays in the adoption of *ICD-10* resulted from concerns about the financial burden and readiness for the switch among providers and insurers, as well as concerns about the increased complexity of the system. Fortunately, the transition to the newer system was relatively smooth and none of these concerns came to fruition (Bowman, 2016).

The *ICD* classification assigns a numeric code to a diagnosis, symptom, or cause of death. Health facilities and providers use these codes to identify a condition or health challenge that a patient faces. For example, if the patient is identified with primary hypertension, the appropriate *ICD-10* code would be I10, whereas the patient with concomitant heart failure would be correctly coded as I11.0. In contrast, a woman who develops hypertension in her first trimester of pregnancy would receive a diagnosis code of O13.1. Numerous online and text-based sources are available to help NPs learn diagnosis codes. Furthermore, many service sites generate billing sheets listing the most commonly seen disorders so that the provider merely has to circle the appropriate diagnoses.

The *ICD* code is used by insurers to assign payment in the prospective payment system, as well as by providers to identify the rationale for care. Agencies such as the Centers for Disease Control and Prevention (CDC) track use of these codes to examine trends and patterns of disease as well as causes of death. Governmental agencies use *ICD* information to plan and fund disease-focused programs. Because these codes are internationally used, global health issues can be identified and tracked.

In addition to understanding *ICD* and *CPT* codes, NPs must understand what makes their services financially beneficial or deleterious to a practice. Most NPs and other advanced practice programs focus on the clinical skills needed for practice; assessment, disease management, and pharmacology are the cornerstones of programs. However, business skills allow NPs to survive individually and as a profession.

■ BUSINESS SKILLS

One of the most important skills for an NP to acquire is the ability to assess the contribution he or she makes to a practice. Without this knowledge, it is impossible to judge whether your compensation is adequate and whether your position has long-term viability. In order to determine your worth to a practice, you will need to track the services you provide over a representative sample of time.

CALCULATING WORTH OF AN NP

To calculate an NP's financial contribution to a practice, an assessment of services delivered is required. This is accomplished by tracking the number of patients seen per day as well as the *CPT* codes used to bill these services. Because there may be day-to-day variations, it is best to examine data for a period of time. For example, if the NP is the only provider seeing patients on Wednesdays, this may be his or her busiest day. However, when other providers are also present, the daily schedule may be lighter. Select a typical week to track number of visits and E&M codes either concurrently or by retrospective review.

First, identify the number of times each billing code is used for services in the week and then determine the billing rates for these services. To determine the billing rate, the NP must coordinate with the billing department. Knowing the amount at which services are billed is not sufficient. Instead, it is important to determine the average reimbursement for each E&M code. Frequently, practices enter into contractual arrangements with payers that result in discounted charges. For example, a visit that would normally bill at $100 is offered to a contracted group for $75. In return for discounting, payers funnel patients to the practice (Keegan, 2012). Most billing professionals can readily tell you about reimbursement rates based on insurance provider, as well as your typical payer mix. However, it is important to determine whether the NP payer mix is similar or distinct from the patient mix seen by other providers in the practice. For instance, if the NP sees a younger patient mix than other providers in the practice, the insurance coverage and average reimbursement may be different from that of other providers. Spend time talking with the billing agent to determine whether it is appropriate to use the average reimbursement or whether additional work is needed to determine the typical reimbursement for the NP's patient population. In addition, inquire whether billing is done under the NP's provider number or under a physician billing number. Recall that NPs are reimbursed at 85% of physician rates under Medicare and many commercial carriers.

Once the average reimbursement per E&M level visit and the usual number of each type of visit per week is known, it is easy to calculate the amount of revenue generated per week. Multiply the reimbursement amount by the number of visits. This amount represents cash flow into the practice. It is does not represent income. To determine actual income into the practice, you will need to explore overhead costs.

OVERHEAD

Overhead costs represent the cost of doing business. Included in this amount are the salaries of support staff, cost of benefits, facility fees, utilities, and licensing. Exhibit 5.1 delineates the typical overhead charges seen in an office practice. Hospital- or facility-based practices may have unique variations. For example, many facility-based providers do not have separate office facilities. Instead, they provide services where the patients are housed. This eliminates a number of high overhead costs. Keegan (2012) found that overhead in family practice or internal medicine offices can be as high as 60% to 70% of revenue, whereas surgical practices, which rely on external space such as hospitals and surgery centers for many of their patient interactions, have lower overhead—closer to 45%. Efficient offices that keep support staff busy with the work of the business and are busy with patients when open will have a lower overhead rate. On the other hand, many offices employ support staff who are only periodically busy. Offices that maintain traditional paper charts, for example, may employ a clerk to pull charts and refile material after use. In contrast, practices that utilize electronic health records will not have this cost, but they will have fees associated with maintenance of the charting system, computer server, and computer equipment used by providers.

Support staff needs will vary based on the type of practice, the needs of a provider, the layout of the facility, the expertise of staff, and the amount of work contracted to outside groups. Many specialists can function with less support staff, but those who conduct in-office procedures may have unique needs for support personnel (Nelson, 2010). Consider the case of a cardiology practice. If the practice conducts noninvasive testing on-site, personnel will need to be hired for this purpose. However, this testing will markedly increase the revenue generated by the practice. Facility-based practices, such as hospitalist groups, have hospital staff available at no charge to the practice. This limits the cost of doing business.

EXHIBIT 5.1 Typical Overhead Charges for a Medical Practice

Salaries for office staff
Salaries for medical assistants
Salaries for providers
Malpractice insurance
Health insurance coverage fees
Disability/life insurance
License renewal costs
Rent
Telephone and computer expenses
Electronic health records systems and backup
Utilities
Office supplies
Medical and lab supplies
Business insurance
Legal services
Billing services (if performed by outside agency)
Dues for professional organizations
Continuing education
Marketing

Source: Adapted from L. G. Moore and Wasson (2007) and McNeill (2016).

Providers also have unique needs. Male providers who see female patients for gynecology or urologic exams require a chaperone for examinations. Therefore, the medical assistant is unavailable for other tasks when chaperoning (Nelson, 2010). Also, some providers are more independent; they are able to perform examinations or procedures without support staff, whereas others desire support at all times. Providers who are highly organized are able to move patients through the system and complete documentation. Others require assistance with referrals and completing chart notes. Providers with high patient volumes may need more support in order to keep patient flow in and out of rooms from being delayed.

Office layout may dictate support staff needs. Compact facilities with adjoining rooms allow providers and staff to spend more time with patients, but facilities on multiple levels or with distinct care pod areas require more staff. Furthermore, satellite sites may require duplication of staff. This often occurs when a practice sees patients in distinct settings. If a practice has an office in the city as well as the suburbs, there is rent and overhead for both sites. Often, providers move between sites, but staff may be distinct. If both sites are open at the same time, it is impossible to have staff rotate with providers.

Staff expertise also affects overhead. Experienced medical assistants and clerical staff are usually more efficient. If there is high turnover of office personnel, a substantial amount of time is spent in training mode. New employees require more time to complete tasks and need more assistance to complete work. If the percentage of employees who have been with the practice less than 1 year is 30% or more, efforts should be directed at recruiting and retaining experienced personnel (Reeves, 2002).

Finally, the amount of work contracted to outside groups will affect overhead costs. Many practices employ outside agencies for billing, computer maintenance, janitorial services, or marketing. The key question is whether contracting is advantageous to a practice. For example, outside billing agents often operate by taking a percentage of revenue received. As a result, the billing agent is incentivized to follow up on unpaid balances or to seek contracts with insurance providers that are more lucrative to the practice. Although the initial cost of an outside agent may appear higher, these incentives may generate more revenue for the practice.

To calculate overhead, examine all of these features to determine whether the practice has high or low overhead. The billing agent or bookkeeper is an important resource in this calculation. Knowing this information is valuable not only for examining NP worth to a practice, but it also may identify areas for potential improvement in the practice.

WHAT DOES THE NP CONTRIBUTE?

Perhaps the best way to examine NP worth to a practice is to look at an example. Table 5.4 delineates an office-based example for an NP working 4 days per week and seeing on average 20 patients per day. The NP's typical billing pattern is used to calculate the revenue generated from patient encounters. In consultation with the billing agent, he or she determines the average reimbursement rate for these visits as well as the percentage of revenue used to cover overhead.

In addition to calculating revenue from NP–patient encounters, consider whether the NP contributes to the practice in other ways. Possible contributions include coordination of office staff; review of lab tests; prescription renewal management; response to patient calls or emails; and coordination of patient care with other health agencies, such as home health, SNFs, or specialists for other providers. This work ensures successful flow of patient care and the running of the practice. It also frees up other providers so that they can be more productive with generating revenue. As a result, all NPs should consider the amount of time they spend in practice-related business. If the NP schedule calls for an 8-hour day, of which 3 hours are spent managing and coordinating the practice, the NP is generating income for 5 hours but is pulled away from visits for 3 hours. It is difficult to quantify the value of this work. In fact, many practices consider this time as an expense for the business. However, if the NP services are crucial for the practice to

TABLE 5.4 Calculating the NP's Contribution to a Practice

	Percentage of Visits	Average Reimbursement per Visit	Amount Reimbursed per Week
Problem-focused level	10% of 80 = 8/week	$35	$280/week
Expanded problem-focused level	35% of 80 = 28/week	$50	$1,400/week
Detailed	35% of 80 = 28/week	$75	$1,400/week
Comprehensive	20% of 80 = 16/week	$90	$1,440/week
Totals	80 visits/week	Average reimbursement/ visit $56.50	$4,520[a]/week

Jane Doe is employed at an office-based practice 4 days per week. On average, she sees 20 patients per day. Her average weekly number of visits is 80.

[a]Additional revenue may be received in the form of co-payments at each visit. This will vary widely based on insurance coverage of patients.

Allowing for 2 weeks of vacation per year, plus an additional 2 weeks of time for holidays, Jane works on average 48 weeks/year. As a result, the revenue she generates is: 48 weeks × $4,520 of reimbursement/week—$216,960 per year. Her office employs multiple support staff per provider. The billing agent estimates that overhead (the cost of doing business) consumes 50% of revenue. As a result, $108,480 of her revenue is used to cover the cost of support staff, licensing, rent, benefits, and so forth. An additional $108,480 is available for salary and profits.

operate, they should be factored in when computing salary. Consideration should also be given as to whether these tasks can be performed by others so that the NP is able to see patients instead.

OPPORTUNITIES

Knowledge of how revenue is generated and spent is key to understanding how the NP and a practice can be financially successful. Self-reflection as well as honest appraisal of the strengths and weaknesses of a practice will identify areas for improvement or enhancement.

The first task is to determine whether billing is actually being done in the name of the NP or under a physician provider. Although practices may want to bill under the physician to receive higher reimbursement, recognition of the NP is lost. Given the looming shortage of physicians entering primary care or internal medicine, coupled with a steady rise in NPs and other APRNs entering practice, there is substantial momentum for NPs to be recognized as providers (Huff, 2016; Naylor & Kurtzman, 2010). Billing the work of the NP under the name of the NP allows others—payers, employers, legal and regulatory bodies—to see the value of NPs. In order to do this, NPs must be nationally certified and obtain a national provider identifier (NPI), a unique health care provider identifier, which is part of a national registry. The NPI was mandated in the Health Insurance Portability and Accountability Act (HIPAA) of 1996 (National Plan and Provider Enumeration System, 2011), and, as of May 2008, is required for all billing and health information transmittal. An NPI can be obtained online at https://nppes.cms.hhs.gov. NPs working in acute care must also meet with finance and billing personnel to remove NPs from the cost reports that are submitted to Medicare, thereby allowing NPs to bill under Medicare Part B. A change in this status paves the way for billing to private insurance, as well.

Next, it is essential to examine billing patterns. Billing is based on documentation of care. If the NP is obtaining histories and performing examinations but limiting charting, billing will occur at a lower rate than what the work warrants. Catch-all phrases, such as *within normal limits* and *noncontributory*, lower the level of the visit, because they do not indicate the depth to which a symptom was explored. Consider forms or charting systems that can aid with documentation. Electronic health records may be valuable for improving documentation, because they allow development of templates. Forms or templates can be developed that can be used at all visits or can address specific diagnoses (e.g., diabetes mellitus, congestive heart failure) or purpose for a visit (e.g., well-child check, women's health examination). Improved documentation will result in a direct increase in revenue and money available for salary and profits.

Examination of work flow, need for support staff, and setting of care can present opportunities for decreasing overhead and enhancing revenue. For example, reassigning examination rooms used by each provider may improve flow. Offering early morning and/or evening appointments creates opportunities to capture visits that may be lost to clinics, emergency rooms, or other providers. Altering staff and provider hours to parallel busy times improves efficiency and may significantly reduce overhead. The more the NP knows about the practice, the more he or she can offer suggestions to the practice.

Finally, understanding the politics regarding reimbursement also provides opportunities for delivering care. For example, recent attempts to control the rising cost of health care have focused on preventing hospital readmissions, moving toward reimbursement based on health outcomes and patient satisfaction, and bundling reimbursement for services based on conditions and procedures (Medicare Payment Advisory Commission, 2017). NPs are in an ideal position to develop care innovations that provide quality and satisfaction in a cost-efficient manner.

NEGOTIATIONS

Being knowledgeable about the amount of revenue you generate for a practice is a necessity when entering negotiations for salary and benefits. For example, the NP depicted in Table 5.4 would be foolhardy if he or she asked for a salary of $125,000 per year. This would represent a loss to the practice and would most certainly be denied. However, it may be completely appropriate to ask for a salary greater than the amount generated through patient visits if the NP contributes to the practice in other ways besides direct practice. If the NP provides coverage for colleagues who allow him or her to generate income and removes himself or herself from potential revenue-generating patient visits, it would be reasonable to request compensation that includes this value-added dimension of his or her practice. The NP who is informed about practicing financial issues is in the best position to negotiate.

A successful contract specifies the intent of the contract and matches the personal goals, needs, and wants of the NP. First to consider is the type of contract. Determine whether the contract is an employer-to-employee contract versus an independent contractor offer. Many medical groups prefer to offer independent contractor status as it shifts responsibility for paying taxes, benefits, and malpractice to the NP (Brown & Dolan, 2016). Next consider what services will be provided. It is important to know how many days per week the NP will see patients; if there are an expected number of patients to be seen per day; what are the expectations of the physician with regard to collaboration; and what, if any, nonpatient care duties are expected of the NP. Time to review labs and diagnostics, document care, and communicate with patients and other providers is crucial for patient care, so it is worthwhile to investigate whether there is time allotted for this in the workday.

Once this information is obtained, it is important to examine the salary structure. Discover whether the salary is set, determined by productivity, or based on actual reimbursement. Finally, look at benefits and terms. Benefits include continuing education, health care coverage, and malpractice insurance. Be sure to examine the type of malpractice coverage offered. Occurrence-based policies protect the NP if the policy was in effect when the incident occurred, whereas claims-made policies must be in effect at the time of the incident *and* at the time of the claim. NPs should consider negotiating for "tail coverage" if the latter is in place in order to protect them if they are no longer employed at the site when a claim is made. A typical contract is 1 year in length with a 30-day notice period for termination. Increasingly, NP contracts contain non-compete clauses. These clauses restrict NPs from working in a competitive practice. Be wary of these clauses because they may substantially inhibit career mobility (Brown & Dolan, 2016).

If the NP is applying to a new position, identify what is attractive about the position and how it will fit with personal goals. These goals may not always be practice related. An NP may want to work less in order to pursue a hobby or spend more time with family or friends. Honest self-reflection about goals is important before discussing financial matters with a practice manager. Consider the importance of time off as well as salary and benefits. Being able to articulate personal desires to a practice manager is integral to continue to match the goals and interests of the practice. If the NP is interested in working only half-time but the practice is very busy and is hoping for additional hours, conflict may arise. Be sure to clarify the interests and directions of the practice and realistically consider whether an alternative proposal, a third solution or compromise, will address the needs of both parties.

◼ CONCLUSION

The APRN has become increasingly more important in the United States because of the limited availability of primary care physicians, coupled with a growing body of research that documents excellent outcomes with care provided by APRNs (Institute of Medicine [IOM], 2010). NPs constitute the bulk of APRNs, although few operate their practice in an entrepreneurial manner. However, these are the skills that are necessary to allow a knowledgeable clinician to flourish in a highly competitive, cost-conscious clinical environment. Knowledge about financial transactions and billing matters will enable NPs to become partners in health care practices and to contribute valuable suggestions for steering care toward approaches that are financially viable and contribute to improved patient outcomes. NPs must take on a greater role in the financial and business aspects of care if they wish the profession to flourish.

CRITICAL THINKING EXERCISES

1. Examine the Nurse Practice Act in your state. How are the NP and other APRN roles described? Is there opportunity for independence or does the law require supervision and collaboration? Can an NP develop an independent business in your state?

2a. What is your current contribution to the practice you are involved with? Calculate the revenue you generate. Also, evaluate the overhead in your practice site.

2b. Based on your revenue calculations, what amounts of funds are left for salary and profit? How does this correlate with your current salary?

3. What opportunities exist in your practice that add value to your services and improve patient care quality?

4. Identify your ideal NP position. Consider setting, hours, patient population, benefits, and terms. Compare your current position with your ideal position and determine what career advancement you should consider.

REFERENCES

Allen, K. R., Reinke, C. B., Pohl, J. M., Martyn, K. K., & McIntosh, E. P. (2003). Nurse practitioner coding practices in primary care: A retrospective chart review. *Journal of the American Academy of Nurse Practitioners, 15*(5), 231–236.

American Academy of Nurse Practitioners. (2013). *Position statement on nurse practitioner curriculum*. Washington, DC: Author.

American Association of Colleges of Nursing. (2006). *The essentials of doctoral education for advanced nursing practice*. Retrieved from http://www.aacnnursing.org/DNP/DNP-Essentials

American Medical Association. (2017). *CPT 2017: Professional edition*. Chicago, IL: American Medical Association Press.

Balen, B. A. (2014). "Incident to" billing: Is it worth it for medical practices? [Web log post]. Retrieved from http://www.physicianspractice.com/blog/incident-to-billing-it-worth-it-medical-practices

Bodenheimer, T. S., & Grumbach, K. (2016). *Understanding health policy: A clinical approach* (7th ed.). New York, NY: McGraw-Hill.

Bowman, S. (2016). Look back on the *ICD-10* transition: Crisis averted or imaginary? *Journal of American Health Information Management Association*, 87(8), 24–31.

Brown, L. A., & Dolan, C. (2016). Employment contracting basics for the nurse practitioner. *Journal for Nurse Practitioners*, 12(2), e45–e50.

Buppert, C. (2015). *Nurse practitioner's business practice and legal guide* (5th ed.). Burlington, MA: Jones & Bartlett.

Centers for Medicare and Medicaid Services. (2016). *Advanced practice registered nurses, anesthesiologist assistants, and physician assistants*. Washington, DC: Author.

Clack, C. A., Freeman, R., & Lewis, L. (2017, January 17). Provider's condensed resource for revenue cycle, coding tools, and more. *Journal of American Health Information Management* (1), 44–47.

Department of Health and Human Services. (2016). *Evaluation and management services*. Washington, DC: Author. Retrieved from https://www.cms.gov/Outreach-and-Education/Medicare-Learning-Network-MLN/MLNProducts/Downloads/eval-mgmt-serv-guide-ICN006764.pdf

Diers, D. (1991). Nurse-midwives and nurse anesthetists: The cutting edge in specialist practice. In L. H. Aiken & C. M. Fagin (Eds.), *Charting nursing's future: Agenda for the '90's* (pp. 159–180). Philadelphia, PA: J. B. Lippincott.

Frontier Nursing Service. (2000). *The frontier nursing service: A history*. Wendover, KY: Author.

Hoffman, L. A., & Guttendorf, J. (2014). Integrating nurse practitioners into the critical care team. Retrieved from https://www.ahcmedia.com/articles/31424-integrating-nurse-practitioners-into-the-critical-care-team

Huff, C. (2016). Solving the nation's primary care shortage: Increasing the number of U.S. physicians means tracking many complicated issues on numerous fronts. *Medical Economics*, 93(24), 42–45.

Institute of Medicine. (2010). *The future of nursing: Focus on education* (pp. 1–8). Retrieved from http://www.iom.edu/~/media/Files/Report%20Files/2010/The-Future-of-Nursing/Nursing%20Education%202010%20Brief.pdf

Keegan, D. W. (2012). Five key benchmarks that could make or break your practice. Retrieved from http://www.medscape.com/viewarticle/765783

LaSala, C. A., Connors, P. M., Pedro, J. T., & Phipps, M. (2007). The role of the clinical nurse specialist in promoting evidence-based practice and effecting positive patient outcomes. *Journal of Continuing Education in Nursing*, 38(6), 262–270.

McNeill, S. M. (2016). Lower your overhead with a patient portal. *Family Practice Management*, 23(2), 21–25.

Medicare Payment Advisory Commission. (2017). Report on Medicare payment policy. Retrieved from http://www.medpac.gov/docs/default-source/press-releases/mar17_medpac_report_newsrelease.pdf?sfvrsn=0

Moore, K. J. (2010). Documenting history in compliance with Medicare's guidelines. *Family Practice Management*, 17(2), 22–27.

Moore, L. G., & Wasson, J. H. (2007). The ideal medical practice: Improving efficiency, quality, and the doctor-patient relationship. *Family Practice Management*, 14(8), 20–24.

Moriyama, I. M., Loy, R. M., & Robb-Smith, A. H. T. (2011). *History of the statistical classification of diseases and causes of death*. Hyattsville, MD: National Center for Health Statistics.

National Nursing Centers Consortium. (2014). *NNCC's state-by-state guide to laws regarding nurse practitioner prescriptive authority and physician practice*. Philadelphia, PA: Author.

National Plan and Provider Enumeration System. (2011). The national plan and provider enumerations system. Retrieved from https://nppes.cms.hhs.gov/NPPES/Welcome.do

Naylor, M. D., & Kurtzman, E. T. (2010). The role of nurse practitioners in reinventing primary care. *Health Affairs*, 29(5), 893–899.

Nelson, R. (2010). FTEs per doctor—More than a number. Retrieved from http://www.medpagetoday.com/Columns/22099

O'Brien, J. M. (2003). How nurse practitioners obtained provider status: Lessons for pharmacists. *American Journal of Health-System Pharmacy, 60*(15), 2301–2307.

Phillips, S. J. (2017). 29th annual APRN legislative update. *The Nurse Practitioner Journal, 42*(1), 18–46.

Reeves, C. S. (2002). How many staff members do you need? *Family Practice Management, 9*(8), 45–49.

Savrin, C. (2009). Growth and development of the nurse practitioner role around the globe. *Journal of Pediatric Health Care, 23*(5), 310–314. doi:10.1016/j.pedhc.2008.10.005

WOCN (Wound, Ostomy, and Continence Nurses Society) Reimbursement Task Force and APRN Work Group. (2012). Reimbursement of advanced practice registered nurse services: A fact sheet. *Journal of Wound, Ostomy and Continence Nurses Society, 39*(25), S7–S16.

Yee, T., Boukus, E., Cross, D., & Samuel, D. (2013). *Primary care workforce shortages: Nurse practitioner scope-of-practice laws and payment policies.* Washington, DC: National Institute for Health Care Reform. Retrieved from http://nihcr.org/wp-content/uploads/2015/03/NIHCR_Research_Brief_No._13.pdf

6 Strategic Planning and Capital Budgeting

Mikhail Shneyder

As doctor of nursing practice (DNP) graduates are prepared to practice in a variety of roles, *The Essentials of Doctoral Education for Advanced Nursing Practice* calls for the development of "organizational and systems leadership" (American Association of Colleges of Nursing [AACN], 2006, p. 8) expertise. "Assessing organizations, identifying systems' issues, and facilitating organization-wide changes" (p. 10) are just a few attributes of a successful nurse leader. While preparing a DNP graduate to design, evaluate, and navigate complex organizational structures and develop "systems thinking and the business and financial acumen," (p. 10), this chapter addresses many requisite elements of the *DNP Essentials* and answers a variety of practice questions (AACN, 2006).

In the world of always-competing priorities, ever-increasing complexity, and persistent uncertainty, how do organizations manage to stay on track, move forward, evolve, and even succeed? What drives nurse executives and managers to make certain decisions, select one project over another, or lead their respective institutions and units? With thousands of employees, seemingly disconnected from each other, why do some large companies manage to function as single cohesive organisms? Who provides the proverbial glue to hold it all together at the core?

In this chapter, we explore the answers to these and other questions that arise when observing organizations, both large and small. The first part of the chapter is dedicated to discussing a sample organizational framework that allows nurse executives and managers to lead and stay on course. Here, we introduce the concepts of strategy, alignment, organizational planning, executing, and monitoring as well as provide sample tools for accomplishing these important leadership functions. The second part looks at capital budgeting, project feasibility, evaluation, and selection and provides a sample model for financial decision making. Although the concepts and tools contained herein are widely applicable to many industries, we concentrate on nursing services and nursing education.

▨ STRATEGY PROCESS

Having its roots in the military, the term *strategy* is generally defined as the process of carefully devising and executing plans to achieve particular goals ("Strategy," n.d., para 2b). Many business

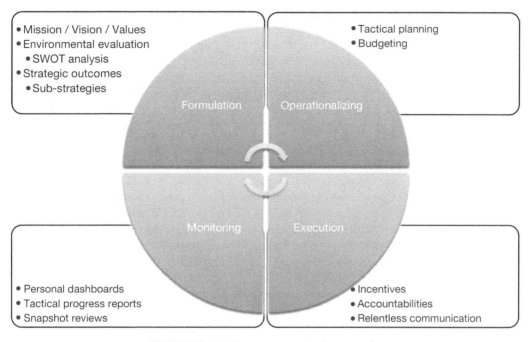

FIGURE 6.1 Strategy process framework.

SWOT, strengths, weaknesses, opportunities, threats.

schools dedicate entire academic courses to exploring the concept of strategy, and numerous in-depth texts have been devoted to this topic. Here we offer a sample framework for strategy process in organizations. It is meant as a practical and somewhat simplified overview and not as an exhaustive exploration of organizational strategy.

Not unlike a nurse utilizing the nursing process to care for patients, leaders rely on systematic, cyclical, dynamic, broad-based approaches to ensure the continual health and success of their organizations. Although there are numerous variations of approaches and frameworks for strategy, the principal elements of the cycle remain fairly constant: assessment, planning, implementation, and evaluation. To differentiate our sample framework from the nursing process, we define the four stages in the strategy process as *formulation, operationalizing, execution,* and *monitoring.* All elements of the strategy process are interconnected. The relationship between them is illustrated in Figure 6.1.

We define each of the stages, break them down into elements, and provide tools a nurse executive or manager could use in establishing, implementing, and monitoring the organization's strategy.

STRATEGY FORMULATION

The strategy process in an organization commences and culminates with its *governing board,* frequently referred to as *board of directors, board of managers,* or *board of trustees,* which delegates strategy responsibilities to the executive leadership. The board is then engaged mainly as the final approver, ultimately sanctioning both the strategic plan and the budget every year. This approach ensures suitable involvement by the board while permitting for broad engagement across the entire organization. To focus the strategy process, an organization's leadership often establishes a *strategy committee,* mainly consisting of members of executive management and department heads.

Moreover, a *director of strategy* is usually named. In large organizations, this frequently is a full-time position reporting directly to the president or CEO, whereas smaller firms assign the task to a member of the management team. The director of strategy and strategy committee lead the strategy process and determine the timing of each of its components.

The strategy formulation begins annually with executives, managers, staff, and the strategy committee reviewing, engaging in widespread dialogue about, and, if needed, recommending revisions to the organization's *mission, vision, values,* and *strategic goals statements.*

Mission

At large, an organization's *mission* is its reason for existing. A firm expresses its mission in a succinct, precise declaration that is known as the *mission statement,* or a present-oriented passage that describes what the organization is and does. Mission statements should be stable and long lasting. However, as an organization evolves, so could its mission. Hence, mission statements should be periodically evaluated for their fit with the overall organizational trajectory and adjusted as needed. Following are a few examples of actual mission statements from health care and higher education organizations.

Cleveland Clinic—"The mission of Cleveland Clinic centers on improving patient care, researching diseases, and further developing healthcare professionals" (The Cleveland Clinic, 2017).

Mayo Clinic—"To inspire hope and contribute to health and well-being by providing the best care to every patient through integrated clinical practice, education and research" (Mayo Clinic, 1998–2017).

Johns Hopkins Medicine—"Johns Hopkins Medicine strives to elevate health of local communities and the world while promoting diversity and inclusiveness in educating the next generation of doctors, allied health professionals and health researchers" (Johns Hopkins Medicine, 2017).

Nightingale College—"Guided by the principles of confidence, competence, and compassion, Nightingale College is committed to creating pathways to educational and professional success for its learners, alumni, and collaborators; to improving the communities it serves; and to elevating health care" (Nightingale College, 2017).

Vision

John Naisbitt, a world-renowned business author and speaker, asserted "strategic planning is worthless—unless there is first a strategic vision" (Naisbitt, 1982, p. 94). Strategy is what takes an organization from where it is today, living its mission, to where it wants to be, realizing its *vision.* Therefore, a *vision statement* is a forward-looking pronouncement that describes what a firm aspires to be and do. In some organizations, a charismatic leader at the helm specifies the vision statement, whereas others develop organically within the firm and then surface at the top. In either case, executive leadership and governing boards have the responsibility of clearly stating the organization's vision. Vision statements must inspire all in the organization to perform and achieve. They are motivational in nature but also measurable and actionable. Here are a few examples.

Cleveland Clinic—"Cleveland Clinic envisions being in the global vanguard of patient care and outcomes as well as clinical research and education" (The Cleveland Clinic, 2017).

Vanderbilt University School of Nursing—"The Vanderbilt University School of Nursing will continuously reinvent itself in ways that distinguishes the School among its peers, with innovations in academics, faculty practice, research, and informatics and an unparalleled focus on activities that benefit the community and society at large" (Vanderbilt University School of Nursing, 2017).

Nightingale College—"Better Health & Better Humanity for a Better World" (Nightingale College, 2017).

Values

Organizational *values* provide a framework that allows all within a firm to evaluate their decisions, take pride in their institution's work, and make commitments. Values serve as criteria for prioritization, problem solving, conflict resolution, and strategy development. Much like mission and vision statements, values must be supported by the firm's leadership, openly stated, modeled, and followed. In the absence of clearly articulated organizational values, every employee's bias would serve as a compass for decision making, thus rendering cohesive functioning of the institution impossible. Often, *core values statements* include explanations of the individual value components. Following are examples of values statements.

Mayo Clinic:

"Primary value: The needs of the patient come first.

Respect: Treat everyone in our diverse community, including patients, their families and colleagues, with dignity.

Compassion: Provide the best care, treating patients and family members with sensitivity and empathy.

Integrity: Adhere to the highest standards of professionalism, ethics and personal responsibility, worthy of the trust our patients place in us.

Healing: Inspire hope and nurture the well-being of the whole person, respecting physical, emotional and spiritual needs.

Teamwork: Value the contributions of all, blending the skills of individual staff members in unsurpassed collaboration.

Excellence: Deliver the best outcomes and highest quality service through the dedicated effort of every team member.

Innovation: Infuse and energize the organization, enhancing the lives of those we serve, through the creative ideas and unique talents of each employee.

Stewardship: Sustain and reinvest in our mission and extended communities by wisely managing our human, natural and material resources." (Mayo Clinic, 1998–2017)

Johns Hopkins Medicine:

"Excellence and Discovery, Leadership and Integrity, Diversity and Inclusion, Respect and Collegiality." (Johns Hopkins Medicine, 2017)

Vanderbilt University School of Nursing:

"The Vanderbilt University School of Nursing values innovation in preserving and advancing the art and science of nursing in academics, faculty practice, research and informatics. These values are demonstrated through transactions that integrate technology and embrace cultural and academic diversity" (Vanderbilt University School of Nursing, 2017).

Nightingale College:

"Florence Nightingale, the founder of modern nursing, lit the way for success with her unwavering values. Today and always, we commit to following her path of going beyond self with excellence, integrity, respecting humanity, collaboration, continuous improvement, and accountability.

- Beyond self: A commitment to selflessly serving others.
- Excellence: A commitment to actualizing all potentials.
- Integrity: A commitment to doing what is right.
- Respecting humanity: A commitment to honoring and accepting every individual.
- Collaboration: A commitment to building synergy and succeeding together.
- Continuous improvement: A commitment to evolving relentlessly.
- Accountability: A commitment to fulfilling all commitments." (Nightingale College, 2017)

Mission, vision, and values are at the core of institutions' day-to-day lives, strategic planning, decisions, dialogue, and public persona. However, in order to be impactful, these principles must be relentlessly communicated throughout the organization. This responsibility falls on executives and managers. Through posters, banners, wallet cards, computer screen savers, and numerous other means, these important core components of the organization must be made visible and accessible to all. New employees' assimilation into an institution must commence with an in-depth discussion of the organizational history, mission, vision, and values. Ongoing, company-wide application and evaluation of these pillars must permeate the day-to-day work lives and provide a compelling basis for employees' *alignment*, a concept we discuss later in this chapter. Only then would there be a solid foundation for strategy and organizational success. The director of strategy facilitates the annual company-wide dialogue about the mission, vision, and values and then consolidates the feedback from constituents, whose participation is critical, and presents it to the strategy committee. Soliciting input from throughout the organization can be done in various formats: individual interviews, team meetings, and internal and external advisory committees. Thorough documentation is an essential part of this process. In turn, the strategy committee meets and reviews the input, ultimately deciding whether to recommend any alterations to the governing board. Organizational mission, vision, and values tend to be stable over time; however, significant changes in either the internal or external environment may prompt revisions to the established statements. The final recommendations of the strategy committee, if any, with regard to the mission, vision, and values are presented to the board for review and approval.

Alignment

According to Abraham Maslow's widely accepted theory of human needs, human drive to self-actualize, or "the tendency to become actually in what he is potentially: to become everything that one is capable of becoming," is universal (Maslow, 1943, pp. 382–383). Per Maslow, self-actualizing individuals display several common characteristics, such as perceiving reality efficiently, tolerating uncertainty, accepting themselves and others for what they are, being problem-centered rather than self-centered, and concerned for the welfare of humanity, among others (Maslow, 1970). Considering these attributes, it is not difficult to imagine the positive impacts that employing self-actualizing individuals would have on organizations. Because the clear majority of individuals devote a significant portion of their lives to work in order to support themselves and their families, organizations must ensure that employees have ample opportunities to elevate toward self-actualizing while meeting all lower level needs along the way.

". . . [P]roper management of the work lives of human beings, of the way in which they earn their living, can improve them and improve the world . . ." (Maslow, 1998, p. 1). Therefore, an organization's mission, vision, and values must inform the company's culture and speak to employees' deeply held beliefs about the world while continually satisfying the desire for meaningful contributions and growth. In the absence of such meaning, institutions find it more difficult to attract and retain employees and, therefore, to succeed strategically and financially. Fortunately, nursing services and education are largely perceived as generating public good rather than harm and, hence, their employees find it easier to align themselves with the stated missions, visions, and values than those who work, for example, in the tobacco industry. This, however, does not happen by accident: systems and processes leading to alignment must be carefully designed, and all employees should understand and be able to verbalize the connection between who they are and what they do on a daily basis and their institution continually living its mission and moving closer to realizing its vision.

An employee's alignment matures along three distinct dimensions: cultural, role, and developmental. *Cultural alignment* refers to the degree employees subscribe to, accept, and model their employer's mission, vision, and values. *Role alignment* encompasses the extent to which an employee's job matches his or her passions and the level of skills and knowledge he or she possesses to be successful in the job. Finally, *developmental alignment* speaks to an employee's level of satisfying his or her needs along Maslow's hierarchy. We discuss these concepts more in-depth later in this chapter.

Strategic Goals

Having its roots in the popular framework, developed in the early 1990s and first published in *The Balanced Scorecard: Translating Strategy Into Action* (Kaplan & Norton, 1996), this approach provides a sample method for linking the organization's mission, vision, and day-to-day operations. To begin, an institution develops a set of *strategic goals* or *strategic outcomes*. These are broad, high-level statements that set targets for and describe how a firm progresses from the state of its present mission to the state of its desired vision. The road to identifying strategic goals begins with a comprehensive *environmental evaluation* both within and outside the organization.

Environmental Evaluation

An environmental evaluation is performed annually at each of the institution's functional departments and operating units by *evaluation teams* comprised of managers and staff. The goal of these exercises is to pinpoint where each department, unit, and, cumulatively, the entire firm stand in regard to the stated mission, vision, and existing strategic outcomes and how they should proceed forward. Of course, an even more effective approach to the environmental evaluation processes would be continual institutional assessment.

To inform their research and determinations, evaluation teams mine data from various sources of operational, financial, and market information such as client and employee surveys, company and regulatory agency reports, internal financial statements and projections, institutional performance measures, research conducted and published by universities and governmental agencies, program review results (in academic establishments), and community surveys and interviews. In many organizations, the distinct functional department of *institutional research* plays a significant role in providing data for the environmental evaluation.

Staff and client feedback may be collected in a variety of ways. Numerous reliable survey tools and companies exist to assist organizations with these tasks. Additionally, internal listening sessions may be conducted, in which clients and employees are afforded the opportunity to comment on the strategic direction of the organization. Limited in the number of participants (normally 10 to 20), these invitation-only sessions seek input concerning individuals' vision for the organization, their take on the strategic goals, and suggestions for the future. In similar fashion, advisory committee meetings are conducted with representatives of local communities and other stakeholders. Additionally, in organizations with strong communication cultures, top executives lead periodic "town hall" meetings. These gatherings are open to all employees, allowing the leaders to solicit direct input from the internal constituents. Documentation from all forms of listening sessions serves as a basis for the work of evaluation teams.

Evaluation teams examine and synthesize the various data and uncover trends; then, based on the findings, create comprehensive *SWOT analyses*, and make recommendations concerning unit- and organization-level strategic goals to the strategy committee.

SWOT Analysis

Referring to an organization's strengths, weaknesses, opportunities, and threats, the acronym *SWOT* was coined in the 1960s (Learned, Christensen, Andrews, & Guth, 1965) and is a commonly used tool for analyzing a firm's strategic capabilities and positioning. To minimize bias, SWOTs should be derived not based on individual opinions, but rather on comprehensive data sets from broad-based environmental evaluations. In SWOT, the strengths and weaknesses refer to the trends in the company's internal environment, whereas external forces drive the opportunities and threats. Many free SWOT resources and templates are available to the executives and managers today. Table 6.1 illustrates a generic SWOT template and sample probing questions.

On completion of SWOT analyses, evaluation teams meet, discuss findings, and formulate recommendations for strategic goals and outcomes, which, ultimately, must align with the current mission, move the institution closer to achieving its stated vision, and be consistent with the set of organizational values. Subsequently, functional departments and operating units' leaders present the SWOT analyses along with recommendations to the strategy committee, which, in turn, may request that units and departments act on specific conclusions and/or report back with additional information. At the conclusion of this process, the strategy committee makes its final decision to include findings and recommendations in its strategic outcomes and *substrategies*, which are subsequently presented to the board.

Strategic Outcomes and Substrategies

Once the board approves the mission, vision, and values, the strategy committee works to review and, if necessary, revise the company's strategic outcomes. Normally, an organization chooses to pursue a handful of high-level strategic outcomes at any one time. In choosing and prioritizing the outcomes to include in the annual and long-term plans, strategic leadership considers the potential operational and financial impacts of each; evaluates their alignment with the mission, vision, and values; and sets measurable, well-defined targets within the outcomes. Often, top strategic

TABLE 6.1 Sample SWOT Template and Questions

Strengths	Weaknesses
In what aspects does our unit/organization excel?	In what aspects does our unit/organization fall short?
What makes our unit/organization attractive to customers?	Which areas of our operations may be vulnerable?
	Why are we underperforming in certain areas of our operations?
What differentiates our unit/organization from the other players in the industry?	
Opportunities	**Threats**
Are there new market developments that could offer our unit/organization opportunities to grow?	Is there a proposed regulation that could significantly affect the way we operate?
	Has a new direct competitor emerged?
Are there any underserved geographical areas?	Are our offerings still relevant to the customers and markets we serve?
Could our core competencies allow us to create and offer a new service?	

SWOT, strengths, weaknesses, opportunities, threats.

goals include improvements to the organization's core business outcomes. In a hospital, for example, patient-centered outcomes aimed at quality and cost of care would be at the core of the strategic plan, whereas a nursing school would concentrate on several student achievement measures, such as learning outcomes, graduation rates, and licensure examination results.

People Outcomes

As we discussed earlier in this chapter, an organization's strategic and financial success as well as the achievement of its mission rely heavily on the alignment of its employees and their ability to experience continual professional and personal growth in the context of work. Yet, most companies pay no or very little attention to their *people outcomes* as part of the strategic analyses and planning, and even fewer have specific human resources (HR)-targeted narratives within their mission and vision statements. In service organizations, human capital is the most essential and costly asset; hence, it must be one of the main focal points within the strategy process. As mentioned earlier in this chapter, employees' alignment and, hence, their company's people outcomes lie along three distinct dimensions: cultural, role, and developmental, concepts discussed next.

Cultural Alignment and Outcomes

Recall that cultural alignment refers to the degree employees subscribe to, accept, and model their employer's mission, vision, and values. Hence, institutions should continually evaluate cultural alignment of employees and develop systems and processes to strengthen it. For example, to assess its collaborators' alignment, Nightingale College utilizes periodic built-in self-reflection and dialoguing throughout the organization. Everyone at the college is invited to contemplate, record, and discuss with others answers to various questions. What are you doing personally and professionally to align with the college's vision? How do you contribute to the college's mission on a daily basis? In some companies, the focus on cultural alignment begins well before a new employee is invited to join the organization. These firms clearly communicate their cultural pillars and expectations in employment advertising and throughout the candidate selection process. Many also undertake culture benchmarking through several psychometric products available on the market and incorporate these tools into preemployment cultural alignment screenings. Finally, through employee surveys, companies can gauge the aggregate level of cultural alignment. However, the best indicators for positive cultural alignment are low turnover, high levels of productivity, and strong internal employment referral base.

Role Alignment and Outcomes

Organizations cannot succeed strategically without having the right people in the right jobs, or sound role alignment, throughout the firm. For every employee, the role alignment lies in the convergence of his or her technical expertise and his or her enthusiasm toward performing the duties of the job. Of course, professional knowledge and skills are important for success in fulfilling the responsibilities of any job. However, these attributes alone cannot sustain productivity and effectiveness in the long term; passion for what one does must always permeate day-to-day duties for endured success. The more *passion skills* an employee utilizes in execution of everyday responsibilities, the better outcomes he or she will achieve in his or her role. Therefore, an organization's outcomes in role alignment could be classified into two categories: continual professional development of skills and knowledge and personal job match. The concepts of continual professional development and lifelong learning are widely accepted in the nursing profession, and many organizations invest heavily in this arena. However, only a few firms purposely assess their employees' levels of expertise, as related to specific role responsibilities, and engage the workforce in individually focused professional development. Furthermore, most organizations do not gauge their employees' zeal for impact along with aspirations and consequently do not direct resources toward modifying role responsibilities and organizational structures to fully capitalize on and further build each person's unique set of passion skills. Quite oppositely, many institutions inadvertently create hostile work environments while driving the culture of excellence, through their focus on punitive rather than developmental approaches to performance management. As the result, most employees spend inordinate amounts of time "covering up their weaknesses, managing other people's impressions of them, showing themselves to their best advantage, playing politics, hiding their inadequacies, hiding their uncertainties, hiding their limitations," resulting in tremendous negative economic impact to their companies (Kegan & Lahey, 2016, p. 1). Reflection and dialoguing are, once again, important tools to solicit employees' self-assessment on the topic of role alignment and strengthen the corresponding people outcomes, such as job satisfaction, engagement, and effectiveness. In the context of reflection, employees should contemplate the degree to which their current level of expertise matches the specific role competencies and transparently communicate any perceived deficiencies to their managers. In addition, they should self-assess the alignment of their passion skills with current and, if applicable, aspirational roles. Conversely, employers must commit to creating safe environments for employees' continual professional growth and set aside ample resources within strategic planning and budgeting for the workforce development and organizational fluidity.

Developmental Alignment and Outcomes

Another way to address the issue of people outcomes within organizations is through utilization of Maslow's hierarchy of needs model (Maslow, 1943, pp. 370–396). In this context, an institution's people development and outcomes could be broadly divided into four categories: *health and wellness* (basic physiological needs), *company environment* (safety and security), *relationships* (love and belonging), and *achievement and recognition* (esteem). Over the last decade, the focus on HR personal growth along Maslow's hierarchy and other humanistic psychology theories of adult development led a few pioneering companies across different industries to become deliberately developmental organizations (DDOs). A DDO is organized around the idea that "organizations will best prosper when they are more deeply aligned with people's strongest motive, which is to grow" (Kegan & Lahey, 2016, blurb). Notably, DDOs deliberately focus on and invest in continual personal development of their people at all levels of the organization and consequently experience higher levels of employee engagement and satisfaction, very stable workforces, and significantly better business outcomes across the board, as compared to their peers, including greater profitability, better error detection in operational and strategic design, reduction in cost structures, and political maneuvering (Kegan & Lahey, 2016, pp. 1–2). Published in 2016, *An Everyone Culture: Becoming a Deliberately Developmental Organization* takes a closer look at the theories behind and practical applications of the DDO movement in three U.S companies: Next Jump—an e-commerce tech company; the Decurion Corporation—a parent to several operating subsidiaries, including Pacific Theatres, Robertson Properties Group (RPG), ArcLight Cinemas, and Hollybrook Senior Living; and Bridgewater—the world's best-performing hedge fund (Kegan & Lahey, 2016). Nightingale College is one of the examples of a DDO in nursing education; maintaining a comprehensive health and wellness program and elevating performance through leadership and professional development, mentorship programs, and performance recognition are samples of its people developmental alignment outcomes.

People outcomes should be explicitly incorporated into an organization's strategies and receive the management's attention on par with other institutional priorities. In other words, a company should look at its "culture as itself a business strategy" and the "relationship between realizing human potential and organizational potential . . . [a]s dialectic, not a trade-off" (Kegan & Lahey, 2016, p. 6). In the strategy formulation stage, it is necessary to develop *substrategies*, or methods, for achieving the broad strategic goals. Each substrategy must retain the measurability and explicit target aspects of the strategic objective it serves. Customarily, specific metrics, data-gathering

TABLE 6.2 Sample Strategic Outcomes and Substrategies

Strategic Outcome	Substrategies
Be the brand of choice for adult nursing services in our geographical area	• Establish internal quality benchmarks based on the NDNQI data and strive for the 90th-percentile ranking minimum on all indicators • Enhance promotional materials' quality and seek new distribution channels • Improve availability of services across the system • Create strong communications culture with referring physicians
Invest in long-term growth initiatives	• Pursue strategic acquisitions • Open two new clinic branches per year • Further diversify service offerings
Achieve a 10% year-over-year increase in profit margin	• Decrease the average length of stay • Increase ED throughput • Educate staff nurses regarding the cost of care factors

ED, emergency department; NDNQI, National Database of Nursing Quality Indicators.

methods, and evaluation techniques are described within the substrategies. In addition, accountability for achieving each substrategy could be assigned to a member of the executive team. Table 6.2 represents sample strategic outcomes with the corresponding substrategies.

Strategic outcomes and substrategies tend to be more fluid than the mission, vision, and values: over time, outcomes are accomplished and strategic priorities may change. As they arise from the mission, vision, and values, strategic goals would likely change, should there be overarching transformations in these core organizational pillars.

Ample time should be allocated each year for the strategy committee members to work on formulating strategic outcomes and substrategies during the scheduled multiday strategy sessions. The completed product of the strategy formulation process, including mission, vision, values, strategic outcomes, and substrategies, is then presented to the board for approval. After the board resolves to accept the strategic plan, the revised strategic summary document is disseminated throughout the organization and the operationalizing and execution stages of the strategy process begin.

STRATEGY OPERATIONALIZING

After the strategy formulation stage is complete, each functional department and operating unit as well as the organization at large must *operationalize*, or translate, their environmental evaluations, SWOT findings, strategic outcomes, and substrategies into concrete, executable tasks and project the costs associated with these undertakings. Hence, the operationalizing stage of the strategy process consists of two distinct components: *tactical planning* and *budgeting*.

Tactical Planning

Tactics are the planned activities undertaken to meet the stated strategic outcomes. On receiving approval from the board for the company's strategic plan, the director of strategy initiates the tactical planning process by distributing the tactical planning packet, including tactical map template, instructions for completion, and timelines, to all unit and department heads. In turn, these leaders facilitate the process within their respective operating and functional areas, involving staff in developing the plans.

TABLE 6.3 Tactical Map Template

Strategic Objective #1					
Substrategy 1.1	Tactic	Owner	Cost and timing	Complete by	Quarterly status update
Substrategy 1.2	Tactic	Owner	Cost and timing	Complete by	Quarterly status update
Substrategy 1.3	Tactic	Owner	Cost and timing	Complete by	Quarterly status update

Linking day-to-day work functions to the strategic plan, *tactical maps* present the tactics to be performed by units, departments, teams, and individual employees within an organization. In addition to including tasks targeted to achieving relevant company-level strategic outcomes and substrategies, operating units and functional departments incorporate actionable items from the respective environmental evaluations, SWOT analyses, and people outcomes into their tactical plans for the upcoming fiscal year. Each tactic must be associated with a substrategy, carry a target completion deadline, and be assigned an "owner." Furthermore, if a tactic requires any financial expenditure, the map must indicate its amount and timing for budgeting purposes. Tactical maps' alignment with the overall organizational strategy is of paramount importance. An example of a tactical map template is presented in Table 6.3.

After tactical maps are complete, operating and functional leaders present them to the strategy committee and company executives during interactive planning and budgeting review meetings, where tactics approval, denial, deferral, or revision decisions are made. The maps are then finalized and recommended to the board for approval. Once approved, execution of the tactical plans begins on the first day of the fiscal year.

Budgeting

Organizations normally undertake *budgeting*, or a financial planning process, over several months during the second half of each fiscal year. New budgets become effective on the first day of a new fiscal year. The budgeting stage of the strategy process runs in conjunction with the tactical planning. As tactics are approved, the budgetary concerns associated with them become approved as well. Tactical plans carry embedded expenses that belong to either *operating* or *capital* budgets. Although every organization establishes its own classification for budget entries, usually items with the total outlay of $1,000 or more are considered *capital expenditures*, commonly abbreviated as *CapEx*. Budgeting for operations is explored in depth in Chapters 3 and 4 of this textbook, whereas CapEx budgeting is discussed later in the second part of this chapter.

STRATEGY EXECUTION AND MONITORING

"However beautiful the strategy, you should occasionally look at the results."

—Winston Churchill

After all of the methodical planning, lack of sound strategy execution and monitoring may become the pitfall, preventing a company from realizing its mission and achieving the vision. Strategy cannot be a separately compartmentalized function of an organization or simply "another thing to do"; instead, it must be interwoven deep into the fabric of the organization, permeate the day-to-day employee activities, and be "the way of life" in the company. In order to compel employees to perform at the highest possible levels and fulfill the tactics set forth, organizations must first establish strategy-aligned *incentives*, *accountabilities*, and *communication* programs as well as "close-the-loop" systems.

Incentives and Accountabilities

As organizational systems drive employees' focus and behaviors, leadership must ensure that the incentives and accountabilities structures implemented in the organization are geared toward accomplishing strategic outcomes. One of the common methods of enticing employees to achieve and exceed set goals is to tie individual, unit, department, and firm-wide operational, financial, and strategic results to a portion of employees' total compensation. This is accomplished through fiscal year-end cash bonuses, commonly referred to as *gains*, or profit, *sharing*. Many companies hire consultants to assist them in creating these often quite elaborate programs. Most successful incentive plans cover every employee in an organization. Let us explore a sample *incentive compensation* framework.

Gains Sharing

Prior to the start of every fiscal year, the board, in collaboration with the executive leadership, creates a plan outlining the terms for and setting the aggregate dollar amount limits of year-end bonuses to be paid throughout the organization, while retaining the right to modify, adjust up or down, suspend, or even cancel the gain sharing in the event of unforeseen extraordinary events, internal or external. The aggregate limits normally increase as the organization's financial performance is improved, until the maximum aggregate payout is reached. The board then sets the maximum bonus amounts for each of the levels of employees, expressed as a percentage of the annual salary. The maximum percentage levels tend to increase toward the top echelons of leadership in the company. For example, a staff nurse may have an opportunity to earn a bonus in the amount of 5% of his or her salary, whereas a chief nursing officer (CNO) could receive up to 25% of his or hers.

TABLE 6.4 Employee Bonus Criteria Decision Matrix

Results Level	Strategic (1/3)	Operational (1/3)	Financial (1/3)
Company (1/2)	Outcomes	Critical quality and operating targets	EBITDA
Department/Unit (1/4)	Tactics and outcomes	Critical quality and operating targets	EBITDA
Individual (1/4)	Tactics[a]	Individual goals[a]	Individual contribution

[a]When an employee does not bear any direct responsibility over revenue or expenses, strategic and operational results are weighted equally at ½.

EBITDA, earnings before interest, taxes, depreciation, and amortization.

After the maximum percentage targets have been set, every employee's actual bonus amount is driven by several factors and is based on specific weighting assigned to each. The decision matrix in Table 6.4 illustrates sample criteria for bonus payouts and proportion weights of each of the line items. Reaching the stated outcomes and goals, fulfilling the assigned tactics, and meeting the budgetary projections at every level of the organization are common determinants of individual incentive compensation.

Certain organizations take the "all-or-nothing" approach for each of the matrix squares, whereas others give some leeway for partial achievements. For example, the board and the leadership might decide that reaching 90% of the budgeted *earnings before interest, taxes, depreciation, and amortization (EBITDA)*, or the difference between a firm's operating revenues and expenses, will trigger a reduced level bonus payout, and then progressively increase to 100% for the criterion. According to Table 6.4, one half of every employee's bonus will depend on how well the company performed during the year. Hence, if the firm fully succeeded in every criterion, the staff nurse mentioned earlier will add a minimum of 2.5% to his or her earnings for the year.

Conversely, in the "all-or-nothing" scenario, where the company did not meet all of its strategic outcomes but achieved the target EBITDA and critical quality and operating targets, the nurse would only earn 1.67% ($= 5\% \times \frac{1}{2} \times (\frac{1}{3} + \frac{1}{3})$, rounded up) of his or her annual salary for the company's performance during the fiscal year. Similar logic is applied to other criteria in the matrix to arrive to the total payout percentage for every staff member.

In order to motivate employees to not only meet the stated goals, outcomes, and projections, but to exceed them as well, the leadership often establishes additional discretionary bonus pools for overachievement and sets "stretch" triggers for payout. For example, if the company outperforms on its financial targets, employees have a chance of doubling their bonuses, as illustrated in Table 6.5. Similarly, bonus reductions could be set for underachieving.

Finally, to help avoid gross underperformance in key strategic outcomes or operational and quality measures, the gains sharing plan must contain caveats that would reduce total bonuses at

TABLE 6.5 Stretch EBITDA Targets With Corresponding Bonus Upsides

Percent of EBITDA Achieved	Percent of Bonus Earned	Percent of EBITDA Achieved	Percent of Bonus Earned	Percent of EBITDA Achieved	Percent of Bonus Earned	Percent of EBITDA Achieved	Percent of Bonus Earned
101	102	114	128	127	154	139	178
102	104	115	130	128	156	140	180
103	106	116	132	129	158	141	182
104	108	117	134	130	160	142	184
105	110	118	136	131	162	143	186
106	112	119	138	132	164	144	188
107	114	120	140	133	166	145	190
108	116	121	142	134	168	146	192
109	118	122	144	135	170	147	194
110	120	123	146	136	172	148	196
111	122	124	148	137	174	149	198
112	124	125	150	138	176	150	200
113	126	126	152				

EBITDA, earnings before interest, taxes, depreciation, and amortization.

certain levels of deficiencies. For example, if the student attrition rate in a nursing school exceeds the target by more than 20%, everyone in the organization loses 10% of his or her respective bonus amounts. In addition, all individual bonus amounts will be prorated down equally if the aggregate payout amount exceeds the established limit at the achieved level of EBITDA.

Although gains sharing plans are excellent tools for attracting, retaining, and rewarding employees, promoting unit cohesion and teamwork as well as improving the firm's performance and achieving the strategic outcomes, organizations must exercise care in ensuring that ample control systems are put in place to prevent any potential cheating or gaming by members of the staff (Prendergast, 1999, pp. 7–63). On the other hand, successes, however small, should be publicly celebrated.

It is worth noticing that incentive compensation does not always need to be monetary to be effective in motivating employees throughout the year, as long as it is perceived to carry meaningful value for each affected individual (Baker et al., 1988, pp. 593–616). Hence, organization-wide achievement recognition programs could be implemented in parallel with the gains sharing. In fact, such mechanisms satisfy employees' innate esteem needs and contribute to their elevation to self-actualizing, thus improving the overall economic state of an institution. For example, at Nightingale College, every collaborator is encouraged to recognize his or her fellows through submitting "values spotlight" notes for anyone exemplifying one or more of the company's values at any time. Every functional and committee meeting also begins and ends with a values spotlight. The college also bestows annual "Flame! Forward!" awards to celebrate collaborators who consistently demonstrate exceptional cultural alignment, and "Founder's Club" awards are given to those who have made significant and lasting contributions toward the achievement of the organization's mission and realization of its vision. These public recognitions take place during annual company-wide collaborator appreciation dinners.

Performance Management

To further drive strategy execution, parallel to the incentives, the leadership establishes accountability, or *performance management*, programs. Counter to the widely utilized performance management mechanisms, DDOs move away from *annual performance appraisals* and *performance improvement plans* toward continual built-in *self-reflection*, ongoing *dialoguing and feedback*, and individualized *development plans*. We discuss both approaches in some detail.

Successful execution of any organizational strategy relies heavily on the comprehensive understanding of, company-wide subscription to, and modeling of its elements: mission, vision, values, and strategic outcomes. In order to be consequential for employees, the alignment with these principles must be a significant part of the annual performance appraisal process. Employees' work results and behaviors must be evaluated according to the observable and measurable components of the strategic pillars. For example, if service excellence is one of the clinic's core values, staff nurses might have patient satisfaction survey results incorporated into their appraisals to evaluate the degree to which they act according to this value. Conversely, when the responsibility for tactics is assigned to individual "owners" during the operationalizing stage of the strategy process and the accountability for the substrategies is placed on the respective executives, these employees' annual appraisals must reflect how well the set goals were accomplished.

So as to not find employees blindsided during the annual performance appraisal process, organizations must institute the culture of *periodic feedback*, where managers are required to check in with their staff from time to time during the year and provide feedback, both positive and constructive, whereas individual employees are invited to solicit and welcome such feedback. Similar to the annual appraisal criteria, periodic feedback sessions must carry the elements of organizational strategy and critical quality and operating targets. For managers, one such measure could be providing timely periodic feedback to employees. In DDOs, however, this approach takes the center stage in performance management. Not only leaders are required to continually connect and dialogue with their direct reports in respect to cultural, role, and developmental alignment, but also employees, through weekly, dedicated time allowances, are invited to self-reflect and share their findings on these topics with the leadership. From these reflections and discussions, individualized development plans are made. These plans, at Nightingale College per se, carry specific "elevate points" and pathways for closer alignment, or steps to continual personal and professional development.

In the traditional approach, to be most effective, a constructive *performance improvement plan* should be a collaborative effort between the manager and the staff member, whose work results or behaviors are not on track with the strategic foundation or outcomes. Uncovering the root causes of objectively assessed underperformance and creating concrete, timed tactics for course correction are at the heart of this process. Often, employees' fit with the assigned job duties or tactics are evaluated, so these could be reassigned in a timely manner, if needed, to keep the organization on track for achieving its strategic outcomes. It is worth noticing that performance improvement plans should not be punitive, but rather targeted for finding creative solutions to problems. However, in some cases, when these efforts do not produce the expected results, further corrective actions may be undertaken.

Effective performance and organizational behavior management require leaders to have a specifically unique set of skills. Unfortunately, the overwhelming majority of people in leadership roles do not have the requisite expertise to be effective in this realm. Realizing the fact, organizations devote significant economic resources to periodic leadership development trainings, centered on employee motivation and behavior modification. Unfortunately, the effectiveness of these efforts is marginal, at best. A few pioneering organizations, including Nightingale College, undertake an alternative approach to the problem. Rather than relying on constant management retraining, these companies invest in separation of the technical and behavioral management. Since individuals who elevate to leadership positions usually possess incredible technical expertise, including the ability to effectively modify functional systems and processes for utmost strategic impact, these employees' utilization within organizations must capitalize on their passion skills, without diffusing time and energy to noneffective undertakings, like attempting to affect cultural and developmental alignment attributes of their reports. Consequently, these functions may be split away from the technical management and allocated to individuals whose expertise lies in counseling and coaching. These coaches serve as neutral champions of personal elevation and development for everyone in an organization while effectively mediating management conflicts, leadership challenges, and communication shortcomings. Although as of the day of publication of this work no empirical proof of effectiveness of the *leadership duties separation model* exists, anecdotal evidence suggests a potential revolutionary breakthrough development in the approach to organizational management.

Communication

Without the culture of relentless communication, organizational strategy execution would be dead on arrival. Like the mission, vision, and values, strategic outcomes, substrategies, and tactics must be clearly visible and discussed often throughout the organization. Techniques and tactics, similar to those discussed earlier in this chapter, in conjunction with communications surrounding the organizational pillars, may be used to create awareness of and promote dialogue about the company's strategy and its execution. Strong communication cultures encourage employees' involvement in the lives of their organizations, hence increasing collective pride, promoting better alignment and performance, and helping achieve strategic goals.

Monitoring and Close-the-Loop Tools

At every level of an organization, visibility drives results and that which is closely monitored gets done. When department heads are asked to report weekly on their outcomes and progress in front of the peers and the executives, they are compelled to lead their employees to better performance and achievement of goals. No strategy process would be complete without sound

TABLE 6.6 Sample Personal Dashboard Template

Weekly Achievements			
1.			
2.			

Tactics and Projects			
Tactic or project name	Milestones	Due date	Status
	1.		Green
	2.		Yellow
	3.		Red
	4.		Gray

Critical Quality and Operating Targets (CQOTs)			
Critical performance area	CQOT		Status
	1.		Green
	2.		Yellow
	3.		Red
	4.		White

Issues and Risks		
Issue	Root cause	Mitigation plan
1.		
2.		

Elevate points	
Health and wellness	
1.	
2.	
Environment	
1.	
2	
Relationships	
1.	
2.	
Achievements	
1.	
2.	
Expertise development	
1.	
2.	

Legend	
Red	Major milestone missed or CQOT significantly off target. Tactic or project completion may be in jeopardy. Complete issues section.
Yellow	Timely completion of tactic or project is in jeopardy, or CQOT is slightly off target. Complete issues section.
Green	Milestone is completely on track or CQOT significantly better than the target.
Gray	Milestone is complete.
White	CQOT is on target.

organizational systems that promote outcomes visibility and strategy execution. We discuss a few common approaches that organizations use to monitor performance.

Personal Dashboards

Personal dashboards are widely used tools for intradepartmental communication and alignment monitoring. They allow employees to focus their weekly activities and provide a quick visual snapshot of the status of tactics, projects, *critical quality and operating targets (CQOTs)*, or key indicators of an organization's health, and personal alignment, elevate points, and continual development. There are many different variations of dashboard templates. However, many have a few elements in common: list of accomplishments, color-coded status indicators for achieving milestones within tactics and projects, known issues with mitigation plans, and personal and professional developmental opportunities. A sample personal dashboard template is presented in Table 6.6. Operational and functional department leaders submit their dashboards weekly to the respective supervising executives and, if needed, schedule follow-up meetings. Depending on the level of personal involvement with strategic tactics, major projects, or critical quality and operating targets, other employees could also be required to use weekly dashboards. In DDOs, however, these tools are commonplace throughout.

Snapshot Reviews

A periodic, weekly, or biweekly *snapshot review* is an effective approach for keeping the critical quality and operating targets as well as other strategic indicators continually visible throughout the institution and for driving performance to reach goals. To facilitate the discussion, a performance snapshot report is produced for every functional department, operating unit, region, and division. The snapshot reports present selected performance measures and color-code the results, according to the criteria determined by the executive team. Commonly, red indicates the need for improvement, whereas green points out unique strengths; the absence of color signifies neutral performance. When in-person snapshot review meetings are not feasible, companies utilize teleconferencing capabilities for managers to discuss the areas of performance weaknesses and strengths. Strong performers share best-demonstrated practices and performance know-how with the rest of the team, whereas underachievers report on the root causes and mitigating plans. Depending on the organization's to-date performance and shifting areas of focus, the indicators presented on snapshot reports could change over time.

Tactical Progress Reports

The reporting on the execution of tactical plans happens at the end of every fiscal quarter, when departmental and functional leaders as well as the executives share the status of their planned tactical activities and account for the progress toward achieving the set substrategies. Every "owner" of tactics completes the quarterly status update of his respective tactical map, offering explanations for any variances to plan. At that time, course correction could be set and additional resources allocated, if deemed necessary.

At the end of the fiscal year, the strategy director reviews and aggregates all of the final tactical progress reports, generating an organization-wide tactical results digest, which is, in turn, presented to the strategy committee at its annual meeting. The strategy committee then carries over any necessary tactics into the next year's tactical maps. The digest is also offered for review to the board.

As mentioned earlier, the strategy process is cyclical and dynamic. Although it normally follows an annual cycle, reassessments of organizational pillars or environmental factors and adjustments to strategic plans could happen any time there are significant changes in external and internal environments. Strategy process requires unrelenting commitment, dedicated resources, and sound systems throughout the organization. Only when these factors converge can there be success!

◼ CAPITAL BUDGETS, PROJECTS SELECTION, AND FINANCIAL MODELING

Every year, organizations must use discretion in determining how to allocate limited financial resources between competing capital purchases and projects. Generally, annual CapEx budgets consist of both new and maintenance components, which could be equally important, because many CapEx items arise from the tactical plans and support the institution's overall organizational strategy. In this part of the chapter, we explore a sample framework for capital budgeting and projects selection while introducing several financial concepts.

Suppose an ED director performed a meticulous financial analysis of the proposed department expansion project and determined that there will be a significant return on the invested capital within three years of the expansion. Should the executives approve the project? Although it is an important decision factor, projected financial returns should not be used as the sole selection criterion for capital projects. Other critical questions must be answered before capital investments, large or small, are made. Introduced later in this chapter, our *3-F framework* for capital projects selection includes three equally essential components: *finances*, *fit*, and *feasibility*.

TIME VALUE OF MONEY AND INVESTMENT DECISIONS

What is worth more: $1 today or $1 tomorrow? Is there a difference in the value? There are multiple ways of evaluating the financial feasibility of capital projects and other investments. In this chapter, we concentrate on two of them: *net present value*, or *NPV*, and *internal rate of return*, or *IRR*. In a world without inflation, inherent risk, and other economic pressures, the value of money tomorrow, or 10 years from now, would be absolutely the same as today. In reality, that is not the case. Therefore, your present buying ability with a predetermined sum of money is higher than it would be in the future with the identical amount. In other words, money loses its value over time.

Net Present Value

To understand the concepts of *present value (PV)* and *future value (FV)*, consider the following: the author of this chapter asks you for a loan, promising to repay $1,000 in 1 year. How much would you be willing to lend, assuming you decided to invest your money in some way? The answer would depend on two factors: how risky you think lending to the author would be, or the odds of getting your money back, and your *opportunity cost of capital*, or best-return investment alternative of the same *risk*. Suppose the author is riskless and there is 100% guarantee of the promised payment at the end of the borrowing period. Also, assume that your best alternative is to invest in a certificate of deposit (CD) at your local bank at a 2% return per annum. Because bank deposits are Federal Deposit Insurance Corporation (FDIC)-insured, this investment would not carry any risk either. A simple equation solves for the maximum amount ($X) you would be willing to lend on these terms in order to be paid $1,000 in 1 year:

$$X \times (102\%) = \$1,000$$
$$X = \$1,000 \div 1.02 = \$980.39$$

Therefore, $980.39 is the PV of your future cash inflow and represents the amount you should be willing to lend to the author. For any one-period uncompounded investment, or a single cash outflow today with a single cash inflow in the future, PV could be expressed as: $PV = FV \div (1 + r)$, where r denotes the *discount rate* for the lending period and depends on the inherent *undiversifiable*, or *systemic, risk* of the investment. Adjusting for the timing and risk, PV interrelates present *cash flows* with future cash flows. *NPV* of any investment or project is simply the sum of its *discounted cash flows*. In this lending example, your investment represents a negative cash flow (*outflow*), whereas the payback is a positive cash flow (*inflow*).

Therefore, your NPV of lending to the author is:

$$NPV = -\$980.39 + (\$1,000 \div 1.02) = 0$$

Obviously, one would want the NPV to be larger than zero, hence offering to lend a smaller amount.

Risk-Adjusted NPV

Of course, if you were not 100% certain that the author would not default on repaying the loan, you would have to adjust the discount rate to account for this risk. Say, the probability of default was 20%, then, your expected return, on average, would be 80% of $1,000, or $800, at the end of the lending period. Assuming that your best investment alternative of the same risk is the stock market, which returns 15% on average, the PV and NPV of this investment would be:

$$PV = \$800 \div (1 + 0.15) = \$695.65$$
$$NPV = -\$695.65 + (\$1,000 \times 80\%) / (1 + 0.15) = 0$$

It is worth noting that the NPV of capital market transactions is usually zero. Hence, organizations can create the most value by undertaking projects with the highest positive NPV.

NPV of Projects

Generally, capital projects consist of multiple cash flows: initial and subsequent investment outflows, revenues that are generated as a result of a project, and expenses associated with operating a new venture created by the project. For example, a university that is evaluating the feasibility of adding a BSN program will consider the costs associated with bringing such a program to life as well as projected revenues and expenses that the program will generate in the foreseeable future.

The PV formula in the loan example would be identical for a project with a single cash flow, denoted as C, at the end of year, or period, one. Conversely:

$$PV = C_1 \div (1 + r)$$

or, considering discount rate compounding over time, for a cash flow at some point in time, or period t:

$$PV = C_t \div (1 + r)^t$$

Combining the PVs of the multiple cash flows for the BSN project, the university would use the following formula to determine the NPV and evaluate the feasibility of this undertaking:

$$NPV = C_0 + C_1 \div (1 + r) + C_2 \div (1 + r)^2 + C_3 \div (1 + r)^3 1 \ldots 1 \, C_t \div (1 + r)^t$$

Naturally, if the NPV of a project is negative, it does not make financial sense to proceed with such undertaking. However, as discussed later in this chapter, there may be other compelling reasons for an organization to invest in negative NPV projects. Moreover, as is often the case with maintenance CapEx items that carry seemingly negative NPV, investments might improve customer satisfaction or other operational and/or strategic aspects whose financial impacts are difficult to quantify but could be positive in the long term.

NPV Considerations

NPV is a common method for evaluating financial feasibility of projects and investments. It is straightforward, contingent only on the forecasted cash flows and the suitable discount rate, and easily computed in Excel. Because it is measured in current dollars, NPV allows managers to select more valuable projects when considering a few investment alternatives, irrespective of the timing of returns. However, to arrive at accurate conclusions, managers should remember a few ground rules for NPV utilization.

First, all *sunk costs*, or the dollars already spent on the project, should be disregarded. Only the NPV of future cash flows should be considered. Leaders in organizations often tend to include all previous spending in their consideration of whether to continue with certain projects. This, however, may lead to the erroneous rejection of investments with positive NPVs of future cash flows. Second, whenever possible, cash flow projections and discount rates should be used on the after-tax basis. Third, all organization-wide financial effects of projects should be estimated and taken into account. For example, investing in a new piece of the latest diagnostic equipment might not only bring new direct revenue to the imaging department, but also increase the overall number of client cases for the institution. Fourth, only *incremental*, or additional, cash-based projections should be considered. Do not account for any existing revenues, expenses, or noncash transactions such as depreciation and amortization. Fifth, existing *overhead* costs should not be allocated to the new projects. For instance, an apportioned amount of the salary of the dean of health sciences should not be considered in the new BSN program decision. Finally, *opportunity cost* of the project must be evaluated. In other words, the question of what the company would be giving up by investing its resources in a given project must be answered.

IRR of Projects

IRR is a popular alternative or supplemental measure to NPV for evaluating projects and investments. Producing a correct outcome most of the time, IRR calculation provides an intuitive gauge for the level of return that a project or investment will yield. The IRR is calculated by setting the NPV in the formula previously presented to zero and then solving for the discount rate. In other words, IRR is the discount rate (*r*) at which the NPV of a project or investment equals zero.

$$0 = C_0 + C_1 \div (1+r) + C_2 \div (1+r)^2 + C_3 \div (1+r)^3 + \ldots + C_t \div (1+r)^t, \text{ where IRR} = r$$

Notably, no real mathematical solution exists for such an equation; therefore, a manager would rely on the assistance of an Excel spreadsheet to approximate the answer for *r*. A project should be accepted if its IRR is greater than the organization's set *hurdle*, or minimum acceptable rate of return. Often, the company's *weighted average cost of capital* (WACC) is used as the hurdle rate. WACC is the rate representing the combined risk-adjusted opportunity cost for both the company's debt and equity holders. Simply stated, WACC is the organization's cost of accessing cash for investment. Therefore, undertaking a project makes economic sense only if its IRR is greater than the firm's WACC.

IRR Considerations

On occasion, the IRR calculation could produce a result that would lead to an erroneous project acceptance, rejection, or selection decision. Generally, any alternative approach for financial feasibility evaluation that produces a conclusion different from the NPV result is incorrect! Because IRR only approximates the percentage yield of an investment, it cannot be used to compare projects of different magnitude. Naturally, a very large investment with a smaller IRR would create a greater economic value than a relatively small investment with a larger yield. Moreover, because of shifting economic reality, interest rates, risk, and other factors, hurdle rates vary over time; hence, it is virtually impossible to accurately pinpoint the actual cost of capital at some point in the future. Comparing projects of different duration, consequently, is not feasible by utilizing the IRR method. Finally, a high-order equation that approximates the IRR could produce as many results as there are switches from negative to positive cash flows and vice versa.

In summary, IRR is a widely utilized alternative method for evaluating projects and investments. It produces an accurate decision when considering only a single project with one initial cash outflow followed by a number of cash inflows, where the hurdle rate is the same for all time periods.

3-F: FINANCIAL MODELING FOR CAPITAL BUDGETING DECISIONS

In this day and age, the vast proliferation of computers and financial software streamlines capital budgeting decisions and makes managers' and executives' jobs much easier. There are many varieties of computerized *financial models*: some are available off-the shelf, some commercial products could be customized to fit the needs of a specific organization, and many others are created in-house, utilizing spreadsheet applications such as Excel.

Sample Financial Model

For illustration purposes, we created an Excel financial model to assist our hypothetical university's administration in making the decision regarding developing and rolling out a new generic BSN program. The model consists of three distinct components: 5-year pro-forma income statement, estimated CapEx and operational *cash burn* budget, and project valuation analysis. Both the CapEx and the operational projections require managers to make many assumptions regarding the respective individual model components. These assumptions are not mere guesses; they are based on research, consider past trends, and offer good-faith estimates for the future. We explore the sample model and its assumptions later. Similar financial feasibility analysis models could be created for nursing services.

Pro-Forma Income Statements

In order to determine the future cash flows associated with the new BSN program, we built 5 years worth of *pro-forma income statements*, which forecast revenues, expenses, and profits and/or losses resulting from the program's operations. Recall that in order to correctly estimate the NPV of a project, managers should only use incremental revenues and expenses and not allocate any current amounts to the new project. Case in point: The university has enough existing physical facilities to house the new BSN program; it currently pays rent for this underutilized space. Therefore, the pro-forma statements will exclude rent as well as building and utilities expenses for the purpose of determining the profitability of the proposed educational program. Furthermore, only cash-based incremental revenues and expenses will be considered. Hence, accruals, depreciation and amortization, and any other noncash items are excluded. Table 6.7 illustrates forecasted revenues and expenses for the first year of operating the program.

Of course, both revenue and expenses depend on the size of the student population as well as curriculum hours and its composition. We made the following assumptions to derive the student population "waterfall." First, the board of nursing will approve the program to enroll 40 students four times per year. Second, the university will operate the program year-round and will be able to attract full student cohorts every quarter. Third, the BSN program will be comprised of four academic years of instruction, where every academic year is three calendar quarters long and all instructional quarters will eventually operate concurrently. Fourth, the quarterly attrition rate will be 1.5%, with students withdrawing from the program at the end of each academic quarter; however, the university will be enrolling three replacement students, who have completed all of the necessary prerequisite courses, into the beginning of the fourth quarter of instruction every 3 months, starting with the first time the second academic year commences. Fifth, the overall graduation rate will be 80%. Based on the foregoing assumptions, student population at the end of the first full year of operations will be 155.

To estimate tuition charges, we explored comparable institutions offering generic BSN programs and projected quarterly tuition at $6,000, the median competitor price. This tuition will include all charges such as textbooks and lab fees. Therefore, first-year revenue from operating the new BSN program will be more than $2.3 million. Next, we consider the incremental expenses.

TABLE 6.7 Pro-Forma Income Statement for Generic BSN Program, Year 1

		Q1	Q2	Q3	Q4	YR1
POPULATION	Beginning population	—	39	77	115	—
	New starts (first-year students)	40	40	40	40	160
	Replacement starts (second year)	—	—	—	3	3
	Withdrawals	(1)	(2)	(2)	(3)	(8)
	Graduates	—	—	—	—	—
	Ending population	39	77	115	155	155
	Tuition revenue	$240,000	$474,000	$702,000	$948,000	$2,364,000
STAFFING & COMPENSATION	Instructional FTEs	3	5	7	10	
	Cost of instruction	$70,200	$117,000	$163,800	$234,000	$585,000
	Cost of onboarding	$46,800	$46,800	$70,200	$46,800	$210,600
	Program director	$31,200	$31,200	$31,200	$31,200	$124,800
	Admissions FTEs	2	2	2	2	
	Cost of admission advisors	$31,200	$31,200	$31,200	$31,200	$124,800
	Student services FTEs	1	1	1	1	
	Cost of SS advisors	$15,600	$15,600	$15,600	$15,600	$62,400
	Program coordinator	$13,000	$13,000	$13,000	$13,000	$52,000
	Overtime	$2,652	$3,354	$4,407	$5,109	$15,522
	Salaries and wages	$210,652	$258,154	$329,407	$376,909	$1,175,122
	Taxes and benefits	$52,663	$64,539	$82,352	$94,227	$293,781
	Total compensation	$263,315	$322,693	$411,759	$471,136	$1,468,903
	Recruitment and retention	$4,213	$5,163	$6,588	$7,538	$23,502
	Media advertising	$30,000	$30,000	$30,000	$32,250	$122,250
	Incremental operating expenses	$48,000	$94,800	$140,400	$189,600	$472,800
	Scholarships and waivers	$4,800	$9,480	$14,040	$18,960	$47,280
	Total operating expenses	$350,328	$462,136	$602,787	$719,484	$2,134,735
	EBITDA	$(110,328)	$11,864	$99,213	$228,516	$229,265

EBITDA, earnings before interest, taxes, depreciation, and amortization; FTEs, full-time equivalents; SS, student services.

As compensation is, by far, the largest incremental expense, we first had to determine the appropriate staffing levels for the BSN program. We supposed that the curriculum is comprised of 1,300 theory hours, 1,000 clinical hours, and 500 lab and simulation hours, or the accepted norms yielded by our research. In addition, we discovered that the respective customary instructor-to-students ratios are 1:40, 1:10, and 1:5. We further assumed that each academic quarter will consist of 11 weeks of instruction and that the full-time (FT) faculty's average weekly contact hours will be 30. Combining the data, we arrived at the required faculty staffing levels, presented as instructional full-time equivalents (FTE) in Table 6.7. Furthermore, the university will fill

TABLE 6.8 Projected Wages

Instructional wage	$45.00
Director wage	$60.00
Admissions wage	$30.00
Student services wage	$30.00
Program coordinator wage	$25.00

TABLE 6.9 Operating Expenses Trends

Advertising/enrolled student	$750
Incremental operating expense rate	20.0%
Scholarships and waivers rate	2.0%
Recruitment and retention rate	2.0%

program director and coordinator positions, in addition to increasing admissions and student services staffing, at 1:22 and 1:175 staff-to-students ratios, respectively.

Utilizing market compensation data, from sources such as the Bureau of Labor Statistics, we determined that the weighted average hourly wages for the incremental faculty and staff would be as shown in Table 6.8. Total wages were then calculated based on the FTE staffing levels and considering the cost of onboarding faculty members, each of whom will be brought in for orientation a full quarter ahead of being in front of the students. Total compensation figures also include overtime wages, based on a 1.5% rate, and the benefits and payroll taxes expenses at 25%. Both of these rates are the historically observed trends at the university. Our assumptions led us to project that in the first year of operations the university will spend almost $1.5 million in incremental compensation.

To round off the operating expenses category, we considered the university's historical trends in recruitment, retention, advertising, and other expenses. Table 6.9 depicts these factors. The incremental operating expenses category includes items such as instructional and office supplies, database subscriptions, telecommunications, and so forth.

Finally, subtracting total operating expenses from total revenues, the projected EBITDA for the first year of the BSN program operations will be about $230,000. Tables 6.10 through 6.12 illustrate revenues and expenses for the second, third, and fourth years of operations. Based on our assumptions, the program will reach operational maturity in year 4, with a rotating total population of 424 students and annual EBITDAs of approximately $4.6 million.

Projected CapEx and Cash Burn Budget

This component of the financial model carries the budgetary projections for developing and rolling out the BSN program along with the anticipated timing of expenditures. Table 6.13 illustrates the forecasted expenses.

The CapEx portion represents the estimates of the construction, equipment, and curriculum and program development expenses. In order to correctly project the CapEx cash outlays, quotes were obtained from architectural firms, general contractors, and consultants, utilizing the program assumptions discussed in the previous section. The operating cash burn section represents the program expenses that are incurred before the program's opening and, therefore, ahead of any realized revenue. We determined the timing of the necessary expenditures and, subsequently, applied the underlying assumptions to calculate the total cash burn. Combining the CapEx and cash burn projections, we concluded that, in order to develop and roll out the new generic BSN

TABLE 6.10 Pro-Forma Income Statement for Generic BSN Program, Year 2

		Q1	Q2	Q3	Q4	YR2
POPULATION	Beginning Population	155	195	234	272	155
	New starts (first-year students)	40	40	40	40	160
	Replacement starts (second year)	3	3	3	3	12
	Withdrawals	(3)	(4)	(5)	(5)	(17)
	Graduates	—	—	—	—	—
	Ending population	195	234	272	310	310
	Tuition revenue	$1,188,000	$1,428,000	$1,662,000	$1,890,000	$6,168,000
	Instructional FTEs	12	14	17	19	
	Cost of instruction	$280,800	$327,600	$397,800	$444,600	$1,450,800
	Cost of onboarding	$46,800	$70,200	$46,800	$46,800	$210,600
	Administrator	$31,200	$31,200	$31,200	$31,200	$124,800
	Admissions FTEs	2	2	2	2	
	Cost of admission advisors	$31,200	$31,200	$31,200	$31,200	$124,800
STAFFING & COMPENSATION	Student services FTEs	2	2	2	2	
	Cost of SS advisors	$31,200	$31,200	$31,200	$31,200	$124,800
	Program coordinator	$13,000	$13,000	$13,000	$13,000	$52,000
	Overtime	$6,045	$7,098	$7,800	$8,502	$29,445
	Salaries and wages	$440,245	$511,498	$559,000	$606,502	$2,117,245
	Taxes and benefits	$110,061	$127,875	$139,750	$151,626	$529,312
	Total compensation	$550,306	$639,373	$698,750	$758,128	$2,646,557
	Recruitment and retention	$8,805	$10,230	$11,180	$12,130	$42,345
	Media advertising	$32,250	$32,250	$32,250	$32,250	$129,000
	Incremental operating expenses	$237,600	$285,600	$332,400	$378,000	$1,233,600
	Scholarships and waivers	$23,760	$28,560	$33,240	$37,800	$123,360
	Total operating expenses	$852,721	$996,012	$1,107,820	$1,218,308	$4,174,861
	EBITDA	$335,279	$431,988	$554,180	$671,692	$1,993,139

EBITDA, earnings before interest, taxes, depreciation, and amortization; FTEs, full-time equivalents; SS, student services.

program, the university must spend close to $1.8 million on the project in the year prior to enrolling the first cohort of students.

Project Valuation Analysis
After the amounts of the initial cash outlay and the subsequent earnings have been determined, we complete the financial feasibility model by calculating the NPV and the IRR of the university's

TABLE 6.11 Pro-Forma Income Statement for Generic BSN Program, Year 3

		Q1	Q2	Q3	Q4	YR3
POPULATION	Beginning population	310	347	384	420	310
	New starts (first-year students)	40	40	40	40	160
	Replacement starts (second year)	3	3	3	3	12
	Withdrawals	(6)	(6)	(7)	(7)	(26)
	Graduates	—	—	—	(35)	(35)
	Ending population	347	384	420	421	421
	Tuition revenue	$2,118,000	$2,340,000	$2,562,000	$2,778,000	$9,798,000
	Instructional FTEs	21	23	26	28	
	Cost of instruction	$491,400	$538,200	$608,400	$655,200	$2,293,200
	Cost of onboarding	$46,800	$70,200	$46,800	$-	$163,800
	Administrator	$31,200	$31,200	$31,200	$31,200	$124,800
	Admissions FTEs	2	2	2	2	
	Cost of admission advisors	$31,200	$31,200	$31,200	$31,200	$124,800
STAFFING & COMPENSATION	Student services FTEs	3	3	3	3	
	Cost of SS advisors	$46,800	$46,800	$46,800	$46,800	187,200
	Program coordinator	$13,000	$13,000	$13,000	$13,000	$52,000
	Overtime	$9,438	$10,491	$11,193	$11,193	$42,315
	Salaries and wages	$669,838	$741,091	$788,593	$788,593	$2,988,115
	Taxes and benefits	$167,460	$185,273	$197,148	$197,148	$747,029
	Total compensation	$837,298	$926,364	$985,741	$985,741	$3,735,144
	Recruitment and retention	$13,397	$14,822	$15,772	$15,772	$59,763
	Media advertising	$32,250	$32,250	$32,250	$32,250	$129,000
	Incremental operating expenses	$423,600	$468,000	$512,400	$555,600	$1,959,600
	Scholarships and waivers	$42,360	$46,800	$51,240	$55,560	$195,960
	Total operating expenses	$1,348,904	$1,488,236	$1,597,403	$1,644,923	$6,079,466
	EBITDA	$769,096	$851,764	$964,597	$1,133,077	$3,718,534

EBITDA, earnings before interest, taxes, depreciation, and amortization; FTEs, full-time equivalents; SS, student services.

investment into the new generic BSN program. Table 6.14 illustrates the valuation component of the model.

We start converting the EBITDA figures into after-tax *free cash flows* by first subtracting the noncash depreciation and amortization expenses to determine the basis for the income tax expense. Assuming that the university depreciates its tangible assets and amortizes the intangible holdings over a 10-year period, utilizing a straight-line method, we deduct 10% of the CapEx

TABLE 6.12 Pro-Forma Income Statement for Generic BSN Program, Year 4

		Q1	Q2	Q3	Q4	YR4
POPULATION	Beginning population	421	422	423	424	421
	New starts (first-year students)	40	40	40	40	160
	Replacement starts (second year)	3	3	3	3	12
	Withdrawals	(7)	(7)	(7)	(8)	(29)
	Graduates	(35)	(35)	(35)	(35)	(140)
	Ending population	422	423	424	424	424
	Tuition revenue	$2,784,000	$2,790,000	$2,796,000	$2,802,000	$11,172,000
	Instructional FTEs	28	28	28	28	
	Cost of instruction	$655,200	$655,200	$655,200	$655,200	$2,620,800
	Cost of onboarding	—	—	—	—	—
	Administrator	$31,200	$31,200	$31,200	$31,200	$124,800
	Admissions FTEs	2	2	2	2	
	Cost of admission advisors	$31,200	$31,200	$31,200	$31,200	$124,800
STAFFING & COMPENSATION	Student services FTEs	3	3	3	3	
	Cost of SS advisors	$46,800	$46,800	$46,800	$46,800	$187,200
	Program coordinator	$13,000	$13,000	$13,000	$13,000	$52,000
	Overtime	$11,193	$11,193	$11,193	$11,193	$44,772
	Salaries and wages	$788,593	$788,593	$788,593	$788,593	$3,154,372
	Taxes and benefits	$197,148	$197,148	$197,148	$197,148	$788,592
	Total compensation	$985,741	$985,741	$985,741	$985,741	$3,942,964
	Recruitment and retention	$15,772	$15,772	$15,772	$15,772	$63,088
	Media advertising	$32,250	$32,250	$32,250	$32,250	$129,000
	Incremental operating expenses	$556,800	$558,000	$559,200	$560,400	$2,234,400
	Scholarships and waivers	$55,680	$55,800	$55,920	$56,040	$223,440
	Total operating expenses	$1,646,243	$1,647,563	$1,648,883	$1,650,203	$6,592,892
	EBITDA	$1,137,757	$1,142,437	$1,147,117	$1,151,797	$4,579,108

EBITDA, earnings before interest, taxes, depreciation, and amortization; FTEs, full-time equivalents; SS, student services.

TABLE 6.13 CapEx and Cash Burn Forecast, Generic BSN Development, Year 0

CAPEX	Q1	Q2	Q3	Q4	YR0
Program and curriculum development	$70,000	$70,000	$70,000		$210,000
Nursing labs and Simcenter build-out	$250,000	$250,000	$250,000		$750,000
Science lab build-out and equipment		$75,000	$75,000	$25,000	$175,000
Nursing labs equipment				$270,000	$270,000
Additional classrooms equipment				$50,000	$50,000
Total CapEx	$320,000	$395,000	$395,000	$345,000	$1,455,000
CASH BURN					
Staffing					
Program director			$31,200	$31,200	$62,400
Program coordinator				$13,000	$13,000
Admissions advisors				$31,200	$31,200
Instructors				$70,200	$70,200
Salaries and wages			$31,200	$145,600	$176,800
Taxes and benefits			$7,800	$36,400	$44,200
Total compensation			$39,000	$182,000	$221,000
Recruitment		$15,000	$30,000	$20,000	$65,000
Media advertising				$30,000	$30,000
Total cash burn		$15,000	$69,000	$232,000	$316,000
				Total investment	$1,771,000

expenses from the annual EBITDA for the 10 years following each investment. Notably, the historical trends show that the university spends about 0.5% of its revenues on maintenance CapEx, such as equipment replacements, in the first 2 years following a major expansion project. This amount increases to 0.7% of revenues in subsequent years.

After the taxable earnings have been determined, we apply the 35% corporate tax rate to determine the income tax expense. The after-tax, cash-based profit or loss is calculated by subtracting the income tax expense from EBITDA. Please note that the project's negative EBITDA, or loss, in year 0 will result in proportional tax savings to the university at large, due to the incremental reduction in organization-wide earnings. Free cash flows for the NPV calculation are then determined by combining the after-tax, cash-based income with the CapEx items.

Of course, it would be impractical, if not impossible, to try determining cash flows in perpetuity for the purposes of deriving the NPV of the project. Therefore, we utilize a shortcut known as *terminal value*. Many companies, including our hypothetical university, calculate the terminal value of the project by estimating the overall enterprise value, as if it would be sold after reaching maturity and having a promise of stable financial returns, by applying an industry-comparable earnings multiplier to the last year's EBITDA. As we discussed earlier, the BSN program would reach maturity in year 4. Therefore, its terminal value in year 5 would be five times its EBITDA in year 4. Not to overstate the terminal value of the program, we chose to use a conservative

TABLE 6.14 Project Valuation Analysis for Generic BSN Program

	Year 0	Year 1	Year 2	Year 3	Year 4	
Revenues		$2,364,000	$6,168,000	$9,798,000	$11,172,000	
EBITDA (cash-based)	$(316,000)	$229,265	$1,993,139	$3,718,534	$4,579,108	
Depreciation and amortization		$(145,500)	$(146,682)	$(149,766)	$(156,625)	
Income tax expense	$110,600	$(29,318)	$(646,260)	$(1,249,069)	$(1,547,869)	
After-tax profit/(loss) (cash-based)	$(205,400)	$199,947	$1,346,879	$2,469,465	$3,031,239	
Initial CapEx	$(1,455,000)					
Maintenance CapEx		$(11,820)	$(30,840)	$(68,586)	$(78,204)	Terminal Value
Free cash flows	$(1,660,400)	$188,127	$1,316,039	$2,400,879	$2,953,035	$22,895,538
NPV @ 15% WACC	$12,303,005					
NPV @ 30% WACC	$5,812,467					
IRR	99%					

EBITDA, earnings before interest, taxes, depreciation, and amortization; IRR, internal rate of return; NPV, net present value; WACC, weighted average cost of capital.

earnings multiplier (5) and, as a result, determined it to be about $23 million, hence finding the last cash flow of the project.

After applying the NPV and IRR formulas discussed earlier in this chapter, we determined the NPV of the new generic BSN program to be somewhere between $5.8 and $12.3 million, depending on the discount rate. Based on the NPV, along with a very healthy IRR of 99%, we would recommend the university to undertake this project. Of course, other, nonfinancial considerations should be weighed in before the university's administration sanctions the project.

3-F: ORGANIZATIONAL AND STRATEGIC FIT

Every potential capital project and investment should be evaluated for fit with the strategic outcomes and organizational mission, vision, and values. Even when carrying the promise of great financial return, a project should be accepted only if it advances the mission of the company, or moves it closer to its vision, and is consistent with the core organizational competencies and values. Following this principle allows firms to focus energy and scarce resources on expenditures that synergistically promote overall organizational success.

3-F: FEASIBILITY OF CAPITAL PROJECTS AND INVESTMENTS

Being feasible is a necessary component of any capital expenditure. In the least, financial and HR toll, as well as market viability of a project or investment, should be considered before sanctioning the expenditure. In our new BSN program example, the university must have free access to a minimum of $1.8 million plus the necessary working capital to ensure that the project is successful. It must ensure that the market can bear an additional BSN program in its geographical location by carefully comparing the projected need for RNs with the projected supply of nurses, as well as the current and future demand for baccalaureate nursing education with the existing number of annual student enrollments. The university must also not miscalculate its ability to attract the appropriate numbers of qualified faculty and secure the necessary clinical partnerships, as well as consider the impact that the new program development and operations will have on the existing personnel and the strategic initiatives already underway.

As indicated earlier, every CapEx undertaking diminishes other possibilities, so the administration must look into a proverbial crystal ball to determine the best course of action. Conversely, bringing the new BSN program to life could have such synergies with the current organization as strengthening the university's brand and promoting growth of other health care programs.

CAPITAL BUDGETING PROCESS

Putting it all together in conjunction with the strategy operationalizing, we suggest the following capital budgeting process. Whether capital expenditure recommendations are embedded within the proposed strategic outcomes, substrategies, or tactics or arise from the environmental evaluations and lie outside of the formal organizational strategy, they are considered at the annual interactive tactical planning and budgeting meetings. To be fully ready to present CapEx recommendations, managers and executives should prepare by utilizing the 3-F framework, which anticipates the likely considerations for capital budgeting decisions.

Traditionally, chief financial officers (CFOs) lead the process by providing capital budget templates and guidance to the operational and functional leaders, who, in turn, offer recommendations and justifications for CapEx items. The CFO then compiles the departmental input for the review and refinement by the executive team and the strategy committee who issue the final annual CapEx recommendations, based on which the CFO prepares the CapEx budget for the board's approval, tying expenditures to the strategic outcomes and tactics. On board approval, the CapEx budget is distributed throughout the organization for execution. The budget document also serves as the basis for setting some of the critical quality and operating targets.

CONCLUSION

Although the full responsibility for the strategy process, budgeting, or projects selection may not fall squarely on a nurse leader's shoulders, she or he must be able to masterfully navigate the complex organizational systems or even design and implement them in the absence or failure of existing solutions. Utilizing the tools presented herein, DNP graduates could successfully embody the principles laid forth in the AACN's *Essentials of Doctoral Education for Advanced Nursing Practice*, ultimately strengthening the U.S. health care system by contributing to and leading larger organizations or even building and improving private practices.

Through the science and tools of organizational leadership, like SWOT analyses and environmental evaluations, a nurse leader could "develop and evaluate new practice approaches" (AACN, 2006, p. 9) and "generate evidence . . . to guide improvements in practice and outcomes of care" (p. 12) consistent with the first and the third *DNP Essentials. Essential II* calls for the nurse leader to utilize "advanced communication processes" (p. 11) such as the tactical maps and personal dashboards presented in this chapter, "develop and/or monitor budgets" (p. 11), including CapEx, and "employ principles of finance" (p. 11) such as NPV and IRR. Principles of financial modeling contained here would allow the graduate to further develop *Essential IV's* information technology proficiency requirement to "support practice and administrative decision-making" (p. 13). As envisioned in the *Essential V*, nurse leaders' participation in their respective strategy committees would allow for the influence in developing an implementation of "institutional health policy" (p. 14) to "improve health care delivery and outcomes" (p. 14). Full understanding of the incentives and accountabilities systems would permit the graduate to "facilitate collaborative team functioning and overcome impediments to interprofessional practice" (p. 14) as well as "guide, mentor, and support other nurses to achieve excellence in nursing practice" (p. 17), as stated respectively in the *Essentials VI* and *VIII*. Finally, through influencing the selection of the critical quality and operational targets in an organization, a graduate could engage in the *Essential VII's* "leadership to integrate and institutionalize evidence-based clinical prevention and population health services" (p. 15).

Expert nursing practice leadership is a critical component in striving to improve the health care system in our country. Our hope is that DNP graduates would utilize the information and tools presented in this chapter to the full extent and become extremely successful in leading for change.

CRITICAL THINKING EXERCISES

1. Evaluate your organization's mission, vision, and values statements and determine how well they match the current state of affairs. How well do they describe what your organization is, does, and aspires to be? How is the organization doing in aligning with its stated pillars? How well is the organization aware of its individual contributors' cultural alignment to these strategic pillars?
2. Devise three people outcomes as well as related substrategies and tactics to improve your organization's focus on alignment. Complete the tactical map template. Prepare an

argument in support of your outcomes, substrategies, and tactics to be presented to the strategy committee.

3. Using the data in Tables 6.4 and 6.5, calculate the total year-end bonus amount for a nurse manager who earns $100,000 annually, has a 10% bonus target, meets the individual financial contributions, and completes his or her assigned tactics, but fails to meet some of the individual and unit operational goals, and works in a hospital that has met all of its strategic, operational, and financial goals, achieved 115% of the projected EBITDA, and utilizes the "all-or-nothing" approach to the incentive compensation criteria. Assume that the maximum aggregate bonus amount is set high enough for all to receive the entire individually calculated bonus amounts.

4. Prepare a full 3-F framework for a new family nurse practitioner private practice, or a project of your choosing. Base your assumptions on research and trends, and utilize Excel for financial modeling. Prepare a presentation for the board of trustees or group of investors. Good luck and have fun!

REFERENCES

American Association of Colleges of Nursing. (2006). *The essentials of doctoral education for advanced nursing practice.* Washington, DC: Author.

Baker, G. P., Jensen, M. C., & Murphy, K. J. (1988). Compensation and incentives: Practice vs. theory. *Journal of Finance, 43*(3), 593–616.

The Cleveland Clinic. (2017). Mission, vision, values. Retrieved from http://my.clevelandclinic.org/about -cleveland-clinic/overview/who-we-are/mission-vision-values.aspx

Duke University School of Nursing. (2017). Duke University School of Nursing—About. Retrieved from http://nursing.duke.edu/about/about

Johns Hopkins Medicine. (2017). Johns Hopkins medicine mission. Retrieved from http://www .hopkinsmedicine.org/about/mission.html

Kaplan, R. S., & Norton, D. P. (1996). *The balanced scorecard: Translating strategy into action.* Watertown, MA: Harvard Business Review Press.

Kegan, R., & Lahey, L. L.; with Miller, M. L., Fleming, A., & Helsing, D. (2016). *An everyone culture: Becoming a deliberately developmental organization.* Boston, MA: Harvard Business Review Press.

Learned, E. P., Christensen, C. R., Andrews, K. R., & Guth, W. D. (1965). *Business policy: Text and cases.* Homewood, IL: R. D. Irwin.

Maslow, A. H. (1943). A theory of human motivation. *Psychological Review, 50*(4).

Maslow, A. H. (1970). *Motivation and personality.* New York, NY: Harper & Row.

Maslow, A. H. (1998). *Maslow on management.* New York, NY: John Wiley. (Original work—*Eupsychian management: A journal,* 1965, R. D. Irwin)

Mayo Clinic. (1998–2017). Mayo Clinic mission and values. Retrieved from http://www.mayoclinic.org/ about/missionvalues.html

Naisbitt, J. (1982). *Megatrends: Ten new directions transforming our lives.* New York, NY: Warner Books.

Nightingale College. (2017). Mission, vision and values. Retrieved from http://nightingale.edu/mission -vision-and-values

Prendergast, C. (1999). The provision of incentives in firms. *Journal of Economic Literature, 37*(1), 7–63.

Vanderbilt University School of Nursing. (2017). Our mission, vision and values. Retrieved from https:// nursing.vanderbilt.edu/about/mission.php

Financial Statements and the DNP: Essential Knowledge for Success

Tim Bock, Carlton Abner, KT Waxman, and Juli Maxworthy

KEY TERMS

balance sheet

cash flow statement

departmental operating report

depreciation

expenses

financial statements

generally accepted
  accounting principles
  (GAAP)

income statement

operating revenue

ratio analysis

revenue

variance

In today's rapidly evolving health care market, hospitals face increasingly difficult financial pressures. According to the Congressional Budget Office (CBO), absent improvements in efficiency, the percentage of hospitals operating with negative margins will increase from 27% in 2011 to 60% by 2025 (Hayford, Nelson, & Diorio, 2016). As hospitals necessarily focus on creating value and deriving operational efficiencies, a critical skill set of the successful nurse leader will be the ability to accurately interpret and analyze financial statements.

Financial statements provide a snapshot into the business health of an organization. These documents and reports are prepared by teams of financial experts and distributed to internal leaders based on span of control and levels of operational oversight. As a nursing manager, director, or executive, the successful execution of your responsibilities requires that you regularly review these statements. As an essential steward of the organization's financial assets, you are entrusted with the task of ensuring the financial viability of your department(s). A principal component to monitoring your business performance is the review and analysis of your financial statements and the subsequent decision making that stems from your informed understanding of these documents. Although the basics of financial statements are generally the same throughout the industry, each organization will have a different format based on the individual perspective and background of their chief financial officer (CFO).

While sitting at the table with senior financial executives, you will need an intimate understanding of how to view key decisions from their point of view. Your ability to interpret and analyze financial statements will lay the foundation for your ability to engage a group of providers, senior financial executives, or your own team. Doctor of nursing practice (DNP) leaders must use this knowledge of financial statements to speak to both the business and clinical needs of the organization in a way that is tailored to their audience. Your success with procuring things such as needed equipment, additional staff, or capital investments will hinge upon your understanding of these financial statements and how to use them to your advantage while engaging with a given audience. For the purposes of this chapter, we guide you through the basics of three major financial reports to provide you with a clear understanding of common financial terminology, the business interpretation of these numbers, and how these statements are derived from organizational performance.

■ HEALTH CARE ACCOUNTING

Each organization, whether for-profit or not-for-profit, utilizes generally accepted accounting principles (GAAP) for financial reporting. The U.S. government does not directly set accounting standards, in the belief that the private sector has better knowledge and resources. U.S. GAAP is not written in law, although the U.S. Securities and Exchange Commission (SEC) requires that these standards are followed in financial reporting by publicly traded companies. Currently, the SEC has delegated authority for establishing standards of financial reporting to the Financial Accounting Standards Board (FASB). The FASB is a private organization that serves to enhance and improve financial accounting standards for private sector business. For local and state governments, GAAP is determined by the Governmental Accounting Standards Board (GASB), which operates under a set of assumptions, principles, and constraints different from those of standard private sector GAAP. Financial reporting in federal government entities is regulated by the Federal Accounting Standards Advisory Board (FASAB). GAAP is an evolving set of standards, principles, and practices that serve to guide how financial statements are constructed and organized. Thus, although GAAP provides a common set of accepted processes for an organization's accounting efforts, there remains room for expert interpretation and industry-specific emphasis. Although the principles remain the same, the financial statements that follow from these principles are subject to notable variation.

The basic equation of accounting is Assets = Liabilities + Owner's Equity. Assets are the total resources owned by the organization and expressed in dollar terms. Liabilities and owner equity represent the total capital investment borrowed (liabilities) and owned (equity) used to acquire the organization's assets. Note that for not-for-profit entities such as many health care organizations, owner's equity is more correctly referred to as net assets, referring to those assets remaining after accounting for the total liabilities of the organization (Finkler, Jones, & Kovner, 2013). An accounting of organizational assets and liabilities is reported by the balance sheet, which is discussed later in this chapter.

FINANCIAL STATEMENTS

For a business enterprise, financial statements are relevant financial information presented in a structured manner and in a format that is easy to understand. They typically include three basic financial statements:

1. *Statement of financial position*: also referred to as a balance sheet, reports on a company's assets, liabilities, and equity at any given point in time.
2. *Statement of comprehensive income*: also referred to as profit and loss statement (P&L), it is a report on an institution's income, expenses, and profits over a period of time.
3. *Statement of cash flows*: reports on a company's cash flow activities, particularly operating, investing, and financing activities.

Financial statements are tools that provide consistency between businesses, no matter what services they provide. These statements are compiled by financial managers working under the direction of the CFO. The purpose of financial statements is to convey information about the organization's financial condition and the results of its business operations (Finkler et al., 2013). Along with the included notes and ratio analysis found within these documents, financial statements provide the nurse leader an overview of the organization's financial well-being. As a DNP and leader within your organization, your ability to use the information presented by these statements is essential to your role. Like the translational concept inherent to DNP preparation, nurse leaders understand the need to translate information from financial statements into successful business management decisions.

Statement of Financial Position: Balance Sheet

The balance sheet is a snapshot of the organization's financial position at a given point in time through an accounting of the entity's total assets, liabilities, and net equity. Of the three basic financial statements, the balance sheet is the one statement that applies to a single point in time of the fiscal year. The importance of this document is that it directly affects the organization's credit rating, which impacts the ability to leverage external sources of capital to build facilities, expand services, or grow new market share (Waxman, 2008). The document is a numerological picture of what the organization owes and what it owns. This financial position statement indicates an assessment of total assets for the organization and the financing measures employed to acquire those assets. Given that the balance sheet is a statement in time, the document itself would change daily as liabilities and net assets are utilized to generate additional assets because of daily business operations. Furthermore, industry sectors and participants may experience seasonal fluctuations reflecting core business realities. One would expect changes in the balance sheet for hospital organizations subject to seasonal demand changes associated with flu outbreaks or the winter patient influx experienced by many sun belt providers.

Balance sheets often compare the current year to the previous year (or another reasonable time frame, perhaps quarterly). The snapshot provided by the balance sheet is a decent starting point; however, comparing these statements over time provides a more comprehensive view of the organization's business activities. A common strategy for financial managers is to present the current balance sheet in conjunction with year to date and prior year statements. It is critical to understand the balance sheet and read it carefully. The astute observer will look for signs of strengths and weaknesses and get a clear grasp of whether the unit's or organization's financial performance is improving or declining (Finkler et al., 2013). In this manner, organizational leaders can discern a more accurate understanding of the financial health of business operations and assess the impact of strategic management decisions. Table 7.1 is a sample balance sheet for Hospital System Y. Assets are listed at the top and liabilities at the bottom. Depending on your organization, the assets could be on the left and the liabilities on the right, but for the purposes of this exercise, we will use the former.

Assets are resources that are possessed by the organization that have an economic benefit (Penner, 2004). Most assets are tangible in that they can be measured, such as cash, goods, or services; however, some meaningful assets are considered intangible as they are difficult to quantify, such as reputation. Reputation, although problematic to measure, can have a profound effect on the bottom line of an organization. Assets are generally broken down further into two categories to distinguish current assets from long-term assets (Gapenski, 2012).

Current Assets

Current assets are those resources that are either cash, can be converted to cash, or used up within 1 year of the publication of a particular balance sheet. Cash is the most liquid of all assets and is always listed first. The concept of cash includes cash on hand and items known as cash equivalents such as savings, checking accounts, and some short-term certificates of deposits (Finkler et al., 2013). Other financial instruments including certificate of deposit (CD), investment assets, and marketable securities that could be liquidated to cash within the year are also recorded under current assets. It is important for organizations to have cash on hand to fund the daily operations of the business including timely payment to vendors, payroll, and to serve as a mitigating strategy for operational contingencies. Days cash on hand is an important financial ratio for the organization, serves as an indicator for operational cash flow, and is critically important to bond rating. We discuss aspects of ratio analysis later in this chapter.

Cash and cash equivalents are usually followed by accounts receivable (AR), or patient revenue. AR refers to the money that is owed to the organization from the patient or insurer. The money owed to the organization as a result of core business activities—in this case, patient care operations—is reported on the balance sheet as a current asset. However, to generate the

TABLE 7.1 Sample Balance Sheet

($ in 000's)	3/31/17	3/31/16	Change	1-Year Growth
Current Assets				
Cash and investments (savings/checking)	$80,000	$56,800	$23,200	⬆ 40%
Patient revenue (money owed to hospital)	$472,000	$370,120	$101,880	⬆ 26%
Inventory (on the shelf)	$16,400	$15,200	$1,200	⬆ 8%
Subtotal	$568,400	$442,120	$126,280	⬆ 29%
Less:				
Bad debt	($57,200)	($77,250)	$20,050	⬇ 26%
Charitable allowance	($14,100)	($13,680)	($420)	⬆ 3%
Contractual allowance	($269,300)	($233,750)	($35,550)	⬆ 15%
Subtotal	(340,600)	($324,680)	($15,920)	⬆ 5%
Total Current Assets	$227,800	$117,440	$110,360	⬆ 94%
Fixed Assets				
Land	$29,000	$27,500	$1,500	⬆ 5%
Buildings (plant)	$805,000	$805,000	$0	No Change
Equipment	$610,000	$624,000	($14,000)	⬇ 2%
Construction in progress	$37,000	$28,000	$9,000	⬆ 32%
Total Fixed Assets	$1,481,000	$1,484,500	($3,500)	⬇ 0.2%
Less accumulated depreciation	($880,800)	($810,200)	($70,600)	⬇ 9%
Net Fixed Assets	$600,200	$674,300	($74,100)	⬇ 11%
Total Assets	$828,000	$791,740	$36,260	⬆ 5%
Current Liabilities				
Accounts payable salaries, supplies, pharm	$36,560	$27,600	($8,960)	⬆ 32%
Accrued compensation and benefits	$10,900	$8,280	($2,620)	⬆ 32%
Accrued liabilities (interest, physician contracts)	$2,520	$2,960	$440	⬇ 15%
Current portion of long-term debt	$8,350	$9,000	$650	⬇ 7%
Subtotal	$58,330	$47,840	($10,490)	⬇ 22%
Long-Term Liabilities				
Bonds payable	$38,000	$37,000	($1,000)	⬆ 3%
Mortgage payable	$2,100	$1,900	($200)	⬆ 11%
Subtotal	$40,100	$38,900	($1,200)	⬆ 3%
Total Current Liabilities	$98,430	$86,740	($11,690)	⬆ 13%
Net Worth (Assets–Liabilities)	$729,570	$705,000	$24,570	⬆ 3%
Total Liabilities and Net Worth	$828,000	$791,740	$36,260	⬆ 5%

revenue associated with the provision of care requires a consumption of resources. The hospital must maintain an inventory of various patient care supplies and resources to service daily care activities. Those inventories that will be consumed as a result of clinical operations in the provision of care such as wound dressings, linens, and medications are all considered current assets and are reported accordingly on the balance sheet. These items are presently in the facility and can be thought of as "on-the-shelf" inventory.

The sum of reported cash, AR, and inventories reflects an organization's current gross assets. However, in order to determine net assets, the following must be deducted: bad debt, charitable allowances, and contractual allowances associated with governmental and other payers. *Bad debt* represents payment for care that, although expected to be paid, is in fact not paid. Although organizations can use various measures for collecting these payments, at some point these charges are written off as a loss and thus subtracted from the organization's gross assets. The GAAP process for managing such nonpayments is to include a provision for bad debt on the balance sheet. This provision for bad debt is a prediction of the amount of money owed to the organization by patients and payers (Patient Revenue line in Table 7.1) that will never be collected. The number on this line for bad debt is an estimate derived through an annual assessment of the organization's actual bad debt from the prior year. *Charitable allowances* include care provided to those who have limited resources and are not expected to pay. The accounting for charitable care is managed in a parallel fashion to bad debt and likewise recorded on the balance sheet. Charity care is distinctly different from bad debt based on expectation of payment. Provisions for charity care are based on the known inability to pay on the part of the patient, whereas bad debt is that expected to be paid by those with an ability to pay who do not. Charitable care is free or donated care, whereas bad debt is the result of an unpaid bill. It is important to distinguish bad debt from charity because the latter can be used to demonstrate a financial benefit to the community, whereas the former cannot—a key consideration for not-for-profit providers. In hospitals that have less than optimal payer mixes, there is typically a larger percentage of unfunded and underfunded care provided to the community. Depending on ability to pay, that care may become bad debt or provided as uncompensated charity care. The larger the proportion of bad debt and charity care, the more financial value that must be subtracted from the organization's balance sheet.

Lastly, the *contractual allowance* line in Table 7.1 is most significant. This number reflects the discount to charges accorded to third-party payers by the hospital. These contractual rates are negotiated agreements between the hospital and payer and represent an agreed-on percentage reduction in the gross charges incurred because of an episode of care. Depending on the relationship and contract with the provider, this can be a significant adjustment. Government payers exact more of a contractual allowance than do commercial payers. It is the combination of bad debt, charitable care, and government payments to private payments that perpetuates the vexing problem of cost shifting within health care. Although appreciated on a national and political level, this cost shifting can be discretely visualized within your organization's own balance sheet. Particularly as it pertains to the contractual allowance, a higher proportion of private payers (thus fewer government payments) results in a lower contractual allowance and thus higher retention of gross assets as net assets.

Fixed Assets

Fixed assets (also called property and equipment) are an asset class that cannot be converted to cash within a year (Finkler et al., 2013). Examples are land, building, and equipment owned by the organization. If there is any construction occurring on the campus, the value of that construction would also be considered a fixed asset. Fixed assets are listed on the balance sheet using the historical purchase price minus the accumulated depreciation for the assets. Fixed assets are used to generate revenues over time and we need to account for their usefulness accordingly. Furthermore, if we ascribed the purchase price of fixed assets to a single year without expensing the cost over time, we would have a disproportionately negative impact on profitability for the year of acquisition (Gapenski, 2012). To account for the long-term utility of a fixed asset, the initial cost of an asset is spread over time as an expense, which is termed *depreciation*. The rate of depreciation is determined by the organization, but GAAP principles are adhered to for any such calculations. This depreciation expense accounts for lost value on the original price of the organization's fixed assets.

Liabilities

Liabilities are shown on the balance sheet as current and long-term liabilities. *Current liabilities* are those obligations that must be paid off within the year, whereas long-term liabilities are those that will be paid off in a time period longer than a year (Finkler et al., 2013). The biggest liability for any health care organization is salaries and is reflected under accounts payable. This number accounts for salaries owed to employees. Other accounts payable liabilities include money owed, but not yet paid to suppliers and pharmaceutical companies. *Accrued compensation* includes non-salary liabilities such as vacation time, sick time, and benefits. *Accrued liabilities* are short-term obligations that will need to be paid by the organization and include interest, certain physician contract requirements, and Social Security payments. If the organization has any long-term debts that are to be paid off within the year, these would also be found in this section. *Long-term liabilities* include bonds and mortgage payables, should the organization have an outstanding bond or mortgage. Once the liabilities are totaled, the net worth (or owner's equity) is the difference between the total assets and total liabilities. The goal, of course, is for total liabilities to be less than total assets.

Statement of Comprehensive Income: Income Statement

The income statement is also referred to as the P&L statement or operating statement (Table 7.2). This important document summarizes organizational and departmental revenue and expenses, or credits and debits. The purpose of the income statement is to show managers and investors whether the company made or lost money during the period being reported. It is usually a monthly document for each department as well as the entire organization. In larger organizations, this report can be compiled by individual division or service line. As a nurse leader, you will frequently encounter ideas and opportunities to improve patient care. Whatever the proposed program or project under consideration for improving care delivery, your understanding of operating statements will allow you to realistically evaluate resources needed to support new programs. Your ability to demonstrate to senior financial leaders that your proposed project or program will not threaten existing obligations is critical to gaining the necessary approvals to move forward. The first step in gaining that level of confidence is through developing a clear and articulate understanding of your organization's income statements.

Using GAAP principles, the revenue from patients is listed first. Remember that gross revenue is what is charged to the patient or insurer rather than pure cash. Gross revenue, charges to payers, is quite different from paid reimbursement, the cash payments collected for services. As mentioned previously, the charges are adjusted based on contracts with insurers (contractual allowance) and are listed under "Deductions From Revenue" within the income statement.

Gross patient revenue can be broken down into several categories: routine services, inpatient ancillary, outpatient ancillary, and other revenue. Routine services include charges associated with standard patient care needs such as room charges, food, and medication. Inpatient ancillary revenue includes charges incurred during the course of an inpatient stay for individual treatments, procedures, and tests performed by departments such as respiratory therapy, radiology, laboratory, physical therapy, and so forth. These departments are commonly referred to as ancillary departments. Outpatient ancillary revenue includes charges associated with individual treatments, tests, and procedures associated with care not provided during an inpatient

TABLE 7.2 Income Statement (Profit and Loss)

($ in 000's)	3/17	3/16	Change	1-Year Growth
Gross Patient Revenues				
Routine services	$150,000	$142,500	$7,500	↑ 5%
Inpatient ancillary	$62,500	$49,350	$13,150	↑ 27%
Outpatient ancillary	$118,000	$96,500	$21,500	↑ 22%
Other revenue	$2,500	$2,150	$350	↑ 16%
Total Gross Revenue	$333,000	$290,500	$42,500	↑ 15%
Deductions From Revenue				
Bad debt	$18,000	$21,500	$3,500	↓ 16%
Government allowance DRG	$71,000	$60,800	($10,200)	↑ 17%
Insurance contracts mgd. care	$35,400	$38,400	$3,000	↓ 8%
Charitable allowances	$13,600	$12,500	($1,100)	↑ 9%
Total Deductions	$138,000	$133,200	($4,800)	↑ 4%
Net Revenue From Patient	$195,000	$157,300	$45,700	↑ 24%
Operating Expenses				
Salaries	$90,250	$79,200	($11,050)	↑ 14%
Benefits	$34,000	$31,800	(2,800)	↑ 7%
Supplies	$27,200	$13,600	($13,600)	↑ 100%
Medical fees	$4,300	$3,200	($1,100)	↑ 34%
Purchased services	$8,400	$5,520	($2,880)	↑ 52%
Maintenance	$7,500	$6,200	($1,300)	↑ 21%
Professional liability	$1,400	$1,350	($50)	↑ 4%
Other	$700	$350	($350)	↑ 100%
Depreciation	$7,400	$6,200	($1,200)	↑ 19%
Financing costs	$6,400	$6,100	($300)	↑ 5%
Total Operating Expenses	$187,550	$153,520	$34,030	↑ 22%
Net Income From Operations (pretax)	$7,450	$3,780	$3,670	↑ 97%
% of Net Revenue (Margin) (Net Income/Net Revenue)	3.82%	2.40%	1.42%	

DRG, diagnosis-related group.

admission. Lastly, there may be other revenue that comes into the organization by way of a gift shop or cafeteria.

Once the total charges are added up, we must account for bad debt, contractual allowances for both governmental and other payers, and charity care. This will result in net revenue from patient care, sometimes referred to as *operating revenue*. This is the amount of cash generated through the organization's clinical operations during the accounting cycle. This cash will be used to pay salaries, buy supplies, purchase services, and maintain the physical plant. For purposes of the income statement, we need to account for these operational expenses before we can derive the organization's net income.

Operating Expenses

Operating expenses are listed on the bottom of the income statement in this case, but other formats may report expenses on the right side of the statement with revenues recorded on the left. The first line item under this section is salaries, because it is the largest expense departmentally and organizationally. Followed by benefits, this is usually between 20% and 40% depending on the region in which the facility resides. Supplies, medical fees, maintenance, and professional liability expenses follow. All purchased services are also found under operating expenses and can be a large number depending on what services the organization outsources. For example, if housekeeping or nutritional services are an outsourced service, the fees would be found here. If the organization uses traveling nurses, they would be found here as well. Any depreciation and financing costs would fall under expenses and, once totaled, the difference between revenue and expenses would be the net income. This is pretax; thus, for-profit organizations would need to pay taxes on this amount, which would need to be deducted from this number.

One important indicator of financial performance is the organization's net revenue percentage, also known as the "margin." This number can be found by dividing the net income by the net revenue. Hopefully this number is greater than zero. Within the current health care environment margins between 0% and 5% are common, whereas 20 years ago we were seeing much larger margins. To maintain or improve margins, one can appreciate from the income statement why organizations develop discrete strategies to either increase revenue or reduce costs. As a DNP and organizational leader, you are well served to understand proposed budget changes and their subsequent impact on specific lines of the income statement.

Statement of Cash Flows: Cash Flow Statement

A *cash flow statement*, also known as statement of cash flows or funds flow statement, is a financial statement that shows an organization's cash inflows and outflows (Table 7.3). This document

TABLE 7.3 Cash Flow Statement

($ in 000's)	January 1, 2016 to December 31, 2016
Net income	$131,000
Depreciation and amortization	$70,000
Decrease (increase) in inventories	($20,000)
Decrease (increase) in accounts receivable	$20,000
Increase (decrease) in accounts payable	$30,000
Cash Flows From Operations	$231,000
Capital expenditures	($40,000)
Cash Flows From Investing	($40,000)
Increase in bank loans	$0
Increase in long-term debt	$2,000
Increase in paid-in capital	$0
Cash Flows From Financing	$2,000
Net increase (decrease) in cash and equivalents	$193,000
Cash at beginning of year	$80,000
Cash at end of year	$273,000

provides details as to the sources of cash and how the organization uses this cash; information not available through either the balance sheet or the income statement. The statement of cash flows is broken down into three constituent parts: operating, investing, and financing activities. Essentially, the cash flow statement is concerned with the flow of cash in and out of the business and explains year over year changes in the organization's cash position. The statement captures both the current operating results and the accompanying changes in the balance sheet. It is an analytical tool and useful in determining the short-term viability of a company as well as reporting on the profitability of core business operations. In health care facilities, cash flow statements contain information that is reviewed with the board of directors, especially if facing financial challenges or if it is a for-profit entity. If you invest in stocks, you periodically receive financial reports from these organizations demonstrating their ability to pay their debts and distribute dividends to shareholders. The statements of cash flows will also indicate if core business activities are self-sustaining, or if the organization must pull in cash from other resources to cover operations.

Note that for the cash flow statement, the organization's depreciation is added back into the analysis. Recall that in the income statement we subtract depreciation from gross revenues as part of the accounting mechanism to derive net revenue. The cash flow statement is an analysis of cash flows into and out of the organization and is not a report on net income. A simplification is that the cash flow for the organization is the result of net operating income plus noncash expenses (Gapenski, 2012). Thus, for purposes of analysis we add back our charge for depreciation as well as adjust for considerations of inventories, receivables, and accounts payable to fully understand the flow of cash into and out of our organization.

Financial Ratios and Ratio Analysis

Looking at each individual number or line item from the financial statements (Table 7.3) provides valuable insight. However, when key numbers within the financial statements are compared with others, we are given insight into the finances of the organization that we would not have had when looking at individual numbers alone. This evaluation of business performance using accounting data is referred to as ratio analysis. Ratios should be compared over a given time frame and are more valuable when also compared to state, regional, and/or national benchmarks for the same ratio. The most common types of ratios include:

- Liquidity ratios, which provide insight into an organization's ability to meet its obligation over the next year
- Solvency ratios, which provide insight into an organization's ability to meet its obligation in the long term
- Common size ratios, which provide an indication of the relative size of the organization
- Profitability ratios, which provide insight into an organization's ability to produce profits and cash flow
- Efficiency ratios, which provide insight into how efficiently an organization is using its resources

Table 7.4 provides a closer look at common financial ratios used in health care organizations and how to calculate them.

▨ DEPARTMENTAL/UNIT TOPICS

DEPARTMENTAL OPERATING REPORT

The *departmental operating report*, also known as the cost center report, contains relevant information about a particular department or operating unit. Usually available on a monthly basis, this

TABLE 7.4 Additional Financial Ratios

Current Ratio

What it is	The current ratio is an indicator of whether a hospital has enough resources to pay its debts over the next 12 months. It compares current assets to current liabilities.
How it is used	The current ratio helps investors and creditors understand the liquidity of an organization and how well that organization is managing its liabilities. A higher current ratio is more favorable than a lower current ratio because it shows that the organization can easily manage its current debt.
How it is calculated	$$\text{Current ratio} = \frac{\text{Current assets}}{\text{Current liabilities}}$$

Quick Ratio (Acid Test)

What it is	Measures the dollars of current assets (not including inventories) per dollar of current liabilities.
How it is used	The quick ratio is a more stringent measure of liquidity than the current ratio because it removes the least liquid of assets, inventories, from the calculation.
How it is calculated	$$\text{Quick ratio (Acid test)} = \frac{\text{Current assets} - \text{Inventories}}{\text{Current liabilities}}$$

Debt Ratio

What it is	The debt to equity ratio is another analysis of liquidity that compares an organization's total debt to total equity.
How it is used	The debt ratio defines debt as all interest bearing and noninterest bearing liabilities, making it the most inclusive of the capitalization ratios. The debt ratio shows the percentage of financing that comes from creditors and investors. The higher the debt ratio, the greater the amount of debt financing.
How it is calculated	$$\text{Debt ratio} = \frac{\text{Total debt}}{\text{Total assets}} \times 100$$

Total Margin (%)

What it is	Net income divided by total revenue.
How it is used	Calculates an organization's ability to control expenses by measuring the total profitability as a percentage of total revenues. The higher the total margin, the better it is. Note that total margin includes both operating and nonoperating revenue, so an organization could be operating at a loss but, if nonoperating revenue were large enough, still have a positive total margin.
How it is calculated	$$\text{Total margin} = \frac{\text{Net income}}{\text{Total revenues}} \times 100$$

Return on Assets (%)

What it is	This ratio is a profitability ratio that measures total profitability as a percentage of total assets. It provides guidance on how efficiently an organization uses it to generate income.

(continued)

TABLE 7.4 Additional Financial Ratios (*continued*)

Return on Assets (%)

How it is used	Often referred to as the return on total assets, the higher the ratio the more favorable the organization is to investors as it shows more effective management of assets to produce greater amounts of net income. A positive ratio usually indicates an upward profit trend as well.
How it is calculated	$$\text{Return on assets} = \frac{\text{Net income}}{\text{Total assets}} \times 100$$

Days Cash on Hand

What it is	Days cash on hand measures the number of days that an organization could continue to pay its daily cash obligations without new cash resources.
How it is used	Higher values imply higher liquidity and are viewed favorably by creditors. However, organizations should avoid holding excess amounts of cash and short-term investments because they typically provide a lower return than long-term investments.
How it is calculated	$$\text{Days Cash on Hand} = \frac{\text{Cash} + \text{short-term investments}}{(\text{Total expenses} - \text{Depreciation}) / 365}$$

Days in Accounts Receivable

What it is	Days in accounts receivable (AR) is a measure of the average time it takes an organization to collect what it is owed (receivables).
How it is used	Provides insight into how effective an organization is at managing its receivables. The shorter the average collection period, the lower the dollar amount of receivables, which leads to a lower carrying cost.
How it is calculated	$$\text{Days in AR} = \frac{\text{Net patient accounts receivable}}{(\text{Net patient service revenue} / 365)}$$

Average Age of Plant

What it is	Average age of plant is the average age (in years) of an organization's fixed assets.
How it is used	Provides an indication of how "distressed" an organization's fixed assets are. A low average age usually indicates that an organization will not require large capital expenditures in the near future. Empirical studies show an association between financial status, bond ratings, and net operating revenue projections with an organization's average age of plant and equipment.
How it is calculated	$$\text{Average age of plant} = \frac{\text{Accumulated depreciation}}{\text{Depreciation expense}}$$

Average Daily Census

What it is	The average daily census is the average number of inpatients treated during a given period of time.
How it is used	Provides a measure of inpatient volume on the basis of number of patients. Because a higher number spreads fixed costs over a greater number of patients, a higher average daily census is considered beneficial as it tends to indicate higher profitability.

(*continued*)

TABLE 7.4 Additional Financial Ratios (*continued*)

Average Daily Census

How it is calculated	$$\text{Average daily census} = \frac{\text{Total number of inpatient services for a given period}}{\text{Total number of days in the same period}}$$

Inpatient Bed Occupancy Rate/Bed Utilization Rate

What it is	The occupancy rate is the actual number of inpatient beds occupied by patients over a given time. It is expressed as a percentage of the total number of available beds.
How it is used	This ratio is used to gauge the appropriate balance between the demand for inpatient care and the number of beds available to provide inpatient care. The occupancy rate is a calculation used to show the actual utilization of an inpatient health facility for a given time period.
How it is calculated	$$\text{Occupancy rate} = \frac{\text{Total number of inpatient beds occupied}}{\text{Total number of inpatient beds available}} \times 100$$

report may contain multiple departments within the same division or report out on a single operating unit. The difference between the departmental report and the income statement is that the departmental reports thoroughly break down revenue and expenses to the individual cost center to help managers keep a close eye on the money going in and out of their units (Waxman, 2008). This report does not contain information regarding contractual allowances, which is addressed at the hospital level. As a result, gross revenue may be monitored at the unit level for purposes of assessing charge capture opportunities and possible patient trends, but not net revenue—thus, the departmental operating report emphasis on expense control and variance reporting.

Many departments, due to changes in volume, have variances that occur when the budget is compared to actual operating expenses. When this occurs, most institutions require the manager of the area to provide explanations of these variances. Many organizations request explanations of variances for both positive and negative outcomes of certain amounts (variances between line items). As an individual with oversight (and responsibility), it is essential to understand each line item of your budget. The "buckets" of items that can occupy each line item can be surprising, and if you are new to your position and your predecessor is not available, you may become mired in the available details. Most organizations have guidelines of what should be placed in each line item of a budget, but there is variability between institutions. A thorough review of these operating or cost center reports will certainly be part of your onboarding to a new role or organization where you have such budgetary authority. If this has not been provided, seek this assistance immediately as you will be held accountable to the operating performance of your department/s. It is strongly recommended that you set regular meetings with your organization's finance program manager to thoroughly understand your operating reports and develop the acumen for proactively detecting trends and issues that you and your teams need to address.

With the digitization of clinical health records, many organizations have begun to utilize data generated for electronic health records (EHRs) to produce clinical and financial information as part of an integrated and enterprise-wide approach to data management. The integration of clinical and financial data provides the ability to capture charges associated with care delivery within the normal flow of patient care and clinical documentation. The benefit of this digitized and enterprise-wide approach is that it often comes with dashboards that provide an at-a-glance view of financial performance. If your organization uses such an approach, you will want to become familiar with how the data is generated and develop a clear understanding of what actions you can take in response to identified trends and issues.

VARIANCE

Variances occur in many ways for many reasons in health care. As far as budgeting is concerned, the variance is the difference between what has been projected for the budget and the actual performance. For the individual who has oversight of the budget, variance analysis is often a monthly exercise, which provides the rationale for why there is a positive or a negative variance in a particular cost center. There are many variables that can affect a variance, and as the individual with oversight, it is critical to know how to articulate and explain these causes.

The terms *positive* and *negative* are utilized when describing a variance. When volume and overtime are both higher than expected, there would be both a positive and negative variance, with the positive referring to the increase in the volume and the negative referring to the overtime. These two variables are often closely linked, and it is the role of the nurse leader to review and adjust staffing if the variability becomes the norm. As a DNP and nurse leader, it is important to be able to explain variances fully and develop action plans to manage these variances. For example, if the volume (patient days) increases in a particular nursing unit, it would be safe to assume that the salaries would increase as well. The example in Exhibit 7.1 shows us that, even though the volume increased, salaries increased more than usual.

Typically, variance reporting involves explanation of variance from target budgets. A target budget is a budget that flexes with volume and adjusts budget variables directly affected by volume. This is a particularly useful accounting tool in health care, where patient volumes may fluctuate for any number of reasons from budgeted volumes. As mentioned, if patient volumes are more than budgeted, the organization can reliably predict that salaries will also be above budget. In the case of a flexing variable such as labor cost, the increase in cost expected should be predictably reliable based on the volume observed. In simple terms, a 5% increase in monthly patient volume may be expected to increase labor costs by 5%; thus, the target labor budget for the month would be 105% of what was initially budgeted by the organization. However, if actual labor budget (labor dollars spent during the month) exceeds this new target, then the manager may be required to explain why the labor costs were higher than expected, after considering the additional volume.

EXHIBIT 7.1 Payroll Variance This Month ($40,000)

	Budget	Actual	Variance
Patient Days	450	500	50 patient days over what was budgeted
Payroll Dollars	$209,854	$249,854	($40,000) over what was budgeted
Cost/Patient Day	$466.34	$499.71	($33.37/patient day) more than budgeted

Analysis of variance

Volume: *What portion of the variance can be explained by the volume increase of 50 patient days?*

50 days × $466.34 per patient day (as budgeted) = $23,317

With the $40,000 variance in payroll, only $23,317 is attributed to volume increase. How will you explain the remaining $16,683? Acuity, transfers, overtime?

Variance reporting at the cost center level is almost exclusively an analysis of productivity (labor, volume, overtime) that compares actual month end results to targeted (volume-adjusted) budgets.

KEY INDICATORS FOR PERFORMANCE

CONTRACTUAL ALLOWANCES

You have learned in previous chapters how providers are reimbursed and why increasing the charges is not a wise move, as we are typically paid on a diagnosis-related group (DRG) basis or flat rate or percentage of charges. An example of an actual Medicare DRG reimbursement for a hospital can be found in Exhibit 7.2.

EXHIBIT 7.2 Sample Medicare DRG Reimbursement

Net Revenue and Profit Calculation/Medicare Acute Admission

		Base Calculation	DRG 127 Heart Failure and Shock $30,758.65
Gross Charge:		(Total Charges Incurred and Billed to Medicare)	
Reimbursement calculation:	Federal standard labor	$3,022.18	
	Wage index	X 0.9793	
	Wage adj. std amt	$2,959.62	
	Nonlabor fed std amt	1,852.31	
	Adjusted base rate	$4,811.03	
	Oper. dispropr. share	$1,654.34	
	Operating IME	548.44	
	Federal capital rate	427.03	
	Large urban factor	X 1.03	
	Geograph. adj. factor	X 0.9858	
	Adj. capital rate	$ 433.60	
	Capital disprop. share	50.82	
	Capital IME	61.74	
	Total base payment	$7,989.91 $7,899.91	
	DRG weight (intensity)	1.0 1.049	
Total Reimbursement	**DRG Payment**	**$7,989.91 $8,381.41**	
		(amount hospital was paid)	
Contractual adjustment—(gross charges less reimbursement)		**$22,377.24** **(amount hospital wrote off)**	

Wage index is a value associated with the Office of Management and Budget's CBSA-based geographical designations, by which the base rate may be adjusted.

CBSA, core-based statistical areas; DRG, diagnosis-related group; IME, independent medical examination.

DEPRECIATION

Depreciation is the loss in value the organization anticipates for its buildings and equipment. As assets age, they become less valuable. From an accounting perspective, buildings and equipment generally wear out over time and their value is lessened; they are said to depreciate in value. To account for the diminished value of the organization's assets, we need to capture depreciation on both the balance sheet and income statement. The depreciation expense is the amount of the original cost of a fixed asset allocated as an expense each year. The current value of the depreciated equipment is found on the balance sheet as an asset. Depreciation is usually not done at the unit level; it is calculated at the hospital level. So unless you are working in the finance department, you most likely won't be involved in calculating it. Where you will be involved is in the planning process for replacing capital assets assigned to your department. Imaging equipment, patient care beds, and telemetry systems are just a few of the many types of assets assigned to your unit that are expected to stay in service for many years. Prematurely replacing capital equipment before it has fully depreciated can result in a significant write down of asset values. Such an action, depending on the size of the write down, can have a profound impact on the income statement and balance sheet. As a manager, you need to be aware of those capital assets listed on your department and work with finance teams to strategically plan an appropriate replacement timeline.

EARNINGS BEFORE INTEREST, TAXES, DEPRECIATION, AND AMORTIZATION (EBITDA)

Earnings before interest, taxes, depreciation, and amortization represent how much money a company earns if it did not have to pay interest, tax, or take depreciation and amortization charges. EBITDA is intended to be an indicator of a company's financial performance without consideration of debt, tax, or asset base. EBITDA calculations enable a comparison of profitability across companies and industries despite variations in individual financing and accounting practices. It is also a useful measure for a company's creditors, as it shows the income available for interest payments. This is becoming a much more common way to determine earnings.

PAID CLAIMS RATIO (PCR)

PCR is the hospital bills versus what they actually collect. This metric is similar to asking what we collect on the dollar. To calculate the PCR, we look at the gross charges and divide it by the actual revenue collected. Here is an example:

Gross charges: $800,409,012

Collectable revenue (due to contractual allowances): $208,027,145

The percentage of revenue versus gross charges can be calculated by dividing the collectable revenue by the gross charges:

$208,027,145/800,409,012 = 26\%$. This means that the PCR is 26%, and that for every dollar billed, the hospital collects 26 cents.

YEAR-TO-DATE (YTD)

YTD is a period starting from the beginning of the current year, and continuing up to the present day. The year usually starts on January 1 (calendar year), but depending on purpose can start also on July 1 (fiscal year). YTD is used in many contexts, mainly for recording results of an activity in the time from an exclusive date, since this day may not yet be "complete" (Dunham-Taylor & Pinczuk, 2010).

CONCLUSION

It is critical that nurse leaders, especially DNPs, are knowledgeable of the elements of financial statements and the implications for practice. As health care potentially becomes more complex in the next decade, with impeding sweeping health care reform, strong financial acumen will be a benefit for both the DNP and the organization.

CRITICAL THINKING EXERCISES

1. The invasive radiology department has just purchased a piece of equipment that enables them to perform many of their procedures faster. One of the results of this improvement is that they are able to schedule 20% more cases on an average weekday. During the preplanning of this improvement, the director of short stay was not included and was told her staffing needs might increase by 10%. After the first month of the use of the new equipment, the short stay unit had the following variances. Which of the following variances are positive and which ones are negative? What does the director need to report to senior leadership as to what has happened and why, and what she is doing to make appropriate adjustments?

	Budget	Actual	Variance
Volume (patients)	1,000	1,200	200
Overtime hours (staffing)	50	75	25
Supplies	5,000	5,100	100

2. Using the information in the table, complete the blank columns provided by calculating the variance (both positive and negative) for each month's patient days and nursing hours. Enter your answer on the table in the blank columns.

	Month	Actual Patient Days	Budgeted Patient Days	Variance	Actual Nursing Hours	Budgeted Nursing Hours	Variance
1	January	1,116	1,116		10,965	10,044	
2	February	1,030	1,008		10,209	9,074	
3	March	974	896		8,060	8,064	
4	April	876	960		8,560	8,640	
5	May	930	868		7,739	7,812	

3. Your hospital replaced its entire inpatient bed fleet 10 years ago (120 months) and the nursing departments are stating they need to be replaced again. The beds were originally purchased for $15,000 each and the replacement beds from the same vendor are now $20,000 each. At the time of the original purchase, the beds were assigned a useful life of 15 years.
   a. What is the net book value (NBV—or remaining depreciation) on the organization's 200 beds?
   b. How would the NBV influence your decision making to support or not support this request?
   c. As a nurse leader responsible for stewardship of financial resources, assuring quality patient outcomes, and maintaining an engaged nursing workforce, how would you proceed in balancing these three requisite responsibilities of your role?

4. Review the income statement provided in Table 7.2 and address the following questions:
   a. From your analysis, you understand that the net margin for the organization has shown strong growth over the past year. What factor/s is/are driving this improved performance?
   b. What concerns do you have regarding current financial performance of this organization? As an executive leader within this organization, what priority issues should this organization address?
   c. Is your impression of the reported financial performance generally favorable or unfavorable? Why?
5. Using the data in Table 7.1 and the definitions from Table 7.4, calculate the current ratio, quick ratio, and the debt ratio.
   a. What information do these ratios provide?
   b. If you were concerned about the result, what could be done to adjust these ratios?
   c. In what ways could these ratios be negatively impacted?
   d. When assessing the results of these ratios, what advice would you have for this organization if it was considering securing financing for a major capital expense?
6. Using the data in Table 7.1 and the definitions from Table 7.4, calculate the days cash on hand.
   a. What information does this financial ratio provide?
   b. If you were concerned about the result, what could be done to positively impact this ratio?
   c. In what ways could this ratio be negatively impacted?
7. Using the information in the following table, calculate the average daily census and the bed utilization rate over the last 3 months for this 395-bed hospital.

Month	July	August	September
Days of service	11,480	10,150	9,765

REFERENCES

Dunham-Taylor, J., & Pinczuk, J. (2010). *Financial management for nurse managers*. Sudbury, MA: Jones & Barlett.

Finkler, S., Jones, C., & Kovner, C. (2013). *Financial management for nurse managers and executives* (4th ed.). St. Louis, MO: Saunders/Elsevier.

Gapenski, L. C. (2012). *Healthcare finance: An introduction to accounting and financial management* (5th ed.). Chicago, IL: Health Administration Press.

Hayford, T., Nelson, L., & Diorio, A. (2016). *Projecting hospitals' profit margins under several illustrative scenarios*. Washington, DC: Congressional Budget Office.

Penner, S. (2004). *Introduction to health care economics and financial management*. Philadelphia, PA: Lippincott Williams & Wilkins.

Waxman, K. T. (2008). *A practical guide to finance and budgeting: Skills for nurse managers* (2nd ed.). Marblehead, MA: HCPro.

8 Quality Initiatives: Building the Business Case for Quality

Juli Maxworthy

KEY TERMS

business case	practice management	risk adjustment
comparative effectiveness	pay for performance	value-based purchasing
cost–benefit analysis	quality-adjusted life year	
cost-effectiveness of care	quality improvement	

What is quality in health care? The National Academy of Medicine—NAM (formally known as the Institute of Medicine [IOM]), which has done extensive research and produced the game-changing health care work *To Err Is Human: Building a Safer Health Care System* in 1999, defines quality in health care as "the degree to which health services for individuals and populations increase the likelihood of desired health outcomes and are consistent with current professional knowledge" (IOM, 1999, p. 211). *To Err Is Human* (IOM, 1999) and, subsequently, *Crossing the Quality Chasm* (IOM, 2001) were reports that rocked the health care industry to its core. How could we be allowing 44,000 to 98,000 people to die in hospitals across the United States due to preventable errors every year? It seemed an impossible statistic. Insurance companies as well as the Centers for Medicare and Medicaid Services (CMS) had up until recent years been paying a hospital no matter what the patient outcomes. Preventable health care outcomes such as pressure ulcers and falls were paid by these payers and it was assumed that it was just part of doing business in health care.

Crossing the Quality Chasm (2001) provided health care with tangible solutions for what appeared to most to be literally a chasm that existed in health care related to ensuring that quality care is provided. The report identified many sources of underuse, misuse, and overuse of our current health care system, which contributes to the overall health care costs by increasing direct, indirect, and opportunity costs (IOM, 2001). The authors of the report identified six important aims for the U.S. health care system. The IOM report (2001) suggests that care should be:

- Safe (avoiding injury to patients)
- Effective (providing care based on scientific knowledge while minimizing the overuse, underuse, or misuse of care)
- Patient centered (being respectful, responsive, and considerate of patient preferences, needs, and values)
- Timely (minimizing delays and wait times)
- Efficient (avoiding waste)
- Equitable (providing care that does not vary based on race, gender, geography, or socioeconomic status)

These straightforward tenets seem reasonable, but, in light of the current state of health care in the United States, also seem at times unattainable. These same elements are woven into several of the essentials of the doctors of nursing practice (DNP; see Appendix 8.A). There is a tremendous need for health care leaders to understand the connection between quality outcomes and the savings that can affect the bottom line. There are a multitude of organizations that are insisting and assisting health care institutions to gain and maintain quality outcomes for the benefit of society. This chapter provides insight and examples of how health care is trying to determine what a positive outcome looks like to both the consumer and the institution. It will explore the delicate relationship in health care between quality and costs and how understanding this relationship can be a critical piece in making a business case for funding initiatives, which can improve the outcomes of our patients. It will also discuss the relationships among health care financing, costs, and quality outcomes and the value of building a business case for quality that can ensure that monies are spent on the right initiatives. By understanding the essential elements of quality and learning how to improve outcomes and incorporating them into an effective business plan, the DNP will have the tools to make the necessary changes to health care.

The Essentials of Doctoral Education for Advanced Nursing Practice (American Association of Colleges of Nursing [AACN], 2006) describes various competencies for the DNP nurse. Those addressed in this chapter are:

- *Essential II*—Organizational and Systems Leadership for Quality Improvement and Systems Thinking
- *Essential III*—Clinical Scholarship and Analytical Methods for Evidence-Based Practice

▓ QUALITY IMPROVEMENT STRATEGIES/TECHNIQUES

STRUCTURE/PROCESS/OUTCOME

There are multiple proven strategies that can be applied to assist with performance improvement activities. It is important to begin with one of the founders of modern quality, Avedis Donabedian. Donabedian defined quality as a function of structures, processes, and outcomes of care (Donabedian, 1966). He described structural aspects of quality as resources used in the provision of care (e.g., physicians, nurses, and other health care providers), process aspects of quality as the activities involved in providing care (e.g., the model of care delivery used and organizational policies and procedures), and outcomes as the consequences of care (e.g., condition-specific results of care and patient satisfaction; Donabedian, 1982). He also identified seven pillars he considered to be attributes of quality (Donabedian, 1990):

- Efficacy: the ability of care to improve health
- Effectiveness: the degree to which attainable health improvements are realized
- Efficiency: the ability to obtain the greatest health improvement at the lowest cost
- Optimality: the most advantageous balancing of costs and benefits
- Acceptability: conformity to patient preferences regarding accessibility, the patient–practitioner relationship, the amenities, the effects of care, and the cost of care
- Legitimacy: conformity to social preferences concerning all of the above
- Equity: fairness in the distribution of care and its effects on health

The similarities between Donadebian's work and that of the Institute for Healthcare Improvement (IHI) regarding the recommendations of the IOM report, *Crossing the Quality Chasm*, should be noted. In the late 1990s, the Nursing Role Effectiveness Model (Irvine, Sidani, & McGillis Hall, 1998), derived from Donabedian's structure–process–outcomes framework, was conceptualized as an approach for measuring and improving quality in nursing. In keeping with Donabedian's approach, this model recognizes that structural and process components affect patient outcomes. Pringle and Doran (2003) identified the following as examples of variables that comprise these three components:

- Structure
  - Patients: age, gender, education, socioeconomic status, type and severity of illness, comorbidities
  - Nurses: education, experience, position, tenure
  - Organization: staffing, staffing mix, workload, and work environment

- Process
  - Nurses' independent role, including patient education and the implementation of nursing interventions
  - Medical care-related activities, including medically directed or prescribed care, and the expanded scope of advanced nursing clinical practice
  - Interdependent role: communication, coordination of care, discharge planning, and case/care management

- Nurse-sensitive outcomes:
  - Functional health outcomes, such as functional status, and self-care ability
  - Clinical outcomes, such as symptom control and pain management
  - Knowledge of disease, treatment, and management; prevention of complications and patient safety
  - Patient satisfaction with care
  - Cost

PLAN-DO-CHECK-ACT (PDCA) OR PLAN-DO-STUDY-ACT (PDSA)

Plan–do–check–act (PDCA) or plan–do–study–act (PDSA) is a successive cycle that starts off small to test potential effects on processes, but then, as the proof of concept is determined, it gradually leads to larger and more targeted change. PDSA/PDCA was made popular by Dr. W. Edwards Deming, who was considered by many to be the father of modern quality control; however, he always referred to it as the "Shewhart cycle." Later in Deming's career, he modified PDCA to PDSA as shown in Figure 8.1 because he felt that "check" emphasized inspection over analysis "study."

The elements of the repetitive process are:

- *Plan*—Establish the objectives and processes necessary to deliver results in accordance with the expected output (the target or goals). By making the expected output the focus, it differs from other techniques in that the completeness and accuracy of the specification is also part of the improvement.
- *Do*—Implement the new processes, often on a small scale, if possible, to test possible effects. It is important to collect data for charting and analysis for the following step.
- *Study*—Measure the new processes and compare the results (collected in "DO" in the figure) against the expected results (targets or goals from the "PLAN") to ascertain any differences. Charting data can make this much easier to see trends in order to convert the collected data into information. Information is what you need for the next step, "ACT."
- *Act*—After analyzing the results, it is important to determine their cause. The determination of causes usually leads to more work to be done. Through this process, it can be determined where to apply changes that will make improvements. When a pass through these four steps does not result in the need to improve, refine the scope to which the cycle of improvement is applied until there is a plan that involves improvement.

A fundamental activity of the method is iteration—once a hypothesis is confirmed (or negated), executing the cycle again will extend the knowledge further. Repeating the cycle can bring the project closer to the goal, usually a perfect combination of operation and output. A PDSA

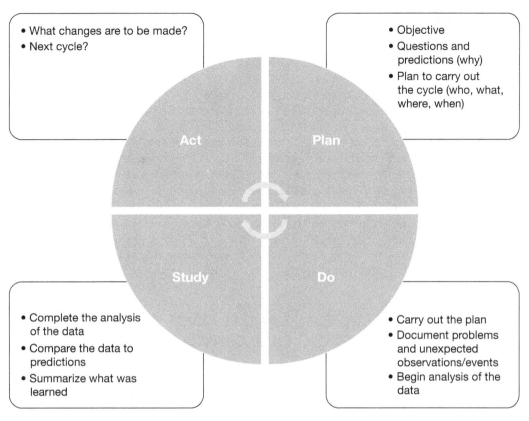

FIGURE 8.1 Plan–do–check/study–act example.

is a well-known and utilized process improvement strategy. A part of ensuring success is to perform small tests of change. The mantra, "one nurse/doctor/pharmacist/tech, one patient, one day," is a way to ensure that efforts are successful and change can happen "real time." It is important to perform these cycles in an organized fashion to be able to ensure proper tracking of findings. Many are often ready to "laminate" their work before it has been thoroughly tested, and this can lead to frustration and a lot of wasted time and effort. In financial terms, the use of the strategy can yield additional insights into the processes that are occurring and what the financial implications may be for the institution.

WHAT'S IN IT FOR ME? (WIIFM)

Another key strategy in securing success in a quality improvement initiative is to ensure that those involved with the improvement are part of the solution. Providing the "why" to a new initiative is critical for success. For nurses in particular, it is important to provide them the critical rationale for why a change needs to occur. In many situations, nurses are the ones who have to institute changes and more often than not they are expected not to ask why but to just "do it" because it is expected. By explaining the "big picture" and how the initiative fits, and what is in it for them and what the desired outcome is for the organization, can create "buy-in." Performing small tests of change and having those involved regroup regularly and discuss how to improve the processes can prove fruitful and help avoid additional steps. Those involved individuals can become the biggest champions of the proposed changes because they understand why the change needs to happen and are part of the solution.

PRACTICE MANAGEMENT

Practice management is the continuum of processes, often unique for each practice, that impact the provision of patient care. These processes include staffing, scheduling, billing, and quality improvement practices. The goal of quality management in this area is to not only improve the outcomes of individuals in the department but also improve the systems or processes in the practice. For example, the nurse practitioner (NP) needs to understand how his or her role impacts the outcomes of the practice, both from a quality and financial perspective. In recent years, these two elements, quality and finance, have become more intertwined, as payers are insisting that proof of positive outcomes will be the ones that will be paid. For the nurse executive who works in concert with practitioners and allied health partners to provide optimal care, it is essential to work together so that the institution will receive optimal reimbursement and perhaps even a bonus for proven excellent care. In many states, practitioners and allied health professionals are employees of the facility or system, which in many ways can make it easier for the hospital to manage and remedy those who do not adhere to guidelines. In states in which laws currently exist that prohibit practitioners from being employees of the institution, there is a need to utilize influence to ensure that they provide exceptional care and quality outcomes.

■ PRINCIPLES OF ECONOMICS AND FINANCE TO REDESIGN EFFECTIVE AND REALISTIC CARE DELIVERY STRATEGIES

PAY FOR PERFORMANCE

Pay-for-performance systems link compensation to measures of work quality or goals. As of 2005, 75% of all U.S. companies connected at least part of an employee's pay to measures of performance, and in health care, more than 100 private and federal pilot programs were underway. Current methods of health care payment may actually reward less safe care, since some insurance companies will not pay for new practices to reduce errors, while physicians and hospitals can bill for additional services that are needed when patients are injured by mistakes (Leape & Berwick, 2005). However, early studies showed little gain in quality for the money spent (Rosenthal, Frank, Zhonghe, & Epstein, 2005), as well as evidence suggesting unintended consequences, such as the avoidance of high-risk patients, when payment was linked to outcome improvements (Rosenthal & Frank, 2006).

The 2006 IOM report *Preventing Medication Errors* recommended "incentives . . . so that profitability of hospitals, clinics, pharmacies, insurance companies, and manufacturers (are) aligned with patient safety goals . . . (to) strengthen the business case for quality and safety" (IOM, 2006a, p. 349). A second IOM report, *Rewarding Provider Performance: Aligning Incentives in Medicare* (2006b), stated, "The existing systems do not reflect the relative value of health care services in important aspects of quality, such as clinical quality, patient-centeredness, and efficiency . . . nor recognize or reward care coordination . . . (in) prevention and the treatment of chronic conditions" (p. 1). The report recommends pay-for-performance programs as an "immediate opportunity" to align incentives for performance improvement (IOM, 2006b). However, significant limitations exist in current clinical information systems in use by hospitals and health care providers, which are often not designed to collect valid data for quality assessment.

In 2001, Ken Kizer, MD, the former CEO of the National Quality Forum (NQF), was credited in coining the term *never event* in reference to medical errors that should never occur to a patient. In 2002, NQF defined 27 types of events under six categories: surgical, product or device, patient protection, care management, environmental, and criminal. The list was revised and expanded in 2006 and again in 2011 to identify adverse events that are unambiguous (clearly identifiable and measurable), serious (resulting in death or significant disability), and usually preventable.

Many of these "never events" are no longer being paid for by CMS when they occur. Many other payers are following their lead and are not paying for care that is associated with this type of event. These areas are good places to start when one is trying to decide what issue to address in a business plan.

VALUE-BASED PROGRAMS

A statement a decade ago from the CMS *Report to Congress: Plan to Implement a Medicare Hospital Value-Based Purchasing Program* (CMS, 2007) stated value-based purchasing (VBP) "which links payment to performance, is a key policy mechanism that CMS is proposing to transform Medicare from a passive payer of claims to an active purchaser of care" (p. 2).

No one will argue the importance of quality, especially in health care, but the critical financial question is, what is the cost of added quality? If a hospital can take actions that will improve its quality score and realize an additional $1 million in payment, should it do so if it costs $2 million to realize those improvements? Some argue that quality improvements will actually reduce costs. However, quality enhancements often require additional resources once production efficiency has been reached. Simple economics will then dictate that improvements in quality are not possible if they are not compensated at levels commensurate with required cost increases. This economic reality runs counter to the public's perspective, which demands quality improvements regardless of cost. Ultimately, however, hospitals need to ensure that high-quality services are provided and that long-term financial viability is not sacrificed.

Since the implementation of the Affordable Care Act (ACA), CMS has developed multiple programs as a mechanism to pay for quality care. These value-based programs that reward (via incentive payments) providers were instituted as part of their overarching quality strategy to reform the processes by which health care is delivered and paid. The value-based programs have three aims (CMS, 2017):

- Better care for individuals
- Better health for populations
- Lower cost

CMS values these programs because they see them as a way to pay providers who provide high-quality care and do not base their payments on volume, which they had been doing in the past. CMS started with four original value-based programs with the goal of linking provider performance of quality measures to provider payment. Those initial programs included:

- Hospital Value-Based Purchasing (HVBP) Program
- Hospital Readmission Reduction (HRR) Program
- Value Modifier (VM) Program (also called the Physician Value-Based Modifier or PVBM)
- Hospital-Acquired Conditions (HAC) Program

CMS also initiated several other value-based programs that were not hospital based. Those programs include:

- End-Stage Renal Disease (ESRD) Quality Initiative Program
- Skilled Nursing Facility Value-Based Program (SNFVBP)
- Home Health Value-Based Program (HHVBP)

As a framework for their journey, CMS has developed a quality strategy for their improvement activities. Their vision for improving health delivery can be said in three words: better, smarter, and healthier (CMS, 2017). They are focusing on:

- Using incentives to improve care
- Tying payment to value through new payment models

- Changing how care is given through:
  - Better teamwork
  - Better coordination across health care settings
  - More attention to population health
  - Putting the power of health care information to work

The strategy is coordinated with the six priorities from the Agency for Healthcare Research and Quality's (AHRQ) National Quality Strategy—NQS (which can be found later in this chapter). CMS's quality strategy goals are to:

- Make care safer by reducing harm caused while care is delivered.
  - Improve support for a culture of safety.
  - Reduce inappropriate and unnecessary care.
  - Prevent or minimize harm in all settings.
- Help patients and their families be involved as partners in their care.
- Promote effective communication and coordination of care.
- Promote effective prevention and treatment of chronic disease.
- Work with communities to help people live healthily.
- Make care affordable.

CMS has four foundational principles to help them meet their goals:

- Eliminate racial and ethnic disparities.
- Strengthen infrastructure and data systems.
- Enable local innovations.
- Foster learning organizations.

CMS has strategically placed their new initiatives over the next several years. Figure 8.2 provides the rollout plan proposed for the implementation of these upcoming programs (through 2019). In 2015, the Medicare Access and CHIP Reauthorization Act (MACRA) was approved by Congress. MACRA will greatly impact the way Medicare payments will be made as the health care industry continues to shift from fee-for-service to value-based care. Under the fee-for-service approach, providers would be paid for their services; therefore, the more services they provided, the more they would be paid. MACRA shifts the focus from volume to value. In this new model, providers will be paid on how well they meet certain quality measures and create value for their patients. MACRA repealed the sustainable growth rate (SGR) formula and replaced it with a new value-based reimbursement system called the Quality Payment Program (QPP). Additionally, it streamlines providers' reporting and gives them two paths to choose from for determining how the value and quality of their care will be measured. The first path is the Merit-Based Incentive Payment System (MIPS) and the other is the advanced Alternative Payment Models (APMs).

The term CMS uses for Medicare Part B providers subject to participation in MIPS is *MIPS eligible clinicians*. During the first performance year, this group includes physicians (MDs/DOs and DMDs/DDSs), physician assistants, NPs, clinical nurse specialists (CNSs), and certified registered nurse anesthetists (CRNAs). In future years, the program may expand the eligibility to include other providers, such as physical or occupational therapists, speech-language pathologists, audiologists, nurse midwives, clinical social workers, clinical psychologists, and dieticians and nutritional professionals.

At least initially, most Medicare providers (CMS estimates between 592,000 and 642,000 for the first performance year) will participate in the QPP by reporting through MIPS (CMS, 2017). MIPS improves and consolidates the Physician Quality Reporting System (PQRS), the Value-Based Modifier (VBM) Program, and the Medicare EHR Incentive Program into one scoring system designed to measure the care given to Medicare patients. When reporting through MIPS, payments are determined by how well providers demonstrate success in four performance

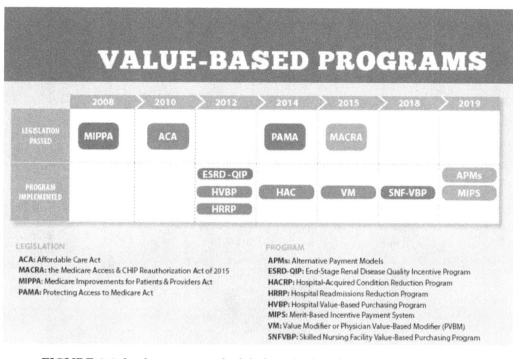

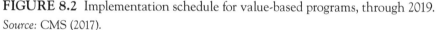

FIGURE 8.2 Implementation schedule for value-based programs, through 2019.
Source: CMS (2017).

categories: quality, improvement activities, advancing care information, and cost. These four categories are weighted to determine a provider's MIPS Composite Performance Score (CPS) of up to 100 points. This score will be used to measure a provider's overall care delivery and compute a positive, negative, or neutral adjustment to his or her future Medicare payments as appropriate (CMS, 2017).

According to CMS, an APM is a payment approach that gives added incentive payments to provide high-quality and cost-efficient care. APMs can apply to a specific clinical condition, a care episode, or a population. Advanced APMs are a subset of APMs, and will let practices earn more for taking on some risk related to their patients' outcomes (CMS, 2017). In the case of reporting through the QPP as an advanced APM, providers can earn a 5% incentive payment in 2019 for advanced APM participation in 2017 if they receive 25% of their Medicare Part B payments through an advanced APM or see 20% of their Medicare patients through an advanced APM.

With all the changes happening within CMS, Figure 8.3 might be helpful. It shows all the CMS-approved programs and their associated activities.

With the recent changes to the administration in Washington, there have been concerns that there will be potentially massive overhauls to CMS. All indications point out that the quality train has long left the station and won't be coming back anytime soon due to all the savings that have been realized with these new initiatives.

■ HEALTH CARE QUALITY/FINANCE CONCEPTS

BENCHMARKING

Benchmarking is a method that assists in comparing outcomes of two or more entities. The entity can consist of another provider, facility, country, and so forth. Benchmarking is an excellent tool

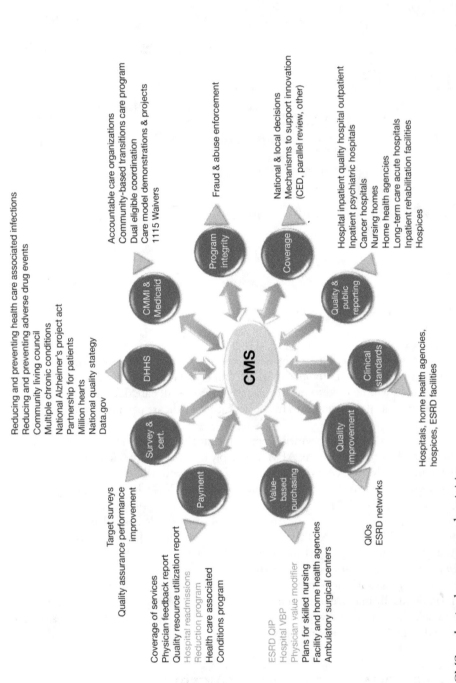

FIGURE 8.3 CMS-authorized programs and activities.

CED, coverage with evidence development; CMMI, Center for Medicare and Medicaid Innovation; CMS, Centers for Medicare and Medicaid Services; DHHS, Department of Health and Human Services; ESRD QIP, End-Stage Renal Disease Quality Initiative Program; QIOs, quality improvement organizations; VBP, value-based purchasing.

Source: CMS (2017).

to share improvements not only in a particular place or time but also how the improvement compares to others. Most vendors who submit data to The Joint Commission or CMS can provide benchmarks of a facility's data as compared to the others in their pool of clients. As demonstrated in Example 8.1 at the end of this chapter, utilizing a benchmark can assist in providing a goal for attainment.

COST-BENEFIT ANALYSIS

Cost–benefit analysis is the process of analyzing health care resource expenditures relative to their possible benefit. This analysis may be helpful and necessary as a mechanism to setting priorities when choices must be made in the face of limited resources. This analysis is used in determining the degree of access to, or benefits of, health care to be provided. Clarity of the decision-making process demands that cost–benefit analysis be separated and differentiated from risk–benefit analysis as well as from determinations of efficient and cost-effective medical care during medical decision making. Those involved in the analysis always need to keep quality and patient safety a priority in the final decisions.

COST-EFFECTIVENESS ANALYSIS

The central purpose of cost-effectiveness analysis (CEA) is to compare the costs and the values of different health care interventions in creating better health and longer life. As with any system financing health care, there are often limited budgets and a vast number of potential spending options. Choices must be made as to how this limited budget is spent. Many new medical devices, procedures, diagnostic tests, and prescription drugs are expensive; CEA can help to evaluate whether the improvement in health care outcomes justifies the expenditures relative to other choices.

COMPARATIVE EFFECTIVENESS

The primary purpose of comparative effectiveness research is to properly inform health care-related decisions. Although comparative effectiveness can be a valuable tool to inform the decision making of the clinician and the patient, it cannot provide simple "one-size-fits-all" answers. There is no standard definition of comparative effectiveness. The IOM, in *Learning What Works Best: The Nation's Need for Evidence on Comparative Effectiveness in Health Care* (IOM, 2007), describes comparative effectiveness as "the comparison of one diagnostic or treatment option to one or more others." Conclusions utilize inferential adjustments based on the relative effect of each intervention to a specific comparison, often a placebo.

COST PER ENCOUNTER

Cost per encounter can be expressed simply as the product of three key cost drivers:

- Intensity of services
- Productivity/efficiency
- Resource prices/salaries and wages

The mix and quantity of services that are combined to produce the encounter of care define the intensity of services. For example, a 5-day inpatient stay for pneumonia includes 5 days of nursing care, a series of drugs, laboratory procedures, and ancillary services. There are often wide variations in the intensity of services across patients and across hospital providers. Although many intensity factors are physician driven, health care managers can and do play an instrumental role in explaining the relative costs associated with alternative treatment protocols. Lowering intensity of services for a defined encounter of care can lead to reductions in total cost per encounter—again, the primary goal.

The costs incurred to produce a specific procedure that is part of an overall encounter of care represent productivity or efficiency. For example, what staffing mix and levels are used to produce a day of nursing care in specific nursing units? Although intensity and productivity are related, they are different. To make the distinction, nursing intensity would involve the number of nursing days involved in the patient stay. Nursing productivity would measure the number of hours nurses worked to provide 1-day of nursing care. Cost efficiency is usually associated with specific cost centers or departments, and the cost per unit of service in that cost center (e.g., cost per laboratory procedure) is often referred to as the departmental measure of efficiency. Lowering the unit costs of departmental products that together constitute a patient encounter can reduce the total cost of the encounter.

As the price paid to hire staff or purchase supplies and drugs increases, the encounter of care becomes more expensive. For example, a hospital can minimize the length of stay (LOS) associated with an inpatient encounter and maintain low nurse staffing ratios, but if it pays its nurses salaries that are 25% higher than those paid by its peers, its overall costs may still be high.

The three drivers of cost per encounter are fairly basic and understood by most health care financial executives. However, the relationships among them are more easily missed. Lowering costs in any given area can produce an adverse effect in one of the other two areas. For example, a hospital may have an all-RN staff, which increases the cost per day of nursing care but may not increase the overall cost per encounter. Perhaps the all-RN staff reduces the LOS and drives the total cost per encounter down. It is the cost per encounter that is of ultimate concern—not the specific cost of any intermediate procedure produced in a cost center. Similarly, it is possible to have a high cost per unit of operating room time, but low total operating room costs because of reduced operating room intensity. The lesson to be learned is a simple one. Focus first on the cost per encounter, not on salaries, staffing, or use of ancillaries. There are trade-offs that can and do exist among all three areas.

Quality of care is also important. If cost per encounter is high and yields a higher quality product, then the higher cost can be justified. However, the existence of higher cost without any objective evidence of quality enhancement needs to be seriously challenged by health care executives who are charged with maintaining the financial solvency of their organizations.

DATA

Data is the basic element by which many critical decisions are based. It cannot be stressed enough the importance of providing data to support an initiative. Another important element to this is ensuring data integrity. It is essential to ensure that whatever data is provided to backup an identified need has been thoroughly examined to ensure its accuracy and integrity. Many a project has been rejected because of data that were not completely analyzed correctly. There are many who will pick apart (question) data that is presented because it is a way to provide some doubt as to its integrity and can invalidate the request or at least suspend it until it can be validated.

Throughout the world of quality and patient safety, the quote "In God we trust; all others must bring data" has been utilized and been linked to both Deming and Robert W. Hayden. Hastie, Tibshirani, and Friedman, coauthors of *The Elements of Statistical Learning* (2009), in the Preface to the Second Edition, have a footnote that reads: "On the Web, this quote has been widely attributed to both Deming and Robert W. Hayden; however Professor Hayden told us that he can claim no credit for this quote, and ironically we could find no 'data' confirming Deming actually said this" (p. vii). It is ironic that such a popular quote about providing data does not have data linking it to the original source.

INCREMENTAL COST-EFFECTIVENESS RATIO

Incremental cost-effectiveness ratio (ICER) of an intervention in health care is a term used in CEA in health economics. It is defined as the ratio of the change in costs of a therapeutic intervention compared to the alternative, such as doing nothing or using the best available alternative treatment to the change in effects of the intervention.

The term does not have the standard economic meaning. Normally, the effects of an incremental change refer to the effect of an additional unit of a specific measurement—for example, the effect of an additional dollar spent on a public health awareness campaign. However, in this case, we are not comparing the effects of an incremental change in some intervention, but rather the effect of switching interventions. Often, the change in effects is measured in terms of the number of quality-adjusted life years (QALYs) gained by the intervention. This includes both health differences during the time alive, and years gained/lost due to a different time of death.

MEASUREMENT

A measurement is a standard, a basis for comparison, a reference point against which other things can be evaluated. How do patients know whether their health care is good care? How do providers pinpoint the steps that need to be improved for better patient outcomes? And how do insurers and employers determine whether they are paying for the best care that science, skill, and compassion can provide? Measurement provides us a way to assess health care against recognized standards. The science of measuring health care performance has made enormous progress over the last decade, and it continues to evolve. The high stakes demand our collective perseverance. Measures represent a critical component in the national endeavor to ensure that all patients receive appropriate and high-quality care.

QUALITY-ADJUSTED LIFE YEAR

The QALY is a measure of disease burden, including both the quality and the quantity of life lived (National Institute for Health and Clinical Excellence [NICE], 2010). QALYs were invented by two health economists in 1956: Christopher Condell and Carlos McCartney. The QALY model requires the utility of independent, risk neutral, and constant proportional trade-off behavior. The QALY is based on the number of years of life that would be added by the intervention. Each year in perfect health is assigned the value of 1.0 down to a value of 0.0 for death. If the extra years would not be lived in full health—for example, if the patient develops a debilitating illness such as pancreatic cancer, loses a limb, becomes blind, or has to use a wheelchair—then the extra life years are given a value between 0 and 1 to account for this. The QALY is often used in cost utility analysis to calculate the ratio of cost to QALYs saved for a particular health care intervention. This data is then used to allocate health care resources, with an intervention with a lower cost to QALY saved (incremental cost-effectiveness) ratio.

The usefulness and meaning of the QALY is fiercely debated (Prieto & Sacristán, 2003). The term *perfect health* is hard, if not impossible, to define. Some may argue that there are health states worse than death, and therefore there should be negative values possible on the health spectrum (some health economists have incorporated negative values into calculations). Determining the level of health depends on measures that some argue place disproportionate importance on physical pain or disability over mental health. The effects of a patient's health on the quality of life of others (e.g., caregivers or family) can be significant and are not figured into these calculations. In Example 8.2 at the end of the chapter, there is a demonstration of how QALY can be applied to a situation. Once a determination is made, the individuals who are affected need to make a choice, which, for some, can have a more significant financial impact than for others.

Theoretically, it might be possible to develop a table of all possible treatments sorted by increasing the cost per QALY gained. Those treatments with lowest cost per QALY gained would appear at the top of the table and deliver the most benefit per value spent and would be easiest to justify funding. Those where the delivered benefit is low and the cost is high would appear at the bottom of the list. Decision makers would, theoretically, work down the table, adopting services that are the most cost-effective.

As one could imagine, there has been much debate on utilizing the principles of QALY in making health care decisions. The method of ranking interventions on grounds of their cost per QALY gained ratio (or ICER) is controversial because it implies quasi-utilitarian principles to determine who will or will not receive treatment. However, its supporters argue that since health care resources are inevitably limited, this method enables them to be allocated in the way that is approximately optimal for society, including most patients. Another concern is that it does not take into account equity issues such as the overall distribution of health states. Also, many would argue that, all else being equal, patients with more severe illness should be prioritized over patients with less severe illness if both would get the same absolute increase in utility.

RISK ADJUSTMENT

Risk adjustment first requires strict definition of each specific outcome. Then each risk factor is measured and weighted accordingly. Severity of illness scores are a special form of risk adjustment. The mechanics of score development include item selection, definition, collection, and potential biases. The process of weighting risk factors usually involves building multivariate models. Issues of derivation, validation, discrimination, calibration, and reliability affect the utility of all scores. Once a comparison is appropriately risk adjusted, there are important cautions about interpretation, including the source of the reference (benchmark) population, sample size, and biases from incomplete risk adjustment. Nonetheless, this data can spur quality improvement efforts that can lead to dramatic, system-wide improvements in outcomes.

RISK-BENEFIT ANALYSIS

Risk–benefit analysis weighs the potential for undesirable outcomes and side effects against the potential for positive outcomes of a treatment and is an integral part of the process of determining medical necessity in the delivery of quality medical care. The process comprises a constellation of methods, drawn from many disciplines, and addresses the question of whether a risk is "acceptable" (Wilson & Crouch, 2001). Whether this question is raised in the context of clinical decision making or public policy, the principles are the same: The analysis requires a comprehensive estimation and evaluation of risks and benefits, highlighting the trade-offs between the two that inform a policy decision. Such analysis also entails a careful quantification of the costs associated with a proposed program for reducing or avoiding risks.

■ HEALTH CARE QUALITY/VALUE ORGANIZATIONS

AGENCY FOR HEALTHCARE RESEARCH AND QUALITY (AHRQ)

The mission of AHRQ is to "produce evidence to make health care safer, higher quality, more accessible, equitable, and affordable, and to work within the U.S. Department of Health and Human Services and with other partners to make sure that the evidence is understood and used" (Agency for Healthcare Quality and Research [AHRQ], 2017). Their efforts have extended into the financial arena in many ways.

Currently, there are two important areas within AHRQ that should be important to a DNP-prepared nurse. One is the Healthcare Cost and Utilization Project (HCUP), one of the most comprehensive sources of hospital data. The database includes information on inpatient, ambulatory, and emergency visits. HCUP assists researchers, insurers, policy makers, and others to study health care delivery and patient outcomes over time, and at the local and national levels. The other program is the Medical Expenditure Panel Survey (MEPS). The MEPS is the only national data source that is measuring how Americans use and pay for their medical care, health insurance, and out-of-pocket spending. It assesses this information by performing annual surveys of individuals and families, as well as their health care providers. The program in turn provides data on health status, the use of medical services, charges, insurance coverage, and satisfaction with care.

The NQS was first published in 2011 and was mandated by the ACA; the NQS was then developed by working with more than 300 groups representing all sectors of the health care industry and the general public. After receiving input from these groups, three overarching aims were identified and they aligned very closely with the IHI Triple Aim. The aims are:

- Better care: improve the overall quality by making health care more patient centered, reliable, accessible, and safe
- Healthy people/healthy communities: improve the health of the U.S. population by supporting proven interventions to address behavioral, social, and environmental determinants of health in addition to delivering higher quality care
- Affordable care: reduce the cost of quality health care for individuals, families, employers, and government

To advance these aims, the NQS focuses on six priorities (AHRQ, 2017):

- Making care safer by reducing harm caused in the delivery of care
- Ensuring that each person and family is engaged as partners in their care
- Promoting effective communication and coordination of care
- Promoting the most effective prevention and treatment practices for the leading causes of mortality, starting with cardiovascular disease
- Working with communities to promote wide use of best practices to enable healthy living
- Making quality care more affordable for individuals, families, employers, and governments by developing and spreading new health care delivery models

Each of the nine NQS levers represents a core business function, resource, and/or action that stakeholders can use to align to the strategy. In many cases, stakeholders may already be using these levers but have not connected these activities to NQS alignment.

- Measurement and feedback: Provide performance feedback to plans and providers to improve care
- Public reporting: Compare treatment results, costs, and patient experience for consumers
- Learning and technical assistance: Foster learning environments that offer training, resources, tools, and guidance to help organizations achieve quality improvement goals
- Certification, accreditation, and regulation: Adopt or adhere to approaches to meet safety and quality standards
- Consumer incentives and benefit designs: Help consumers adopt healthy behaviors and make informed decisions
- Payment: Reward and incentivize providers to deliver high-quality, patient-centered care
- Health information technology: Improve communication, transparency, and efficiency for better coordinated health and health care
- Innovation and diffusion: Foster innovation in health care quality improvement, and facilitate rapid adoption within and across organizations and communities
- Workforce development: Investing in people to prepare the next generation of health care professionals and support lifelong learning for providers

The NQS has aligned its measurements with others within the Department of Health and Human Services (DHHS) as a means to decrease provider burden. The DHHS Measurement Policy Council has so far (as of late 2016) nine topics to date: hypertension control, hospital-acquired conditions/patient safety, Hospital Consumer Assessment of Healthcare Providers and Systems (HCAHPS), smoking cessation, depression screening and care coordination, HIV/AIDS, perinatal, and obesity/body mass index (BMI; AHRQ, 2017).

CENTERS FOR MEDICARE AND MEDICAID SERVICES

There are several programs supported by CMS to ensure that quality is a priority for health care. Being the largest health care payer in the United States, CMS has the power to influence outcomes with their checkbooks. The concept of a "market basket" is a term utilized by CMS to hold on to funds to which facilities may be entitled, but if they do not perform to the recommended standards they may lose the funds, which in many cases go to facilities who are top performers.

QUALITYNET

QualityNet provides health care quality improvement news, resources, and data-reporting tools and applications used by health care providers and others. QualityNet is the only CMS-approved website for secure communications and health care quality data exchange between quality improvement organizations (QIOs), hospitals, physician offices, nursing homes, ESRD networks and facilities, and data vendors.

HOSPITAL COMPARE

The Hospital Compare Database (www.hospitalcompare.org) and its metrics are the result of data submissions by participating hospitals and patients. Over the past several years, the number of hospitals reporting their metrics has increased as well as the quality of the data. Hospital Compare is a consumer-oriented website that provides information on how well hospitals provide recommended care to their patients. On this site, the consumer can see the recommended care that an adult should get if being treated for a heart attack, heart failure, or pneumonia or having surgery. The performance rates for this website generally reflect care provided to all U.S. adults with the exception of the 30-day risk-adjusted death and readmission measures and the Hospital Outpatient Medical Imaging measures that only include data from Medicare beneficiaries. In March 2008, data from a patient satisfaction survey, the HCAHPS survey, was added to Hospital Compare. HCAHPS provides a standardized instrument and data collection methodology for measuring patients' perspectives on hospital care. Hospital Compare was created through the efforts of the CMS, along with the Hospital Quality Alliance (HQA). The HQA, created in December 2002, is a public–private collaboration established to promote reporting on hospital quality of care. The HQA consists of organizations that represent consumers, hospitals, doctors, employers, accrediting organizations, and federal agencies. The HQA effort is intended to make it easier for the consumer to make informed health care decisions, and to support efforts to improve quality in U.S. hospitals.

PHYSICIAN COMPARE

CMS created Physician Compare as required by the ACA of 2010. Physician Compare shows performance information from clinicians and group practices, giving patients the best recommended care so that they can make informed decisions and encourage clinicians to provide quality care. The performance scores on Physician Compare are divided into these categories:

- Preventive care: general health
- Preventive care: cancer screening
- Patient safety
- Care planning
- Referral and follow-up
- Diabetes
- Cancer
- Heart disease
- Kidney disease
- Respiratory diseases
- Stroke
- Behavioral health
- Ear and sinus care
- Eye care
- Orthopedics
- Immunology and communicable diseases

These performance scores come from the PQRS program. Additional performance scores may be available for clinicians who reported information to Medicare through a qualified clinical data registry (QCDR). A QCDR is a Medicare partner organization that is committed to improving the quality of care for patients and is generally focused on a specific area or type of care.

INSTITUTE FOR HEALTHCARE IMPROVEMENT

The IHI has worked tirelessly over the past two decades to move health care in the direction of providing vehicles by which hospitals can work collaboratively in preventing patient harm. The 18-month 100,000 Lives Campaign launched in late 2004/early 2005 encouraged hospitals to implement six initiatives:

- *Deploy rapid response teams*—Prevent death in patients who are progressively failing outside the ICU by implementing rapid response teams.
- *Deliver reliable, evidence-based care for acute myocardial infarction (AMI)*—Prevent deaths among patients hospitalized for AMI by ensuring the reliable delivery of evidence-based care.
- *Prevent adverse drug events*—Prevent deaths by implementing medication reconciliation procedures.
- *Prevent central line infections*—Prevent deaths by implementing a set of interventions to reduce catheter infection rates.
- *Prevent surgical site infections*—Prevent deaths by implementing a reliable set of interventions that help choose and appropriately time perioperative antibiotics.
- *Prevent ventilator-associated pneumonia*—Prevent deaths by implementing a set of interventions known as the "ventilator bundle."

Hospitals were given the option to adopt and implement one to six of these initiatives. More than 3,000 hospitals joined the campaign, which proved that health care had the capacity to work together for a common goal. These initiatives provided a framework that has over time built relationships between hospitals that at one time were in competition, as was the tendency, to hide best practices instead of sharing them. After the success of the 100,000 Lives Campaign, IHI launched the 5 Million Lives from preventable harm campaign, which again proved successful as most health care facilities across the United States participated as a way to improve their outcomes. Today in health care, there are very few hospitals that have not participated in some national performance improvement activity that has benefited not only their organization but others as well. The work of the IHI has shown to health care in the United States and the world that collectively we can make huge gains, whereas in the past we were just competing against each other and patients were dying.

NATIONAL QUALITY FORUM

The NQF was created in 1999 by a coalition of public and private sector leaders in response to the recommendation of the Advisory Commission on Consumer Protection and Quality in the Health Care Industry. In its final report, published in 1998, the commission concluded that an organization such as NQF was needed to promote and ensure patient protections and health care quality through measurement and public reporting (NQF, 2012). Moving ahead to August 2004, NQF published 15 voluntary consensus standards for nursing-sensitive care, including evidence-based–nursing-sensitive performance measures, a framework for measuring nursing-sensitive care, and related research recommendations. The project was funded by the Robert Woods Johnson Foundation. The project was performed due to an identified gap in the work of nurses. At over three million strong, nursing is the largest health care profession in the United States, with nurses serving as the principal caregivers in hospitals and other institutional care settings. Nursing time constitutes the single largest operational expense in any health care delivery system. It was felt that there was a need for national standardized performance measures to assess the extent to which nurses in acute care hospitals contribute to patient safety, health care quality, and a professional work environment (NQF, 2007). The areas that were identified included:

- Patient-centered outcome measures
  - Death among surgical inpatients with treatable serious complications (failure to rescue)
  - Pressure ulcer prevalence
  - Falls prevalence
  - Falls with injury
  - Restraint prevalence (vest and limb only)
  - Urinary catheter-associated urinary tract infection for ICU patients
  - Central line catheter-associated bloodstream infection rate for ICU and high-risk nursery (HRN) patients
  - Ventilator-associated pneumonia for ICU and HRN patients

- Nursing-centered intervention measure
  - Smoking cessation counseling for AMI
  - Smoking cessation counseling for heart failure
  - Smoking cessation counseling for pneumonia

- System-centered measures
  - Skill mix (RN, licensed vocational nurse/licensed practical nurse [LVN/LPN], unlicensed assistive personnel [UAP], and contract)
  - Nursing care hours per patient day—HPPD (RN, LPN, and UAP)
  - Practice Environment Scale—Nurse Work Index (composite and five subscales)
  - Voluntary turnover

One of the recommendations for accelerating the adoption of the NQF-Endorsed National Voluntary Consensus Standards for Nursing-Sensitive Care was to encourage entities to build a business case for nursing quality measurement and the nursing-sensitive consensus standards as a means to get to positive outcomes. Building a strong business case will require dedicated investments within the research, business, and performance measurement/quality improvement communities to test, conceptually and empirically, the links between nursing care, as measured through the NQF consensus standards and patient outcomes in safety and quality. It is important to utilize consumer research, such as patient satisfaction scores, to portray the value these measures provide to our patients and their families. Exceptional outcomes will provide additional revenues to those institutions that can show their sustained improvements and patients will show their support by their choice of provider and health care facility. It was suggested in the report that it was important to hold nurses and nursing accountable for providing high-quality care through the use of public reporting and incentive systems (NQF, 2012).

Over the past decade, NQF has become the "connector" by positioning itself as the one organization in health care that provides direction for the science of health care measurement. To that end, NQF's 2016–2019 strategic plan answers an unmet need for its organization to lead, prioritize, and collaborate to drive measurement that can result in better, safer, and more affordable health care for patients' providers and payers. Its plan also aims to reduce the redundancy and cost of measurement.

NATIONAL INSTITUTE FOR HEALTH AND CLINICAL EXCELLENCE

The NICE is a special health authority by the National Health Service (NHS) in England and Wales. It was established initially as the National Institute for Clinical Excellence in 1999 and in 2005 merged with the Health Development Agency to become the institute for which it is currently named. The work in which NICE is involved attracts the attention of many groups, including physicians, the pharmaceutical industry, and patients. NICE is often associated with controversy, because the need to make decisions at a national level can conflict with what is (or is believed to be) in the best interests of an individual patient. From an individual's perspective, it can sometimes seem that NICE is denying access to certain treatments, but this is not so. Patients are freely able to get access to the treatment but may have to contribute to the cost. For example, approved cancer drugs and treatments such as radiotherapy and chemotherapy are funded by the NHS without any financial contribution being taken from the patient. But certain cancer drugs not approved by NICE because of cost will be available only if the patient is prepared to pay a co-pay to make up the difference of the NICE-perceived value and the actual cost. Where NICE has approved a treatment, the NHS must fund it. But not all treatments have been assessed by NICE, and these treatments are usually dependent on local NHS decision making. For example, the NHS usually pays for several rounds of treatment for fertility problems, but because NICE has not assessed them, some centers may cap the number of rounds; the patient may then have to pay privately if he or she wishes to continue with fertility treatments beyond the capped level.

PUTTING THE PIECES TOGETHER: EVALUATION OF COST-EFFECTIVENESS OF CARE

Measuring the costs of providing quality care is a challenge. As shown in Figure 8.4, higher/better quality is typically associated with higher costs, but to a point. That point, known as the margin, is defined as the point at which a one-unit increment of input (cost) no longer yields a one-unit increase in output (quality). The one-unit increase in cost increment provides less than a unit increase in quality, which causes the decision maker to question why that last one unit increase in cost was allocated (Dunham-Taylor & Pinczuk, 2010). In short, a measurable commensurate level of quality was not achieved in spending more.

Lowering quality also has costs to the organization. For example, lowering quality of care shown in Figure 8.5 is related potentially to both declining reputation and rising numbers of malpractice cases (and remember, reputation is an asset). Lower quality of measurable care that is

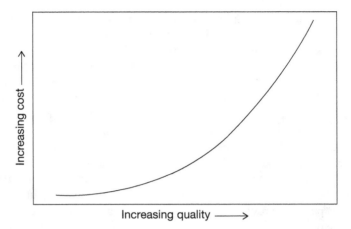

FIGURE 8.4 Evaluation of cost-effectiveness of care. Higher/better quality is typically associated with higher costs, but to a point. That point, known as the margin, is defined as the point at which a one-unit increment of input (cost) no longer yields a one-unit increase in output (quality).

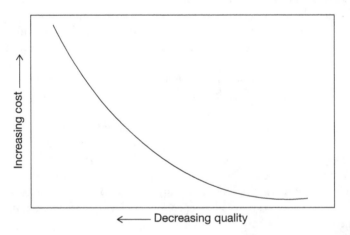

FIGURE 8.5 Evaluation of cost-effectiveness of care. This scenario could be due to both declining reputation and rising numbers of malpractice cases (and remember, reputation is an asset). Lower quality of measurable care that is publicly reported erodes the hospital's competitive position and thus longer term viability.

publicly reported erodes the hospital's competitive position and thus longer term viability (Cleverly & Cleverly, 2011). Where quality and costs intersect (Figure 8.6), one could state there is an acceptable level of quality at a cost that won't close the hospital. As pay for performance and value-based purchasing (VBP) continue to exist and grow in the landscape of health care, the curve will remain but the variables that are affected will be constantly shifting.

MAGNET® DESIGNATION AND QUALITY

Magnet designation is a goal for many nurse executives and their facilities. Does it make dollars and sense (cents) to go on the "magnet journey?" The new Magnet model offers a framework for organizing a nursing service division (Drenkard, 2010). As discussed earlier in the chapter regarding

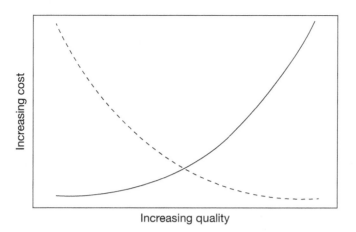

FIGURE 8.6 Evaluation of cost-effectiveness of care. Where quality and costs intersect, there is an acceptable level of quality at a cost that will maintain hospital viability.

the NQF nursing-sensitive indicators, research has shown that Magnet facilities do indeed have decreased pressure ulcers, falls, and increased nurse satisfaction and decreased turnover.

BALANCING PRODUCTIVITY WITH QUALITY OF CARE

By understanding the importance of providing quality care to patients, there is an opportunity to make the business case that providing adequate staffing will ensure quality outcomes. As was discussed in Chapter 4, it is important to obtain the HPPD and compare them with outcomes. If, with a small incremental increase in HPPD, outcomes improve and thereby decrease LOS, one can make the case for increased staffing. When making a determination of whether a change in productivity will increase outcomes, it is essential to determine baseline data prior to making any change. It is also best to start with the change on a small scale.

BUILDING A BUSINESS CASE FOR QUALITY

To build a successful business case for a quality improvement initiative, it is critical to utilize strategies to make your audience understand why they need to do a particular activity besides stating that it is a "regulatory requirement." The proposal needs to show the benefit to the organization from both a financial and outcome-driven perspective. As mentioned earlier in the chapter, it is important to determine the "WIIFM" for each of the key members. The elements of building a business case are covered thoroughly in Chapter 14. Example 8.3 at the end of the chapter provides a common situation by which a nursing leader attends a meeting and comes back with energy about making a difference. It is critical to support the enthusiasm and to direct the energy to make improvements in the system. As you have read throughout this chapter, there are many tools to place in your "toolbox" for making a business case for a quality improvement initiative. Understanding how to do it successfully can make the difference between a "yes" and a "no."

◼ CONCLUSION

Paying for better quality is clearly a reasonable contract feature for both payers and hospitals. The major problem, however, appears to be the measurement of quality. If the metrics used do not lead to actual improvement in health outcomes, then the system fails the patient. Furthermore, if the incentives do not cover the costs to achieve better outcomes, then hospitals will face a dilemma in deciding whether to pursue the quality initiative at the risk of financial distress. This chapter uses the definition of *quality* provided by the NAM (formally known as the IOM): "the degree to which health services for individuals and populations increase the likelihood of desired health outcomes and are consistent with current professional knowledge" (IOM, 1999, p. 211). It should be noted that any business case for nursing quality measurement and reporting will undoubtedly be based on the existing health care reimbursement system. However, current payment practices may not be responsive to improvements in nursing quality—as measured by existing nursing performance measurement activities—and may not support goals for nursing quality. From a policy perspective, current payment models may need to be revisited in the future in order to address this issue. Ultimately, defensible arguments must be formulated, tested, and confirmed that demonstrate the need for measures and the usefulness of the standards in stewardship of resources. In the end, a clear, unambiguous case that supports the primacy of nursing's contribution to improving care as measured that also supports the value of nursing quality performance results in decision making must be made to health care leaders, hospital administrators, nursing executives, and the public. Quality is the ultimate return on investment—especially if it is you or a loved one in the bed.

CRITICAL THINKING EXERCISES

1. As a DNP, you know how providing care that is measurable (at a financial as well as a quality level) can give you the ability to request additional funding. Take a moment and ponder a current project you are working on at your place of work. Could you, if requested, determine the costs associated with your project and what the potential savings to the organization could amount to?
2. If a fictional treatment costs a total of $45,000 at today's value and increases a person's quality of life from 0.5 to 0.6 for the remainder of his or her life from age 70 and onward, and the person's expected life span increases from 73 to 75, what would be the total gain in QALYs and what would be the ICER?
3. With all the changes that are occurring in health care today, what are some of the challenges your environment is facing and what is your organization doing to plan for the financial consequences?
4. What implications do you believe exist with MACRA? Do you believe that moving to a payment for quality over quantity is going to improve patient outcomes? Why?

REFERENCES

Agency for Healthcare Research and Quality. (2017). Retrieved from https://www.ahrq.gov

American Association of Colleges of Nursing. (2006). *The essentials of doctoral education for advanced nursing practice.* Washington, DC: Author. Retrieved from http://www.aacnnursing.org/Portals/42/Publications/DNPEssentials.pdf

Cleverley, W. O., & Cleverley, J. O. (2011). Is there a cost associated with higher quality? *Health Care Financial Management, 65*(1), 96–102.

Centers for Medicare and Medicaid Services, U.S. Department of Health and Human Services. (2007). *Report to Congress: Plan to implement a Medicare hospital value-based purchasing program.* Retrieved from http://www.cms.gov

Centers for Medicare and Medicaid Services, U.S. Department of Health and Human Services. (2017). What are value based programs? Retrieved from https://www.cms.gov/Medicare/Quality-Initiatives-Patient-Assessment-Instruments/Value-Based-Programs/Value-Based-Programs.html

Donabedian, A. (1966). Evaluating the quality of medical care. *Milbank Memorial Fund, Q44*(Suppl. 3), 166–206.

Donabedian, A. (1982). *Explorations in quality assessment and monitoring: Vol. 2. The criteria and standards of care.* Ann Arbor, MI: Health Administration Press.

Donabedian, A. (1990). The seven pillars of quality. *Archives of Pathology and Laboratory Medicine, 114*(11), 1115–1118.

Drenkard, K. (2010). The business case for Magnet. *Journal of Nursing Administration, 40*(6), 263–271.

Dunham-Taylor, J., & Pinczuk, J. Z. (2010). *Financial management for nurse managers* (2nd ed.). Sudbury, MA: Jones & Bartlett.

Hastie, T., Tibshirani, R., & Friedman, J. (2009). *The elements of statistical learning.* New York, NY: Springer.

Institute of Medicine. (1999). *To err is human: Building a safer health system.* Washington, DC: National Academies Press.

Institute of Medicine. (2001). *Crossing the quality chasm: A new health system for the 21st century.* Washington, DC: National Academies Press.

Institute of Medicine. (2006a). *Preventing medication errors.* Washington, DC: National Academies Press.

Institute of Medicine. (2006b). *Rewarding provider performance: Aligning incentives in Medicare.* Washington, DC: National Academies Press.

Institute of Medicine. (2007). *Learning what works best: The nation's need for evidence on comparative effectiveness in health care.* Washington, DC: National Academies Press. Retrieved from https://www.ncbi .nlm.nih.gov/books/NBK64784/

Irvine, D., Sidani, S., & McGillis Hall, L. (1998). Linking outcomes to nurses' role in health care. *Nursing Economic$, 16*(2), 58–64, 87.

Leape, L. L., & Berwick, D. M. (2005). Five years after "To Err Is Human": What have we learned? *JAMA, 293,* 2384–2390.

National Institute for Health and Clinical Excellence. (2010). Measuring effectiveness and cost effectiveness: The QALY. Retrieved from http://www.nice.org.uk/newsroom/features/measuringeffectiveness andcosteffectivenesstheqaly.jsp

National Quality Forum. (2007). Tracking NQF-endorsed consensus standards for nursing-sensitive care: A 15-month study. Retrieved from http://www.qualityforum.org/Publications/2007/07/Tracking_NQF -Endorsed%C2%AE_Consensus_Standards_for_Nursing-Sensitive_Care__A_15-Month_Study.aspx

National Quality Forum. (2012). NQF endorses resource use measures. Retrieved from https://www.quality forum.org/News_And_Resources/Press_Releases/2012/NQF_Endorses_Resource_Use_Measures.aspx

Prieto, L., & Sacristán, J. A. (2003). Problems and solutions in calculating quality-adjusted life years (QALYs). *Health and Quality of Life Outcomes, 1,* 80. doi:10.1186/1477-7525-1-80

Pringle, D., & Doran, D. (2003). Patient outcomes as an accountability. In D. Doran (Ed.), *Nursing-sensitive outcomes: State of the science* (pp. 1–25). Sudbury, MA: Jones & Bartlett.

Rosenthal, M. B., & Frank, R. G. (2006). What is the empirical basis for paying for quality in health care? *Medical Care Research and Review, 63*(2), 135–157.

Rosenthal, M. B., Frank, R. G., Zhonghe, L., & Epstein, A. M. (2005). Early experience with pay-for-performance: From concept to practice. *New England Journal of Medicine, 294*(14), 1788–1793.

Wilson, R., & Crouch, E. A. (2001). *Risk benefit analysis.* Cambridge, MA: Harvard University Press.

◼ APPENDIX 8.A: DNP ESSENTIALS

THE DOCTORS OF NURSING PRACTICE ESSENTIALS RELEVANT TO QUALITY AND FINANCE

There are two essentials that are relevant to the importance of quality and finance. In Essential II: Organizational and Systems Leadership for Quality Improvement and Systems Thinking, it stresses the need for the DNP graduate to "understand principles of practice management, including conceptual and practical strategies for balancing productivity with quality of care . . . DNP graduates must be proficient in quality improvement strategies and in creating and sustaining changes at the organizational and policy levels. Improvements in practice are neither sustainable nor measurable without corresponding changes in organizational arrangements, organizational and professional culture, and the financial structures to support practice. DNP graduates have the ability to evaluate the cost effectiveness of care and use principles of economics and finance to redesign effective and realistic care delivery strategies. . . . In addition, advanced nursing practice requires political skills, systems thinking, and the business and financial acumen needed for the analysis of practice quality and costs" (American Association of Colleges of Nursing [AACN], 2006, p. 10). It is important to understand how quality patient outcomes should drive all activities, for without the patient there would be no need for nurses. The DNP has to have a strong grasp on the tools that are available to implement strategies that will provide sustainability to the facility.

Essential III: Clinical Scholarship and Analytical Methods for Evidence-Based Practice focuses attention to "design and implement processes to evaluate outcomes of practice, practice patterns, and systems of care within a practice setting, health care organization, or community against national benchmarks to determine variances in practice outcomes and population trends. Design, direct, and evaluate quality improvement methodologies to promote safe, timely, effective, efficient, equitable, and patient-centered care" (AACN, 2006, p. 12).

The essentials make it clear that there is a need for the doctorally prepared nurse to have the ability to "employ principles of business, finance, economics, and health policy to develop and implement effective plans for practice-level and/or system-wide practice initiatives that will improve the quality of care delivery. Develop and/or monitor budgets for practice initiatives. Analyze the cost-effectiveness of practice initiatives accounting for risk and improvement of health care outcomes" (AACN, 2006, p. 11). These essentials appear straightforward in theory, but the application can be complex. It will take time and intentionality by the DNP to lay the course and proceed to success.

■ EXAMPLE 8.1: BENCHMARKING

Alpha Beta Hospital located in downtown Los Angeles, California, has a fall rate with injury that is significantly higher than the national benchmark. The CEO has instructed the nursing leadership group that the numbers need to be validated and a plan of action needs to be developed, so outcomes need to be closely monitored to lower the rates.

The plan of action includes:

- Quality management department to work with nursing leadership to review every fall with injury for the past 12 months to ensure that the records were coded correctly and to determine that all the proper fall precautions were instituted for each patient.
- The findings of the review are shared with nursing and administrative leadership.
- The review includes:
  - Identification of units of higher risk
  - Time of day of the falls are shared
  - Medications and other factors that put these patients at risk for falls
  - Developing a huddle model in which a mini-root cause analysis is performed for every fall. Staff gather and determine utilizing a checklist as to whether everything was done appropriately for the patient and additional precautions are instituted
  - Concurrent review of falls and opportunities for improvement are shared with the respective manager of each unit

■ EXAMPLE 8.2: QALY

A patient has a life-threatening condition and is expected to live on average for 1 year receiving the current best treatment, which costs $3,000. A new drug becomes available that will extend the life of the patient by 3 months and improve his or her quality of life, but the new treatment will cost more than three times as much, at $10,000. Patients score their perceived quality of life on a scale from 0 to 1, with 0 being worst possible health and 1 being best possible health. On the standard treatment, quality of life is rated with a score of 0.4 but it improves to 0.6 with the new treatment. Patients on the new treatment on average live an extra 3 months, so 1.25 years in total. The quality of life gained is the product of *life span* and *quality rating* with the new treatment less the same calculation for the old treatment, i.e., (1.25 × 0.6) less (1.0 × 0.4) = 0.35 QALY. The marginal cost of the new treatment to deliver this extra gain is $7,000, so the cost per quality life year gained is $7,000/0.35 or $20,000. This is within the $20,000 to $30,000 ceiling range for funding, so the payer will fund the new treatment.

EXAMPLE 8.3: QUALITY

COST SAVINGS DUE TO IMPLEMENTATION OF QUALITY IMPROVEMENT PROJECT

At Sacred Heart Hospital, the CNO went to a conference where he learned about a new mattress that could decrease pressure ulcers significantly. When he returned, he met with the wound nurse specialist and was told that she had wanted these types of mattresses for some time but the cost was seen as prohibitive. The two of them then met with the vendor, who agreed to loan them three mattresses on trial for 1 month with the expectation that the hospital would purchase at least one (cost $5,000). It was estimated that the cost associated with a stage 3 hospital-acquired pressure ulcer at Sacred Heart was $20,000, which included the extended LOS (average 5 days) and use of antibiotics and additional supplies to treat the wound. Also, the hospital would not be able to charge the payer for the additional care because it was a "never event" per CMS. The hospital would also be obligated to contact the local public health department because the wound had progressed to a stage 3. The hospital on average had a wound progress from a stage 2 to 3 approximately once a quarter. That would make the loss of revenue on an annual basis equal $20,000 × 4 = $80,000.

A protocol was developed to determine the appropriate type of patients to be placed on this special mattress and was approved by the nursing and administration leadership. During the trial month, there were two patients who had met the parameters of the protocol to be placed on the special mattress and neither patient's wounds progressed. The wound nurse took ownership of managing who was placed on the mattress. If she was off when a case came up, she was willing to be paged.

Potential savings:
Prevention of pressure ulcers one/quarter × $20,000/case = $80,000.00
The costs of the project included:
Development of the protocol by the wound specialist $75/hour × 2 hours = $150.00
The purchase of the mattresses $5,000 × 2 = $10,000.00
$10,150.00
Difference = $69,850.00

9

Basic Data Analysis Techniques for DNP Nurse Leaders

Susan Prion

Data analysis differs slightly in its emphasis from *statistics*, the term used to describe the formal mathematical procedures used to organize and comprehend data (Bowen & Weisberg, 1980). As used in this chapter, data analysis includes the following concepts:

- Types of numerical data
- Organizing and tabulating results
- Distinguishing differences
- Quantifying relationships
- Interpreting and applying results

The focus of data analysis is the interpretation and application of statistical results. This necessitates a firm conceptual understanding of quantitative statistical techniques and the assumptions for their use but does not require the nurse leader to be an expert in calculating the various statistical tests.

The Essentials of Doctoral Education for Advanced Nursing Practice (American Association of Colleges of Nursing [AACN], 2006) describes the knowledge, skills, and attitudes necessary for successful doctor of nursing practice (DNP) graduates. These include the following competencies directly related to financial data analysis:

Essential II—Organizational and Systems Leadership for Quality Improvement and Systems Thinking

1. Ensure accountability for quality of health care and patient safety for populations with whom they work.
   a. Use principles of business, finance, economics, and health policy to develop and implement effective plans for practice-level and/or system-wide practice initiatives that will improve the quality of care delivery.
   b. Develop and/or monitor budgets for practice initiatives.

    c. Analyze the cost-effectiveness of practice initiatives, accounting for risk and improvement of health care outcomes.

Essential III—Clinical Scholarship and Analytical Methods for Evidence-Based Practice

    a. Use analytical methods to critically appraise existing literature and other evidence to determine and implement the best evidence for practice.

    b. Design and implement processes to evaluate outcomes of practice, practice patterns, and systems of care within a practice setting, health care organization, or community against national benchmarks to determine variances in practice outcomes and population trends.

Obviously, conceptual and computational mastery of basic data analysis techniques is an "essential" skill for the DNP graduate that can be used in a variety of practice settings. As Henkel (1976) explained, ". . . statistics is a very commonsense approach to obtaining information through the manipulation of numbers" (p. 9).

▦ DATA INTO INFORMATION

Nurse leaders are bombarded with millions of bits of data every day. Any raw or unfiltered fact, figure, number, statistic, opinion, thought, or feeling is a piece of data to be considered for efficient and effective decision making. Unfortunately, not all data are helpful, because they cannot be transformed into useful information to inform the decision-making process. The ability to transform data from various sources into usable information is an important skill for any nurse leader and especially necessary when making financial decisions. Figure 9.1 illustrates the potential dangers of inaccurate data and erroneous information on fiscal decision making.

There are four generally accepted reasons for the importance of understanding data analysis. Bowen and Weisberg (1980, p. 1) list the following as necessary skills for informed consumers:

- Interpretation of research
- Evaluation of research
- Consideration of empirical questions
- Planning research

For financial decision making, skill in the "consideration of empirical questions" is absolutely critical to success. Managers and administrators can theorize about causes and explanations for fiscal events, but Bowen and Weisberg argue that "confronting real data makes one think more systematically" about the information and "think through what would be necessary to prove that causation is involved" (1980, p. 1). Suitable data analysis skills allow the testing of different explanations for those fiscal events and proving or disproving actions and decisions as causative factors.

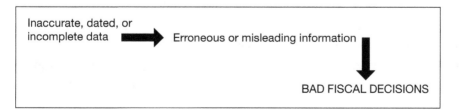

FIGURE 9.1 The influence of erroneous or incomplete data on fiscal decision making.

In this chapter, we review basic quantitative data analysis techniques that are used for financial data manipulation. We will be working exclusively with numerical data, disregarding for the moment the significant contributions of qualitative data such as opinions, narratives, thoughts, and feelings to the overall financial decision-making process.

A large variety of quantitative data analysis techniques are available for use with numerical data. The goal of this chapter is not to explore all of those techniques, because many excellent resources provide a comprehensive and detailed description. The chapter's content has been chosen to assist you in converting potentially useful data into effective and reliable information to inform your financial decision-making processes.

Information is usually preferred over data because information is usable knowledge. Data is by its nature individual bits that are uncategorized and not organized in any usable format. We can differentiate data from information in several general ways (see Table 9.1).

It is important to note that the quality of the data analysis results and its subsequent interpretation depends heavily on the reliability and validity of the raw data; in other words, GIGO or "garbage in, garbage out." Before spending time and energy on data analysis or interpretation, make sure that facts and figures used to generate those results are believable and accurate.

Reliability refers to the consistency and dependability of the data (Carmines & Zeller, 1979). If a measurement of a specific parameter is reliable, then repeated measures of the same thing would give similar results with each measuring. Staff members gathering data do not usually intend to report unreliable information, but it often happens because there are many different factors involved in simple data collection. For example, one of the inpatient adult units routinely lists the number of student nurses per shift as part of their staffing planning. Another unit does not but creatively "adjusts" the recorded staffing plan to accommodate the added workload of a full roster of student nurses requiring staff nurse preceptors. The administrator for both units is trying to determine the financial cost of clinical preceptorships in order to recommend an optimum number of students per rotation. In the absence of a standardized system to document the presence of student nurses and their impact on staffing patterns, any financial decision based on this unreliable data will be flawed.

Validity refers to the level of certainness that the collected data actually represent the concept of interest (Carmines & Zeller, 1979). This is often a concern when using available data rather than collecting new information. The available data may not completely resemble the facts being sought but are the only data available for the topic. In addition, these data may be presumed to be valid but do not actually measure the concept of interest. For example, the results of a patient survey may not always represent the patient's actual experience in the health care facility. A study in 1996 by British researchers compared three different forms of patient surveys and found that (a) levels of satisfaction with physician–patient communication and involvement in decisions were sensitive to changes in wording and (b) asking patients whether they agreed with a negative description of their hospital experience tended to produce greater apparent satisfaction than asking if they agreed with a positive description (Cohen, Forbes, & Garraway, 1996). A more recent

TABLE 9.1 Data Compared With Information

Data	Information
Uncategorized and unorganized	Organized or categorized into useful groupings
Individual facts, figures, numbers, or statistics	Collated facts, figures, numbers, or statistics
Absent/inadequate validity or reliability checks	Subjected to critical analysis and scrutiny
Focus on individual bits of data	Aggregate data more accurately represent the group of data
Undue influence of individual data like outliers	Objective review of summarized data

study (Schoenfelder, Klewer, & Kugler, 2011) of more than 8,000 German patients found that there were 10 determinants of global patient satisfaction. The outcome of treatment was the best predictor of satisfaction scores, followed by nursing kindness as the next most important component. Interestingly, the authors found that the survey items reflecting satisfaction with the amount of information received about the ongoing treatment had very little influence on patient satisfaction.

Data analysis performs a critical role in health care systems administration. Reliable and valid processes can help to evaluate the internal environment, identify problems, reduce performance deficiencies, assess the effectiveness of problem solutions, develop policies and procedures, and make informed decisions that impact daily operations and future strategies of the institution (Broyles, 2006, p. 1). Broyles (2006, pp. 2–3) also identified several key actions for statistical analyses in health care. They include:

- Comparing the expected and actual performance to identify areas of improvement
- Strategic management of the organization's strengths and weaknesses
- Validating the amount and proper flow of resources necessary to provide the expected level of care
- Developing and evaluating alternate scenarios for a variety of clinical and fiscal events
- Measuring operating efficiency and effectiveness
- Monitoring and intervening to promote patient safety and quality of care
- Evaluating cost and quality effectiveness of new processes for delivering care
- Planning for short- and long-term institutional fiscal health
- Using patient and staff satisfaction data to modify care processes

There are many sources of information for data analysis to inform decision making. The organization's financial reporting system collects all of the necessary fiscal data and distributes it to those who are tasked with making operational decisions. Both the income statement and the balance sheet provide rich data for analyzing periodic changes in profitability, debt, liquidity, and asset use (Broyles, 2006). The clinical information system provides information about all types of care delivery, often grouped by patient, diagnostic category, risk group, unit, and department. The meaningful use regulations (Blumenthal & Tavenner, 2010) make available the collection and analysis of real-time, point-of-care data for formative decisions about daily operations. Operational data can be captured through information systems that track resource use and often can pinpoint specific labor and supply needs by area and even individual patient.

Health care organizations also collect data from external sources. These sources include public health alerts, morbidity and mortality reports, governmental reports detailing use of inpatient and outpatient health care, demographics, and institutional rankings along a variety of criteria. Surveys, especially patient satisfaction surveys such as Hospital Consumer Assessment of Healthcare Providers and Systems (HCAPS) or Press Ganey (www.pressganey.com), provide valuable information to administrators about the patient's perceptions of the quality of care. This is a key area for sophisticated understanding, as the results of these surveys are often used for public rankings of health care institutions.

Much of the business of health care involves collecting data. From individual patient assessment data used to deliver care to the overall performance of a large, multisite health care system, billions of bits of data are collected every second. Rather than rely solely on fiscal information analyzed and summarized by others, the DNP-prepared nurse leader has the skills to conduct an informed analysis and make an independent decision about that information. The goal of this chapter and, ultimately, this book is to help nurse leaders transform data into useful information to improve patient care outcomes and enhance the overall quality of health care.

LEVELS OF MEASUREMENT

To effectively convert data into information, it is important to first understand the different levels of numerical measurement. Each level of measurement (Prion & Adamson, 2013a) provides unique knowledge about the phenomenon being evaluated, and it is imperative to understand the contributions and limitations of each type of numerical representation.

NOMINAL

Nominal variables are classifications of data into mutually exclusive categories. By definition, this means that the number used for a nominal variable is arbitrary and functions as a label rather than a quantity amenable to computation. For nominal variables represented as numbers, the numeral indicates neither a meaningful quantity nor any relationship with the other numerals used in a similar fashion. For example, gender, religion, and ethnicity are all nominal variables. Gender can be coded as *"female"* or *"male."* These variables could also be coded as *female* = 1 and *male* = 2. In a creative coding scheme, *female* could be represented as the numeral 272.8 and *male* as −as d be .

The main point to remember about nominal data is that any number used to represent the variable is an arbitrary numerical label that cannot be mathematically manipulated. It does not function as a number but only as an identifier. Common examples of nominal variables include: address, patient room number, race, gender, ethnicity, and education level.

ORDINAL

Ordinal measurements are also known as rankings. We are often asked to rank a certain set of items in order of our preference for or against those items. Ordinal data are ranked against some defined criterion. Although the ranked numbers indicate some ordering, the numerals used are still arbitrary. For example, the following headache ranking scale indicates that 1 = *no pain*, 2 = *slight pain*, 3 = *moderate pain*, and 4 = *significant pain*. A ranking of "significant pain" (4) is more than a "moderate pain" ranking (3), but it is unknown from the scores just how much more pain a ranking of 4 is from a ranking of 3. Similarly, the distance between 1, 2, 3, and 4 ratings may not be equal. Common examples of ordinal variables include Apgar scores, some pain scales, and patient satisfaction surveys.

RATIO/INTERVAL

Ratio/interval data are the most common type of variables that can be mathematically and statistically manipulated. Interval data are ordered, and the distance between each number is identical. This means that $1,000 is exactly two times $500, and that $500 is five times as large as $100. Interval data have an arbitrary zero point. A common example of interval data is temperature. Although Celsius, Fahrenheit, and Kelvin scales have stable distances between numbers, the zero points vary depending on the temperature scale.

Ratio data, like interval data, are ordered and have a constant distance between numbers, but they also have a nonarbitrary zero point. Blood pressure is a good example of ratio data, because the zero point must be the same for all blood pressure scales.

The zero point is usually not significant for calculations using ratio or interval data, so these data are usually treated as one type of variable.

WHY DOES THE LEVEL OF MEASUREMENT MATTER?

The level of measurement determines which statistical techniques can be used to analyze the data. Unfortunately, nominal and ordinal data do not allow for very sophisticated or robust mathematical manipulation. Ratio/interval data are preferred in most instances because the selection of data analysis approaches is much greater, offering more possibilities for understanding the phenomena being explored. This means that the type of analysis planned must be congruent with the level of measurement for the data being collected (Gilbert & Prion, 2016b). Stated more simply, think about what you want to do with the data and what level of data you want before you start collecting! It is often impossible to collect the same data a second time after realizing that is it not in the proper format for use.

▨ TYPES OF DATA

CONTINUOUS AND DISCRETE DATA

The variables that are measured in health care are either continuous or discrete. Just like levels of measurement, the general type of data being collected is important to understand because it helps determine how the data can be analyzed.

Continuous data answer the question "How much?" The precision of continuous data collection is, by definition, dependent on the accuracy of the measuring instrument. The range of possible values is spread along a continuum with an infinite number of "in-between" values. Examples of continuous data include age, serum laboratory values, and length of stay measured in hours or days.

Discrete data answer the question "How many?" These data are frequency or counting values. There are no "in-between" values for discrete data. Examples of discrete data include number of cases of a certain disease, or number of births or deaths.

Now that we have reviewed levels of measurement and distinguished continuous from discrete data, let us look at the different types of data analysis necessary for effective financial decision making.

FREQUENCY DISTRIBUTIONS

A frequency is defined as the number of times a given value occurs. A frequency distribution is a table that shows how many times each given value occurs. It is the most common reporting format for frequency data (Prion & Adamson, 2013a).

There are a variety of different types of frequencies. A *simple* or *absolute frequency* distribution is a table that reports the value and number of times that each value occurs. Although it is interesting to know the actual number of times that each value occurs, it does not tell you how that compares with the overall number of occurrences.

Table 9.2 gives the frequency distributions for a number of identified risk factors for patients at an outpatient clinic in an economically depressed area. The column labeled "absolute frequency" gives information about how many of the patients seen have two to eight identified risk factors. Unfortunately, without the next column ("relative frequency"), the reader is unable to make an evaluation of the importance of 19 patients who were identified with four risk factors.

The relative frequency provides essential information about how the individual value compares to the total group. Relative frequency is reported as the percent occurrence. As you can see from the table, the calculation of relative frequency is quite simple. The number of occurrences of a value is divided by the total number of group occurrences to return the relative frequency.

TABLE 9.2 Frequency Distribution for Cardiac Risk Factors

Score	Frequency	Percent	Cumulative Percent
Variable	Absolute Frequency	Relative Frequency	Cumulative Relative Frequency
2	1	0.8%	0.8%
3	17	14.3%	15.1%
4	19	16.0%	39.1%
5	28	23.5%	54.6%
6	22	18.5%	73.1%
7	21	17.6%	90.8%
8	11	9.2%	100.0%

This number is much more useful than the absolute frequency, as it gives the reviewer a genuine comparison of each individual frequency within the group. From our previous example of 19 patients, we can now report that 16% of the group examined has four identified cardiac risk factors.

Another useful frequency distribution is that of *cumulative percent* or *cumulative relative frequency*. This frequency reports the percentage of occurrences as an additive measure. Table 9.1 demonstrates this approach. If we want to know the number of patients who present with four or fewer cardiac risk factors, we can calculate this using the cumulative relative frequency. The number of patients with two, three, and four risk factors are added together to return a cumulative percentage of 31.1%. Note that the cumulative relative frequency total always equals 100%, because we are calculating the collective contributions of each frequency.

Frequency distributions provide a simple yet very effective format for reporting large amounts of data, but they should be carefully constructed for easy interpretation.

VISUAL REPRESENTATIONS OF DATA

With the ubiquity of desktop and laptop computers, any nurse leader can easily become a data "artist." All spreadsheet software programs allow the user to create graphic representations of most information. Not only can one create a pie chart, but there are options for multicolored, exploding pie charts with continuous animation automatically pointing out the data highlights. Just because one can create an exploding pie chart does not mean that you should create an exploding pie chart.

Unfortunately, most visual representations of data lose significant amounts of precision in the conversion from numbers to graphics. Using Table 9.2 as an example, here are several graphic options for the data.

In reviewing this histogram (see Figure 9.2), we note that the frequencies are different, but it is difficult to determine what the exact numbers are. We also lose the relative frequency information that was so helpful in the frequency distribution table.

Figure 9.3 presents the same data formatted as a pie chart. Note that we again lose the precision of exact frequencies, requiring the reader to "eyeball" the specific frequency information. Like the histogram, this pie chart is visually appealing but is lacking essential information necessary for sound decision making.

Figure 9.4 offers a different graphic representation of the same cardiac risk factors data. This line chart also suffers from a lack of precision in reporting results and also visually implies that there is some continuous relationship among the variables.

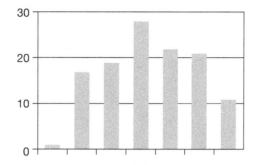

FIGURE 9.2 Frequency histogram of cardiac risk factor data.

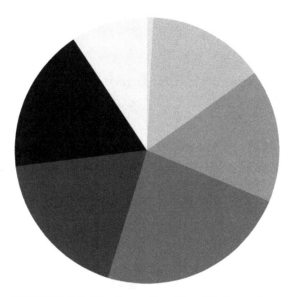

FIGURE 9.3 Pie chart of cardiac risk factor data.

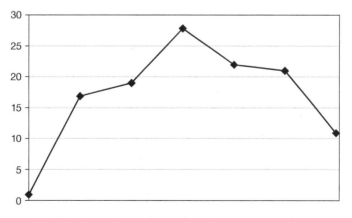

FIGURE 9.4 Line chart of cardiac risk factor data.

It is tempting to want to make lists of numbers more appealing. The ease with which you can create a wide variety of colorful graphic representations of this data makes it even more enticing. However, the smart nurse leader knows that a simple table is the most concise and complete format for presenting most numerical data and allowing readers maximum access to the information.

CONSTRUCTING DATA TABLES

If tables are the most effective format for presenting data, then the organization of those tables is very important. The common convention is to list the individual values or variables along the horizontal rows and the data results in the vertical columns. Table 9.2 follows this format. This allows summary information to be presented at the end of each column and facilitates quick and easy review of the information.

Computers have made easy the process of creating charts and graphs, and have also greatly simplified the construction of tables. Resist the urge to complicate tables with excess formatting (see Figure 9.5) and rely instead on reliable and valid results presented simply and effectively.

MEASURES OF CENTRAL TENDENCY

Measures of the central tendency are probably familiar to most nurse leaders. There are three values that typically summarize the central trends of a group of data: mean, median, and mode (Adamson & Prion, 2013b).

Mean or Average

The mean, also known as the average, is a very common statistical test used to summarize a group of data. The mean is calculated by dividing the sum of each individual value by the total number of values. The result is referred to as the "average" or "mean" value. In mathematical notation, an "X" with a "bar *over it*" represents the mean. This is known as "X bar" to distinguish it from the

Score	Frequency	Percent	Cumulative Percent
Variable	Absolute Frequency	Relative Frequency	Cumulative Relative Frequency
2 (*TWO*)	1	0.8%	0.8%
3 (*THREE*)	17	14.3%	15.1%
4 (*FOUR*)	19	16.0%	39.1%
5 (*FIVE*)	28	23.5%	54.6%
6 (*SIX*)	22	18.5%	73.1%
7 (*SEVEN*)	21	17.6%	90.8%
8 (*EIGHT*)	11	9.2%	100.0%

FIGURE 9.5 Overly formatted data table.

$$\bar{X} = \frac{\sum X}{N}$$

Where $\bar{X}$ = mean, $\sum$ = sum, X = each individual value, and N = the number of values

FIGURE 9.6 Formula for calculating the mean.

X values without the bar. X without a bar over it is the notation for an individual data point. For your reference, the formula for calculating the mean is given in Figure 9.6.

The mean of a group of values can be easily calculated in a readily available spreadsheet software program like Excel. Select the column or row of data points and use the function "=average" to return the mean of that group of values.

Median

The median is the midpoint of a group of results, indicating that 50% of the scores are above the median and 50% are below the median. The median can be a useful statistic to consider when a group of data points are widely dispersed, or there are outliers (values far above or below the group) that pull the mean value in a specific direction. For example, review Table 9.3 with serum glucose levels of a group of adolescents with type 2 diabetes.

In the example, the median is a better summary of the group values than the mean including the outlier (the serum glucose of 180 measured for patient #4). If we exclude this outlier, the mean and median are both fairly accurate representations of the group values.

If there is an odd number of values, then the median is always one of the actual values. In a distribution with n observations, the median is the value of the (n + 1)/2 value. If our example had seven values, then the median would be the (7 + 1)/2, or the fourth value in the distribution.

If there is an even number of values in the distribution, then the median will be the mean of the two middle observations when the data have been arranged in ascending or descending order. The calculation is still the number of observations (n) divided by 2, but the median is not a value that occurs in the distribution. Note that in Table 9.3, the mean both with and without the outlier is *not* a value that occurs in the distribution but instead is between value #3 (125) and value #5 (130).

The median of a group of values can be easily calculated in Excel. Select the column or row of data points and use the function "=median" to return the median value for that distribution.

Mode

The mode is defined as the most frequently occurring value in a distribution. Table 9.4 provides a group of scores indicating the number of days of admission for a group of eight patients.

The mode can be a very useful result because it can be easily applied to ungrouped data. No special organization of values is needed; one only needs to keep track of the most frequently occurring result(s). Many large distributions have more than one mode and are described as "bimodal" (two modes), "trimodal" (three modes), or "multimodal" (more than three modes). The mode can also be used for summarizing qualitative data.

The mode is calculated most easily by visually reviewing the distribution of values when they are arranged in ascending or descending order. It is easy to recognize that "10 days" is the most frequently occurring value in the Table 9.4 example. Note that the mean, median, and mode for this group of patients all provide slightly different information, indicating that the values do not follow a normal curve distribution. Reviewing the values tells us that the scores at the larger end

TABLE 9.3 Serum Glucose Levels

Patient	Serum Glucose Level (mg/dl)
1	125
2	132
3	124
4	180
5	130
6	120
Mean including outlier	135.17
Mean without outlier	126.2
Median	127.5

TABLE 9.4 Time in Days From Admission to Discharge

Patient	Days From Admit to Discharge
1	2
2	3
3	6
4	8
5	10
6	10
7	30
8	32
Mean	12.63
Median	9
Mode	10

of the distribution have more relative influence than those at the smaller end, causing the distribution to be skewed toward the larger values.

The mode for a group of values can be easily calculated in Excel by selecting the column or row of data points and use the function "=mode" to return the most frequently occurring value for that distribution.

MEASURES OF DISPERSION

It is important to know just how alike a group of values are. This is the contribution of the central tendency measures to data result interpretation and application. It is also very useful to have a way to quantify just how different a set of values are, both from the other values in the same group and as a way to compare those data points with another group of values.

The most important data analysis concepts to understand are those of deviation and variation. These two concepts are measures of the dispersion or spread of a data set. Deviation and variation are related ideas, and a thorough understanding of the similarities and differences between the two are the foundation for mastery of data analysis techniques (Adamson & Prion, 2013c).

Range

The range is the simplest measure of dispersion or variation. It is defined as the difference between the largest and the smallest values in a given data distribution. The range is quite easy to calculate, but can be easily misinterpreted and lead to erroneous decisions. The example in Table 9.4 gave the length of stay results for eight patients. To calculate the range, we would subtract the shortest length of stay from the longest. Figure 9.7 provides that calculation.

The range in length of stay for this group of patients was 30 days. But range does not give the entire picture. Consider the following groups of patients and their length of stay information (see Table 9.5).

Note that the lengths of stays are very different among the three units and the nine patients, but the range is the same for all three groups (5). Clearly, there is something influencing length of stay between the 6 south and the 4 west groups, but the range does not reflect this difference.

Deviation

Statistical *deviation* is defined as the amount by which an individual score differs from the group mean. The mean is the arithmetic average of the data set, and usually is the best measure of central tendency. Calculating deviation scores can provide useful information about the distance of each individual data point from the average for the data set.

Because the mean is the average of all the scores of the data set, the sum of all of the deviation scores is zero. This occurs because the spread of scores above the mean is the same as that of scores below the mean: The positive and negative values would cancel each other out and result in a sum of zero.

Range = largest value − smallest value

32 (longest length of stay) − 2 (shortest length of stay) = 30

FIGURE 9.7 Calculating the range.

TABLE 9.5 Length of Stay for Nine Different Patients on Three Units

Patient	Length of Stay	Unit
1	2	8 North
2	2	8 North
3	7	8 North
4	1	6 South
5	1	6 South
6	6	6 South
7	10	4 West
8	11	4 West
9	15	4 West

$$X - \bar{X} = x$$
Where X = individual score, $\bar{X}$ = mean, and x = deviation score

FIGURE 9.8 Calculation of deviation scores.

TABLE 9.6 Nursing Hours per Patient Day (NHPPD) for Five Inpatient Units

Unit	NHPPD
1 West	8.5
1 East	7.0
2 South	9.0
4 North	8.2
4 South	5.5
Average NHPPD	7.64

TABLE 9.7 Deviation Scores for Nursing Care Hours per Patient Day (NHPPD) for Five Inpatient Units

Unit	Deviation Score
1 West	8.5 − 7.64 = +0.86
1 East	7.0 − 7.64 = −0.64
2 South	9.0 − 7.64 = +1.36
4 North	8.2 − 7.64 = +0.56
4 South	5.5 − 7.64 = −2.14
Sum of deviation scores	0

The deviation score calculation is demonstrated in Figure 9.8.

The deviation score of an individual data point is useful to calculate, because it can indicate how close or how far that point is from the group average. For example, Table 9.6 lists the nursing care hours per patient day (NHPPD) for several inpatient nursing units.

The deviation scores can be calculated by subtracting the average NHPPD (7.64) from each individual unit's NHPPD result, shown in Table 9.7.

The deviation score is useful because it gives a quantifiable measure of how much (or how little) each individual value differs from the group mean.

Variance

In contrast to deviation, *variation* refers to the variability of a group of data points (Adamson & Prion, 2013c). In other words, how spread out or close together are the values from the other values within the group? Variation is a measure of the sameness of a group of data points. A group of scores are *homogeneous* if there is little variation among the data points and they are all closely clustered about the mean. A set of scores is considered *heterogeneous*, or highly varied, if there is a lot of spread among the scores.

Variation can be loosely conceptualized as an "average" of all of the deviation scores. Not surprisingly, the formula for variation looks a lot like the formula for the mean. It is calculated as the sum of the deviation scores squared and divided by the number of data points minus one. Because the sum of the individual deviation scores is always zero, those scores are squared to eliminate the positive and negative signs. The results number is always positive and can be divided by the number of data points minus a "fudge factor." The reason for dividing by $n-1$ rather than n (the number of data points) is complicated and involves the difference between population and sample data. The $n-1$ denominator allows an unbiased estimator for the standard deviation and is a common convention. Figure 9.9 provides the formula for variance and also highlights the relationship between variance and standard deviation.

Variation is essential to understanding the distribution of the group data, because it provides a quantifiable measure of the "sameness" or "differentness" of the data that have been grouped together. Sometimes, after reviewing the variation calculation, you may want to reorganize your data into different groupings for a more accurate analysis.

STANDARD DEVIATION

The standard deviation of a data set is the positive square root of the distribution's variance, as calculated in the previous section. The standard deviation is usually a more useful result than the variance, because it is reported in "real" units that correspond to the actual information being collected. Because the variance is a squared value (remember that the numerator is the sum of the deviation scores squared), this number does not correspond to the measurement scale being used for the data. However, the standard deviation can be easily applied to the data because it shares the same measurement scale.

For example, Table 9.6 offered the NHPPD for five inpatient units. The mean NHPPD for the five units was 7.64 hours. If we calculate the standard deviation, the result is 1.40 hours. This tells us that the group was fairly homogenous for NHPPD.

Figure 9.10 illustrates the formula for calculating standard deviation. Note that it is always necessary to provide the standard deviation when reporting a group mean. The mean is a key measure of the central tendency of the distribution of values, but the standard deviation is also necessary to help interpret the amount of variability within the group.

$$\text{Variance} = \frac{\sum X^2}{n-1} = SD^2$$
Where SD = standard deviation

FIGURE 9.9 Variance formula.

$$SD = \sqrt{\frac{\sum X^2}{n-1}}$$

FIGURE 9.10 Formula for standard deviation.

THE NORMAL CURVE

Any discussion of central tendency and variance refers back to the idea of a continuous distribution of data points, often referred to as the normal curve. The normal curve has very specific properties that make it useful for visualizing data analysis techniques and results. The normal curve is symmetrical, and the mean, median, and mode share the same point on the curve.

The standard normal curve incorporates the measurement of standard deviation and defines the parameters for each standard deviation unit. By definition, 34% of the continuous distribution is located between 0 and 1 standard deviation units, meaning that a total of 68% of the total distribution occurs between −1 and +1 standard deviation units (Adamson & Prion, 2014). An additional 14% of the expected distribution falls between −1 and −2, or +1 and +2 standard deviation units from the mean. Obviously, the percentage of the distribution decreases the further away from the mean, meaning that it is more and more unlikely to see data points there. A data point or group of points that are more than −3 or +3 standard deviation units from the mean could be considered an outlier and subjected to a rigorous review to determine if the value will be retained within the group or deleted (see Figure 9.11).

The standard normal curve is an important reference point for quantitative data analysis, as it determines the correct use of parametric or nonparametric statistical tests. A set of results can be examined with a parametric test if it conforms to the assumption of a normal, univariate distribution. By convention, parametric testing is used on a sample to make an inference about the entire population. So, an analysis of lipoprotein levels among a sample of middle-aged nursing executives could be used to predict or infer what those serum lipoprotein levels would be among the population of middle-aged nursing executives. Most parametric statistical tests require ratio/interval data.

Nonparametric statistical testing is used when the set of results do not conform to the assumptions of normal distribution. In fact, there are no assumptions made a priori about the distribution of the results. That means that nonparametric data analysis is less robust than parametric, because

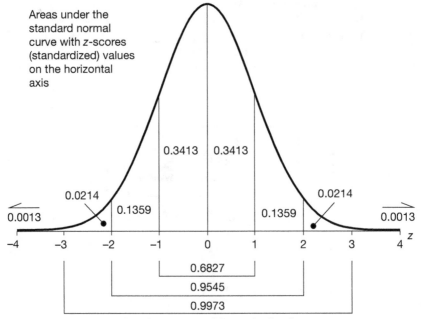

FIGURE 9.11 The standard normal curve.

there is more real and potential variation in the distribution of values and more possible interpretations for the results. Nonparametric statistical tests are used for nominal and ordinal data, and for data that do not meet the stated assumptions for the desired parametric statistical test.

MEASURES OF ASSOCIATION: CORRELATION

Sometimes, one wants to explore whether there is a relationship between two variables of interest. For example, as the chief nursing officer (CNO) you are worried that there is an association between patient satisfaction ratings and the number of nursing students assigned to a particular unit. Correlation does not indicate cause and effect; if you find a relationship, you cannot say that the number of nursing students causes a change in patient ratings. But the correlation coefficient does indicate both the strength and direction of the relationship.

Correlation Coefficient

The most common correlation calculation is the Pearson product moment correlation coefficient (Prion & Adamson, 2014). This calculation can be completed only with ratio/interval data, so you need meaningful numbers. You cannot use nominal or ordinal data for the Pearson correlation, so common demographics data such as ethnicity, race, gender, or medical diagnosis cannot be used (see the next section on chi square for how to calculate associations between two nominal variables). However, the patient age, the number of nursing students assigned to the unit each week, the summary HCAPS score, and the number of medication errors are all ratio/interval data and can be used to calculate a Pearson correlation coefficient.

This requirement for ratio/interval data is important because the correlation coefficient can be visually graphed on an x–y graph. In this example, the number of nursing students is graphed on the y (vertical) axis, and the total patient satisfaction score is graphed on the x (horizontal) axis (Figure 9.12).

From this graph, we can see a rising relationship. We can interpret that as the number of nursing students rises, then the patient satisfaction scores also rise. The patients seem to like having nursing students helping with their care! This would be described as a positive relationship: as one variable rises, so does the other one. A negative correlation would be when one variable rises and the other one falls. Figure 9.13 is the same scatter plot (the name for a graph with dots for

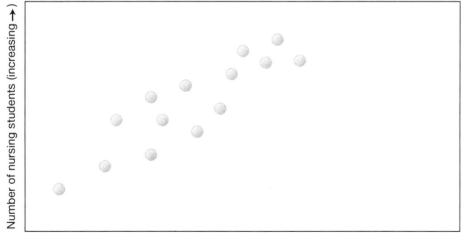

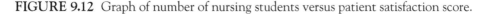

FIGURE 9.12 Graph of number of nursing students versus patient satisfaction score.

each patient satisfaction score–number of nursing students score) with a helpful line added to visualize this positive relationship.

So how much do the patients on this unit like having nursing students care for them? Let us say we calculate a Pearson product moment correlation coefficient of +0.53. This is considered a moderate correlation. The correlation coefficient can be interpreted as in Table 9.8 (Shavelson, 1996; Taylor, 1990).

A correlation coefficient of +0.53 means that there is a moderate relationship between the number of nursing students working on the clinical unit and the patient satisfaction scores. This makes sense, as there are many factors that influence satisfaction scores, but the presence of a helpful, earnest nursing student is memorable for patients and their families and can significantly "color" their inpatient experience.

Chi Square

Chi square, often written as χ^2, is a calculation to test for the association between two nominal (categorical) variables such as gender (male or female) and smoking habit (smoker or nonsmoker). The χ^2 calculation requires a random sample, independent observations, and a cell count of five or more in each cell in the contingency table (Gilbert & Prion, 2016a). Let us examine each of these requirements in more detail.

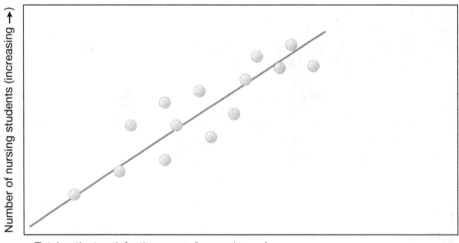

FIGURE 9.13 Graph of number of nursing students versus patient satisfaction score with line indicating positive relationship.

TABLE 9.8 Interpretation of Correlation Coefficients

Correlation Coefficient	Interpretation
0 to ± 0.20	Negligible relationship/association
± 0.21 to ± 0.35	Weak relationship/association
± 0.36 to ± 0.67	Moderate relationship/association
± 0.68 to ± 0.90	Strong relationship/association
± 0.90 to ± 1.00	Very strong relationship/association

TABLE 9.9 2×2 Contingency Table: Smoking Status

Gender	Smoker	Nonsmoker	Total
Male	24 (a)	20 (b)	44 (a + b)
Female	44 (c)	12 (d)	56 (c + d)
Total	68 (a + c)	32 (b + d)	100 (*n*)

Another way of describing the χ^2 calculation is that it allows us to compare expected data with actual data. For example, if we expect to find more male smokers than female smokers, we can compare this expectation with our actual, collected data to determine if there is a significant difference. This significant difference between expected and actual indicates something is unusual or unexpected with our collected data, which makes it different from what we were expecting.

How do we calculate a χ^2 result? The formula uses both the expected data and the observed (collected or actual) data. Once you have calculated the χ^2 value, you can check a chi-square distribution table to determine if the result is significant.

To assist with the χ^2 calculation, we can construct a contingency table. This is a simple two-cell by two-cell representation of our information. Using our smoker example, Table 9.9 is a simple 2×2 contingency table for 100 randomly selected patients. We are hoping to use these results to determine whether smoking status is independent of gender for our 1,000 inpatients.

We can see from reviewing the table that the number of male smokers is almost half that of female smokers, and the number of male nonsmokers is almost double that of female nonsmokers. If we are trying to quantify the significance of this observation, then we use the χ^2 calculation. We determine the test statistic using the observed and expected values, then consult our chi-square distribution table to analyze the size of the difference. It is important to also calculate the degrees of freedom for this data set. Degrees of freedom can be described as the number of parameters in the data set that can be varied. For a 2×2 contingency table, if we are given the sums of each row and column (known as the marginals), we only need one cell to complete the table. The degree of freedom for the 2×2 table is one. Degrees of freedom are important to statisticians because they change the shape of the data distribution and change the critical value—the number that determines whether your result is significant. From any statistics textbook, we can determine that the critical value for a χ^2 distribution with one degree of freedom is 3.841 for alpha ($\alpha = 0.05$). Our calculated value for χ^2 is 28.56, telling us that our data are significantly different from what we expect and that something important is happening with our sample.

■ PRACTICAL, STATISTICAL, AND CLINICAL SIGNIFICANCE

Many students of research methodology and data analysis spend an inordinate amount of their time studying the issues of practical and statistical significance. As a reminder, *statistical significance* is most commonly reported as the *p* value, or the probability that the result occurred because of chance (Adamson & Prion, 2013d). The smaller the *p* value, the less likely the result was random and the more likely there is a real difference. Unfortunately, the *p* value does not provide a measure of the magnitude of the difference among values. That is the function of various measures of practical significance, the most common of which is Cohen's *d*. *Practical significance* reports on the magnitude of the difference between two groups of values as measured in standard deviation units (Adamson & Prion, 2013b).

Statistical and practical significance calculation and interpretation are complicated subjects that require extensive explanations. That information can be found in any of the books listed in the subsequent "Quantitative Data Analysis Resources" section of this chapter. You need to understand the similarities and differences between these two measures of reliability, but also be skeptical in making decisions based only on statistical or practical significance results.

The invaluable expertise that most nurse leaders bring to quantitative data analysis interpretation is that of clinical significance. Clinical significance cannot be calculated nor measured: It is the cumulative assessment of a wide variety of factors that result in the right decision for that environment. After reviewing the quantitative data results, the effective nurse leader makes a fiscal decision that incorporates not only the reported results but also the expert understanding of the characteristics and expectations of the setting in which that decision will be applied. Hopefully, this brief introduction to quantitative data analysis techniques for fiscal decision making will add another tool to your experts' toolbox and enable you to interpret and apply quantitative data to improve patient outcomes.

CONCLUSION

In this chapter, we have reviewed basic quantitative data analysis techniques that are commonly used for informed financial decision making and analysis. These approaches include frequencies, measures of central tendency, measures of dispersion, and measures of association. We differentiated "data analysis" from statistics and emphasized the importance of the nurse leader's comfort and competence to transform data from a variety of sources into usable information, especially for fiscal accountability and responsibility. The chapter also provided some advice about visual representations of data for communicating results.

The interpretation and application of statistical results demands a firm conceptual understanding of quantitative statistical techniques and the assumptions for their use, but does not require the nurse leader to be an expert in calculating the various statistical tests. An understanding of the differences among statistical, practice, and clinical significance is essential for effective financial stewardship and safe patient care.

CRITICAL THINKING EXERCISES

1. The CNO is reviewing patient satisfaction benchmark data from his facility and four similar facilities (see table). What conclusions can he make, given the information? What are the limitations of this information?

Facility	Mean Patient Satisfaction Score (1–40 Scale)	Standard Deviation	Number of Respondents
A	30.85	5.6	256
B	38.56	2.4	84
C	23.31	14.6	1,210
D	30.62	10.8	369
Home facility	31.42	6.6	420

2. A group of nurse practitioners wish to explore the effectiveness of a new treatment approach. As a member of your agency's research and practice committee, you review their proposal. They describe how they will use collected demographic data to statistically test the new treatment against the current treatment. They propose to collect the following patient data: gender,

ethnicity, religion, diagnosis, age measured in decade categories (i.e., 0–10, 11–20, 21–30, 31–40,), and name of medications currently taken. What feedback can you give to them about their choice of variables and proposed statistical manipulation?

3. The oncology inpatient unit has experienced a great amount of nursing staff turnover. In the last 6 months, five of the 22 permanent RN staff have left. In addition, the number of medication errors for the unit has risen from an average of two per month to a high of 11 errors last month. How could you calculate whether there is a significant relationship between staffing and medication safety issues?

4. You complete the calculation of the Pearson product moment correlation coefficient to determine the relationship of number of temporary RNs to the number of medication errors. Remember that correlation does not indicate cause and effect, but only that there is a quantifiable, directional relationship between these two variables. The calculated result is $r = +0.47$. How would you explain this result to your chief financial officer (CFO) to request additional money to hire more permanent staff RNs?

QUANTITATIVE DATA ANALYSIS RESOURCES

The following are useful resources for the reader wanting more detailed descriptions of statistical testing for the health care environment. Also see Prion and Adamson (2015) for a more detailed discussion of helpful resources for data analysis and research methods.

Bartz, A. E. (1998). *Basic statistical concepts.* Upper Saddle River, NJ: Prentice Hall.

Cowell, J. (2007). *Statistics basics: A resource guide for health care managers.* Nashville, TN: HCPro.

Horton, L. (2011). *Calculating and reporting health care statistics* (3rd ed.). Chicago, IL: American Health Information Management Association.

Huck, S. W. (2011). *Reading statistics and research.* Boston, MA: Addison-Wesley.

Lang, T. A., & Cecic, M. (2006). *How to report statistics in medicine: Annotated guidelines for authors, editors, and reviewers* (2nd ed.). New York, NY: American College of Physicians.

Polit, D. (2009). *Statistics and data analysis for nursing research.* Upper Saddle River, NJ: Prentice Hall.

Shavelson, R. J. (1996). *Statistical reasoning for the behavioral sciences* (3rd ed.). Boston, MA: Allyn & Bacon.

Shott, S. (1990). *Statistics for health professionals.* Philadelphia, PA: W. B. Saunders.

REFERENCES

Adamson, K., & Prion, S. K. (2013a). Making sense of methods and measurement: Effect size. *Clinical Simulation in Nursing, 9*(6), e225–e226.

Adamson, K., & Prion, S. K. (2013b). Making sense of methods and measurement: Measures of central tendency. *Clinical Simulation in Nursing, 9*(12), e617–e618.

Adamson, K., & Prion, S. K. (2013c). Making sense of methods and measurement: Statistical power. *Clinical Simulation in Nursing, 9*(10), e477–e478.

Adamson, K., & Prion, S. K. (2013d). Making sense of methods and measurement: Measures of variability. *Clinical Simulation in Nursing, 9*(11), e559–e560.

Adamson, K., & Prion, S. K. (2013e). Making sense of methods and measurement: Significance. *Clinical Simulation in Nursing, 9*(3), e107–e108.

Adamson, K., & Prion, S. K. (2014). Making sense of methods and measurement: Normal curve. *Clinical Simulation in Nursing, 10*(6), e333.

American Association of Colleges of Nursing. (2006). *The essentials of doctoral education for advanced nursing practice.* Washington, DC: Author.

Blumenthal, D., & Tavenner, M. (2010). The "meaningful use" regulation for electronic health records. *New England Journal of Medicine, 363,* 501–504.

Bowen, B. D., & Weisberg, H. E. (1980). *An introduction to data analysis.* San Francisco, CA: W. H. Freeman.

Broyles, R. W. (2006). *Fundamentals of statistics in health administration*. Sudbury, MA: Jones & Bartlett.

Carmines, E. G., & Zeller, R. A. (1979). *Reliability and validity assessment*. Thousand Oaks, CA: Sage.

Cohen, G., Forbes, J., & Garraway, M. (1996). Can different patient satisfaction survey methods yield consistent results? Comparison of three surveys. *British Medical Journal, 313*(5), 841–844.

Gilbert, G. E., & Prion, S. K. (2016a). Making sense of methods and measurement: The chi-square test. *Clinical Simulation in Nursing, 12*(5), 145–146.

Gilbert, G. E., & Prion, S. K. (2016b). Making sense of methods and measurement: Parametric and nonparametric data analysis. *Clinical Simulation in Nursing, 12*(3), 96–97.

Henkel, R. E. (1976). *Tests of significance*. Thousand Oaks, CA: Sage.

Prion, S. K., & Adamson, K. (2013a). Making sense of methods and measurement: Frequencies. *Clinical Simulation in Nursing, 10*(1), e53–e54.

Prion, S. K., & Adamson, K. (2013b). Making sense of methods and measurement: Levels of measurement in quantitative research. *Clinical Simulation in Nursing, 9*(1), e35–e36.

Prion, S. K., & Adamson, K. (2014). Making sense of methods and measurement: Pearson product moment correlation coefficient. *Clinical Simulation in Nursing, 10*(11), 587–588.

Prion, S. K., & Adamson, K. (2015). Making sense of methods and measurement: Helpful resources for research methods and data analysis. *Clinical Simulation in Nursing, 11*(9), 431–432.

Schoenfelder, T., Klewer, J., & Kugler, J. (2011). Determinants of patient satisfaction: A study among 39 hospitals in an in-patient setting in Germany. *International Journal for Quality in Health Care, 23*(5), 503–509.

Shavelson, R. J. (1996). *Statistical reasoning for the behavioral sciences* (3rd ed.). Boston, MA: Allyn & Bacon.

Taylor, R. (1990). Interpretation of the correlation coefficient: A basic review. *Journal of Diagnostic Medical Sonography, 1*, 35–39.

10

Legal, Policy, and Ethical Issues in Health Care Financing

Elena Capella and Judith Lambton

The main part of intellectual education is not the acquisition of facts but learning how to make facts live.

(Oliver Wendell Holmes)

Perhaps nowhere in the trajectory of nursing education is the preceding statement more applicable than to that of the doctor of nursing practice (DNP). At the heart of the DNP is the movement of creative, thoughtful, and novel evidence to practice.

With this notion comes the responsibility of ethical, legal, and appropriate application of both the science and the privilege of managing the financial wellness of individuals and organizations that depend on a complex system of reimbursement. Although a chief financial officer (CFO) holds the fiduciary responsibility for the overall financial health of most organizations, a DNP is educated and indeed is licensed to protect patients from harm. What, then, is ethics? Ethics refers to well-founded standards of right and wrong that prescribe what humans ought to do, usually in terms of rights, obligations, benefits to society, fairness, or specific virtues. Ethical standards also include those that direct the virtues of honesty, compassion, and loyalty. Inherent in the definition of ethics are standards relating to rights, such as the right to life, the right to freedom from injury, and the right to privacy. Such standards are supported by consistent and well-founded reason that has developed along learned societies (Velasquez, Andre, Shanks, & Meyer, 2010).

The underlying theme is that the DNP should become a strong and persuasive advocate who is versed in the ethics that guide learned individuals to stand up to the potential harm that can come when vulnerable individuals, such as patients, or complex systems, such as hospitals, are under pressures exerted by the internal and external forces of political will. This is especially relevant today, at this time when global economic failures influence the quality and delivery of care. To become a strong advocate, it is important to understand the ethical rationales that underlie questions of what is fair and just in the delivery of health care.

In defining the notion of ethics, it is important to speak the same language that is used by professionals. In a seminal discussion by Velasquez et al. (2010), consideration is given to a definition of ethics with two distinct aspects:

The first is a reference to well-founded standards of right and wrong that prescribe what humans ought to do, usually in terms of rights, obligations, benefits to society, fairness, or specific virtues.

The second combines an action, one that requires the continuous effort of studying our own moral beliefs and our moral conduct, and striving to ensure that we, and the institutions we help to shape, live up to standards that are reasonable and solidly-based.

Though distant relatives to ethics, the policy and legal aspects of health care finance must also underlie the DNP practice. To understand the term *policy* is to define the term as directives that serve as documents of decisions about programs, laws, regulations, or legal directives (Milstead, 2012). The law interacts with health policy in several areas that can include individual or group protections, environmental regulation, and laws related to how industry relates to health.

The process of policy making includes an understanding of applicable laws at both the federal and state level that are organized and authored by legal professionals who may or may not seek guidance from strong health care advocates. This is a key point and one that should be of concern for the DNP. The germane question that must be asked is: "Who, if not you, should sit at the table in the debates over health care policy?"

The creation of public policy, as it relates to how to finance in health care, is influenced by the economics of the various constituents that comprise a representative's or senator's district. This is evident when one examines the confounding and convoluted debates regarding health care reform. If one takes the time to view Congressional records (or C-SPAN debates; https://www.c-span.org), it is apparent that the process of policy making is a confluence of special interests and lobbyist efforts that shape the way in which health care is delivered and financed. The debate over whether health care is a "right" (as seen in systems such as France) or a "privilege" (as seen by the U.S. market-driven forces) continues beyond health care reform and was clearly seen in the lines drawn in the debates.

In a thorough and balanced discussion, Kereiakes and Willerson (2012) carefully compare issues of health care as an entitlement or as a privilege. After a review of the Declaration of Independence, the authors ask this important question: Was it the intent of our forefathers to make health care a right for all citizens of the United States?

> For-profit, publicly traded insurance corporations have insinuated themselves between the consumers (patients) and the providers of goods and services (hospitals and physicians). These "corporate proxies" have a fiduciary responsibility to shareholders. They profit by the difference between premiums charged to the consumer and payments made to the providers while adding questionable value to the system. Through double-digit inflation in consumer premiums, these corporate insurers have posted record (32% to 260%) profit gains in 2003, while the number of Americans who remain uninsured continues to climb.

An important feature of our country's health care system is individual access to health services. Equal access to a comprehensive set of health care services is crucial to maintaining optimal health for everyone. In a free enterprise system, nonurgent health care is considered a business transaction between a patient and a physician. Primary care physicians are free to limit the number of uninsured patients they agree to accept into their practices. Most physician practices restrict the number of uninsured patients to a very low percentage of the total number of individuals due to concerns about inadequate cash flow due to nonpayment. This transactional approach to primary care means that individuals without health care coverage have difficulty finding a physician to agree to treat them on an ongoing basis. As a result, individuals without medical care coverage tend to use emergency departments for nonurgent care because they did not have ongoing access to a medical provider.

On March 23, 2010, the Patient Protection and Affordable Care Act (PPACA; Public Law 111–148), also known as the Affordable Care Act (ACA), was introduced to provide coverage to millions of previously uninsured people through the expansion of Medicaid and the establishment of health insurance marketplaces. Measures were included in the ACA to increase health insurance quality as well as affordability. The ACA requires participating insurers to accept all applicants, cover specific conditions, and charge the same rates regardless of preexisting conditions or sex (Kaiser Family Foundation, 2017). An analysis of enrollment data reveals that by the end of 2015, the ACA reduced the number of uninsured nonelderly Americans to 28.5 million, which is a decrease of nearly 13 million since 2013 (Centers for Disease Control and Prevention [CDC], 2015). These coverage gains were most common among those with low incomes living in states that expanded their Medicaid programs under the ACA (Kaiser Family Foundation, 2017).

As the result of the provisions of the ACA, many previously uninsured individuals were able to develop ongoing relationships with a primary care physician because they had insurance. Promoting preventive care to reduce acute exacerbation of chronic disease is a key feature of the ACA and is delivered through the "Patient-Centered Medical Care Home." This type of medical provider commitment to an individual's ongoing health care is widely believed to provide improved preventive care and medical management of chronic conditions (AHRQ, https://pcmh.ahrq.gov/page/defining-pcmh).

The model of the Patient-Centered Medical Care Home was developed in the 1960s for ongoing treatment of chronic pediatric illnesses. In 2000, the conceptualization of a medical home became popular in the treatment of chronic illnesses due to its focus on early management and intervention to prevent acute exacerbation of disease. According to the handbook of the American Association for Ambulatory Health Care (AAAHC, 2016), to qualify as a medical home, a practice must meet specific standards related to ongoing communication, understanding and collaboration between the patient and the provider and health care team, continuity with more than 50% of the patient's medical home visits with the same provider or physician team, comprehensiveness of care that includes preventive as well as end-of-life care, and a process for quality monitoring based on guidelines and established evidence.

With the advent of the ACA, the number of uninsured decreased and more individuals had insurance and access to medical homes that provided preventive care. In 2015, despite the gains in access associated with the implementation of the ACA, many Americans still do not have coverage. As of this writing, health care premiums associated with the ACA have risen due to shrinking insurance markets, making it unaffordable for many Americans (Abelson & Sanger-Katz, 2016).

The issues raised have been debated in the U.S. Congress. Does the "cost" of health care and the advances in technology, delivery, and quality require that Americans agree on a "social contract" in which all individuals carry some load? Congressional efforts to repeal portions of the ACA, undertaken throughout the spring and summer of 2017, revealed the breadth and scope of the national debate on our health care social contract. In March of 2017, the Republicans introduced the American Health Care Act (AHCA). This bill kept many of the features of the ACA, including the ACA exchanges, protections for those with preexisting conditions, and the stipulation that parents could continue to keep their children on their health insurance until they are 26 years of age. The individual and employer mandates in the ACA were intact, although the AHCA canceled the penalties for the individual mandate (Kaiser Family Foundation, 2017).

The AHCA repealed certain features of the ACA, including taxes imposed on health care insurance providers, manufacturers of prescription drugs and medical devices, and the controversial surtax of high-income Americans making more than $250,000 a year. The bill planned to end the requirement that insurers offer plans with specific levels of coverage and left the level of coverage up to the insurer's discretion. The AHCA also included a repeal of the Medicaid expansion program, which it delayed to 2020. Individuals in the expansion plan before 2020 were to be allowed to keep their Medicaid coverage as long as they qualify under the AHCA.

The Congressional Budget Office (CBO) quickly released its analysis of the health plan's impact on the federal budget (CBO, 2017). The analysis showed that premiums would vary depending on the age of the individual. An American who was 64 years old would see premiums rise 20% to 25% over 10 years, whereas an individual who was 40 years old would see premiums drop 8%, and an individual 21 years old would see a drop of 25%. The AHCA allowed insurers to charge older Americans up to five times more than younger ones. In addition, younger individuals would be more likely to buy low-cost plans offering minimal coverage, which would raise costs for the pool of older Americans.

The CBO report indicated that the AHCA would create a significant shift in government spending. Federal funding for Medicaid would be reduced by $880 billion over 10 years. The plan would partially replace that with $100 billion to help states pay for health care. In addition, there would be a significant move to curb the federal deficit by transferring the responsibility for health care costs to the states. Government aid to help individuals obtain health care coverage would be reduced by $312 billion because the ACA tax subsidies, totaling $673 billion, would be replaced by AHCA tax credits, totaling $361 billion. Tax cuts would include repealing the 0.9% Medicare tax on higher income earners, which would be a $117 billion cut; repealing a fee on health insurers, an estimated $145 billion cut; and repealing a 3.8% surcharge on higher incomes, equal to about $154 billion.

Eighteen days after its introduction, the Republicans pulled the bill due to lack of support. This failed attempt to change the ACA demonstrates our nation's conflicting ethics related to health care, particularly on the questions of who can access health care and who is responsible for paying for health care. As of this writing, additional health care reform measures have failed.

It is the issue of "cost" rather than "ethics" that continues to shape the debate. Milstead (2012) insists that nurses who are serious about their role in political influence require contact with legislators and agency directors. During discussion regarding the failed health care reform effort, governors and state lawmakers voiced concern that the AHCA plan was going to be particularly hard on Medicaid, the state–federal program that provides health care services to lower income workers and the poor. Washington State officials reported that starting in 2010, they would have to come up with $1.5 billion a year to keep the same level of coverage for their 600,000 residents who obtain coverage through the ACA Medicaid expansion program. Washington Governor Jay Inslee, a Democrat, noted that the AHCA "would actually leave our nation worse off than before the ACA was implemented," (LaCorte, 2017).

Physicians face the questions of cost regularly in their interactions with their patients. In today's world of electronic and social media, physicians find themselves considering novel patient requests for services, many of which are not included in guidelines and standards of care used by insurers. The question must be asked: "Do Americans expect more in their health care delivery systems?" The anticipation of research developments, such as stem cell therapy, or life-saving surgical interventions are covered comprehensively by the U.S. media. The Internet has allowed many individuals to research potential medical interventions and make requests of their medical providers. The idea that patient demand has not directly increased cost cannot be defended.

In an important paper, Dall, Chen, Siefert, Maddox, and Hogan (2009) suggest that as health care costs increase, efforts to improve both the quality and efficiency of health care delivery rest on the shoulders of professional nurses. An understanding of the legal aspects that guide professional practice is to realize that they are defined mainly by the responsibility to manage the financial affairs of populations and systems. Laws are political entities, designed and shaped by the will of society (Milstead, 2012). That "will" can be influenced in many ways and affects the shape and interpretation of the law—especially when laws are designed to control the cost of health care. Seminal questions must be asked: "Who should pay?" "How should the 'marginalized populations' be supported?" "Can the law be fair to both the rich and the poor?"

■ KEY FINANCIAL ISSUES

FRAUD

To carefully control the monies of vulnerable patients or systems is dependent upon a strong ethical framework that provides for the "respect for persons" necessary to avoid the temptation to commit fraud. The interaction among policy, law, and ethics is in great part dictated by issues related to cost containment and billing and the potential for fraud. The complex billing system that exists under multiple reimbursement structures ranging from public and private insurances gives rise to the notion that it is the provider and billers's conscience that guides the practice of coding and requesting payment. The trust in the insurance entity's process for monitoring each payment request is misguided. What remains, therefore, is the ethical framework under which, as a society, we agree to adhere. The question must be asked: What part of the rising health care costs can be attributed to fraud?

In addition to a strong ethical commitment by the DNP, an understanding of the legal code that underlies fraud becomes prominent. To be specific, in the U.S. legal code, Title 18 Part I Chapter 63 § 1347§ 1347 Health Care Fraud is defined as:

Whoever knowingly and willfully executes, or attempts to execute, a scheme or artifice—

1. To defraud any health care benefit program
2. To obtain, by means of false or fraudulent pretenses, representations, or promises, any of the money or property owned by, or under the custody or control of, any health care benefit program, in connection with the delivery of or payment for health care benefits, items, or services, shall be fined under this title or imprisoned not more than 10 years, or both. If the violation results in serious bodily injury (as defined in section 1365 of this title), such person shall be fined under this title or imprisoned not more than 20 years, or both; and if the violation results in death, such person shall be fined under this title, or imprisoned for any term of years or for life, or both.

THE COST OF MEDICAL ERROR

Since the release of the groundbreaking report of the Institute of Medicine (IOM, 2000) on error, the mitigation and, indeed, the cost of error have been emphasized in broad discussions across multiple disciplines and the lay literature. Estimates by one actuarial study (Society of Actuaries, 2008) were that medical error created a cost to the United States of $19.5 billion. The study was an in-depth review with a very large sample of 24 million people. There were 6.3 million measurable medical injuries in the United States in 2008; of this, it is estimated that 1.5 million were associated with a medical error. The average total cost per error was approximately $13,000.

If not a case of inadvertent error, what is the cost of individuals who deviate from standards and policies that are designed to protect the public? For example, the use of pharmaceutical agents "off label" is a common practice but one that can have serious consequences that lead to expensive legal cases. An example can be found in the prescription of two antiobesity agents (fen-phen) and the subsequent discovery of cardiac ill effect first described in 1996. This type of deviation, although not classified as a medical error, is one exemplar of issues that can occur from a deviation in standard practices.

When thinking about the financial cost of errors alone, one must ask the question: Where does this money come from? In a well-designed analysis of who pays for medical "misadventure," Mello, Studdert, Thomas, Yoon, and Brennan (2007) compared the costs of error that were absorbed by hospitals. Most of the cost was "externalized" to insurance agencies, which then passed on the cost to consumers through higher premiums.

Some errors are classified as "never events," those that are "unacceptable" in occurrence; Medicare, Medicaid, and several private insurers refuse to pay for costs associated with never events. This change in reimbursement has promoted multiple versions of patient safety and surveillance programs, the cost of which is borne by the health care system itself.

In addition, the notion of recovering the cost of error through mechanisms of the law is not sufficient; the tort system is not a good remedy for resolving most cases of medical injury (Berlinger, 2008). So, although medical litigation is one gateway toward reimbursement for medical error, it is often an inefficient one. According to Berlinger, the tort system was designed to affix blame and award damages. As award formulas are based on lost income or earning potential, and as plaintiffs' attorneys are paid out of awards, these attorneys have little financial incentive to take on clients with low incomes or earning potential, including women who do not work outside the home. Empirical research has found that low-income, uninsured, and elderly patients are much less likely to file malpractice suits than are other patients with equivalent medical injuries. Elderly patients, in particular, fear disrupting their relationships with health care providers and tend not to pursue compensation for injuries.

Clearly, the costs of medical errors also mean that less money is available for innovation, research, and technological improvements. The movement toward an understanding of the etiology and corrective actions to suppress the rate is important as both the financial costs and the costs to humans are the subjects of and the causes of medical error and are difficult to measure.

THE COST OF BIRTH AND DEATH

The cost of birth in the United States is affected by the health of the mother; issues related to environmental, genetic-related birth defects; and preterm labor. The annual societal economic burden associated with preterm birth in the United States was at least $26.2 billion in 2005, or $51,600 per infant born preterm. Medical care services contributed $16.9 billion to the total cost, and maternal delivery costs contributed another $1.9 billion. In terms of longer term expenditures, early intervention services cost an estimated $611 million, whereas special education services associated with a higher prevalence of four disabling conditions among premature infants added $1.1 billion. Finally, estimates of lost household and labor market productivity associated with those disabilities contributed $5.7 billion (IOM, Behrman, & Butler, 2007).

In 2001, Raphael and Fowler (2001) summarized estimates of the cost of end-of-life care. According to one estimate, end-of-life care accounts for about 10% to 12% of all health care spending. Annual expenditures for hospice and home care—two health care segments that are closely involved in the provision of end-of-life care—are about $3.5 billion and $29 billion, respectively.

Neither of the two aforementioned financial estimates includes the economic burden experienced by caregivers who must provide care without compensation while managing responsibilities such as employment, other family members, or maintaining their own health and well-being.

The three key areas are not the only financial issues in which law, ethics, and public policy intersect, but ones that relate specifically to the DNP. Two principles, legal and ethical, define the scope of practice for the DNP and are fundamental to the ability for a DNP to remain a strong advocate in the development of health care policy. A discussion of the *DNP Essentials* in relation to those two principles follows.

▨ ESSENTIAL I: SCIENTIFIC UNDERPINNINGS FOR PRACTICE

The American Assembly of Collegiate Schools of Business has fought to include ethics education into the curriculum (Cavaliere, Mulvaney, & Swerdlow, 2010). Teaching ethics in financial management in the DNP curriculum is arguably at least as important in the current health care setting. In a sweeping statement, the IOM boldly advanced the notion that "effective policy making requires better data collection and an improved information infrastructure" (IOM, 2010, p. 3). These two movements compel the DNP to ask important questions, collect evidence, and *transmit* the results among peers to promote ideas that are well anchored within a body of evidence. This is especially true when linking law, policy, and ethics to cost control and, in general, where health care dollars should be spent.

At this writing, the United States faces questions related to how the country can afford and indeed how it will mandate the health care reform. Important in this debate is what type of coverage will be mandated for all individuals and what insurance organizations will be required to provide.

The expansion of coverage both to the actual number of participants and the amount of money that can be spent on each individual has placed increasing pressure on an already burdened system. In 2007, $2.26 trillion was spent on health care and more than 4 billion health insurance claims were processed in the United States; Medicare alone pays 4.4 million claims per day to 1.5 million providers (Saccoccio, 2011). This figure is staggering in its dimension, in light of the 2010 U.S. Census Bureau calculation that 50.7 million Americans were uninsured.

Taking the Medicare system as an example, the growing number of baby boomers who are now classified as Medicare-eligible will further burden the volume of billing requests by providers. For the DNP, whether in the direct billing/provider relationship, or as an executive of a system dependent on reimbursement, the ethical and legal knowledge requirement that underlies financial management becomes a matter of both conscience and law.

ESSENTIAL II: ORGANIZATIONAL AND SYSTEMS LEADERSHIP FOR QUALITY IMPROVEMENT AND SYSTEMS THINKING

Three key issues that face the DNP who is engaged in financial management are the issues of combating health care fraud in a postreform world, the cost of medical error, and the amount of money dedicated to major "life events" for Americans. This means that systems must be designed, monitored, and corrected with conscience, policy, and law in mind. In the case of fraud, it is important to pay close attention to efforts made by the National Health Care Anti-Fraud Association (2010), which suggests seven guiding principles for policy makers. This author takes the position that the role of the DNP must incorporate the following seven principles:

1. *The sharing of antifraud information between private insurers and government programs should be encouraged and enhanced.*

   Though a health care provider may bill Medicare, Medicaid, and several private health insurance plans, no information about the claim is shared among the potential payers. This lack of transparency increases the potential for health care fraud and impairs detection efforts.

2. *Data consolidation and real-time data analysis must be at the forefront of health care detection and prevention.*

   Predictive data models are a significant tool used to combat the fraud.

3. *Prepayment reviews and audits should be increased and strengthened.*

   The claims at high risk for fraud include those made for durable medical equipment, home health services, and "phantom pharmacies." Granting more flexible discretion to auditors for pre- and postpayment audits is a first step to combat fraud.

4. *Public and private health plans should be allowed to protect their enrollees by barring or expelling providers suspected of perpetrating health care fraud.*

Medicare and various states require payers to accept licensed providers into their networks. Additional and enhanced screening of potential providers would identify those individuals who are suspected of health care fraud and bar them from participation in public and private health plans.

5. *Health care providers participating in fraud should be sanctioned by their respective state licensing boards.*

State licensing boards should be encouraged to restrict the licenses of health care providers of individuals determined to have submitted fraudulent claims. The fraudulent providers should be prosecuted, and when convicted, their identities should be revealed in publicly accessible media to deter future work in a health care setting and to protect the public.

6. *Health care provider identifier numbers should be made more secure.*

The current National Provider Identifier, established under the Health Insurance Portability and Accountability Act (HIPAA), is used in claim submissions but *is not* considered sensitive information and is currently widely available to those with Internet access, which makes it vulnerable to abuse.

7. *Investment in innovative health care fraud prevention, detection, and investigation efforts and programs should be encouraged.*

Health care fraud is a crime that directly affects the public trust and health care quality. Since nurses often hold a high level of public trust, the DNP should maintain trust by assisting in prevention techniques.

In the case of medical error, the DNP who is actively engaged in protecting patients and systems can be instrumental in changing practice to include more safety within practice. The use of simulation to study and avoid the "human factors" that contribute to error, and the active employment of "just culture" root cause analysis, should be part of every person who holds responsibility and authority over vulnerable patients and systems. Given the complexity of medical care and the importance of prevention, the development of sound error prevention strategies is critical.

In the last key issue discussed in this chapter, which addresses the cost of life events, the notion that DNPs should be involved in media-related health teaching surfaces to the top. Advanced practice registered nurses (APRNs) should be familiar with the use of Internet search engines to communicate with the public on health care practices. Engagement with electronic and print media must be more carefully engaged so that DNPs can be seen on both local and national stages to discuss how individuals can protect their own health. The DNP is the newest advanced degree that nurses can achieve. Many professionals, including physicians, as well as the public do not understand the scope or potential of this educational preparation. The weight of this novelty hangs heavily on the shoulders of those who hold this degree: to prove its utility in society, each of you must be "above the game" in developing programs to support the public good. The notion that cost might be controlled through better, ethical, lawful policy practice rests in the domain of this degree.

ESSENTIAL III: CLINICAL SCHOLARSHIP AND ANALYTICAL METHODS FOR EVIDENCE-BASED PRACTICE

Any one of the suggested principles could, and indeed it might be argued *should*, be a task that is assumed by the DNP leaders. A collaboration among policy makers, legislators, and business professors that includes those individuals who hold the DNP doctoral degree, as the expertise developed in these individuals by their programs of study, is a natural fit.

This statement requires the due diligence of the DNP in the study and continual refreshment of important data analytical techniques that could be used to model billing and surveillance practices within a variety of organizations. There is a *revolution in analytics* underway today, as massive amounts of data are being captured and stored, and increasingly cheaper and more powerful computers are creating unprecedented opportunities for applying advanced mathematical and statistical techniques. In the business world, successful applications of analytic techniques require expertise in a broad range of disciplines as well as intimate knowledge of the business domain. A partnership between those who can control and interpret sophisticated analytical techniques and the DNP is a complement that can be used to great advantage.

Universities have also picked up on this trend. Several schools have begun to offer graduate degrees in analytics (Boyd, 2011, provides a recent survey). These programs typically involve collaboration between different departments and/or schools within a university. For example, DePaul University's program in Predictive Analytics draws on faculty from several schools, and St. Joseph's University's program in Business Intelligence trains its students in a variety of software, management, and statistics courses. Partnering with universities is a natural way for those in practice to link experts (and their students) with real-world issues in a way that provides important and useful quid pro quo.

■ ESSENTIAL IV: INFORMATION SYSTEMS/TECHNOLOGY AND PATIENT CARE TECHNOLOGY FOR THE IMPROVEMENT AND TRANSFORMATION OF HEALTH CARE

Typically, hospital (and health care) systems receive revenue in a variety of ways that include providing medical services, receiving grants, and through investments (Lane, Longstreth, & Nixon, 2001). Among the potential payers for medical services are public payers (Medicare; Medicaid) and private payers, which include health maintenance organizations (HMOs), preferred provider organizations (PPOs), point-of-service plans, and self-pay.

The myriad of potential payers is made more complex by the amount (and type) of payment methods that include fee-for-service, capitation, and diagnosis-related group (DRG) charges. The requirement that both large systems and small office practices are subjected to the same complex payment and billing systems requires both increased time and emphasis on financial management for professionals. A close analysis of the costs of billing and insurance tasks in a large medical practice found that such tasks consume $85,276 per full-time equivalent physician or 10% of operating revenue. Standardizing health plan benefits and billing procedures would reduce administrative complexity and costs (Sakowski, Kahn, Kronick, Newman, & Luft, 2009). The natural fallout of this time and cost is less service that can be dedicated to any given patient issue.

If a transformation of health care can occur in the United States, who should be at the table to design a system that is both patient centered and socially conscious? The individuals who hold a DNP could, and indeed should, avail themselves of potential grant funding to solve problems related to cost, quality, and outcomes. Health care reform initiatives have set aside major investments in "comparative effectiveness research" that is designed to compare outcomes of one therapeutic approach with those of others to benefit the majority of patients. Although this approach might exclude the "outliers," it is an important direction that uses the existing evidence to guide major decisions. Cost will likely be less if standards, procedures, and policies can be agreed upon.

Nurse practitioners (NPs) who hold close relationships with their patients and nurse executives who manage the costs related to care are key individuals who should be part of well-designed, well-planned comparative effectiveness research.

ESSENTIAL V: HEALTH CARE POLICY FOR ADVOCACY IN HEALTH CARE

Human values shape personal, social, and professional behaviors by signaling desirable ways of behaving (Graf, Van Quaquebeke, & Van Dick, 2011). "Fitting" into any organizational structure includes a complex association with the values and mission. It is the leadership of any given organization that influences the ethics of its mission and enforces the legality of its operation.

Perhaps there is no greater responsibility for the DNP leader than in the shaping and refining of health care policy on handling the fair and equitable distribution of health care dollars. Important ethical and moral questions must be asked and answered. This type of discussion is particularly important in light of the country's conflict regarding health care reform.

WHO SHOULD PAY?

Although many in the United States are in support of specific social welfare programs, such as Medicare, others believe that the "rich do not always have to support the poor." Extending the health care metaphor, what is the appropriate moral prescription for any given society in its distributive justice? An understanding of both sides of any argument is fundamental to any just decision. Though words such as *underserved* and *indigent* are found within any given health care policy and finances discussion, these words often serve to inflame the passions of those on the "opposite side of the aisle," who believe more closely in the theories of "personal responsibility" in important life decisions. From both an ethical and legal argument, both sides must be considered carefully.

HOW LONG SHOULD PAYMENT CONTINUE?

The extension of an ethical and legal requirement for any society to support its weakest members is the important corollary "for how long?" Given someone who is grossly obese, smokes tobacco, and does nothing to support his or her own health, what is the greater societal responsibility to pay for the entire cadre of chronic conditions that surround such a profile? Does this person deserve more or less financial support than the neonate born to a drug-addicted mother? How "old" is too old to perform "elective" surgery on an extreme geriatric patient?

The discussions that precede the development of financial policy with both its attendant legal and ethical considerations require careful attendance to the principles of professional competence of the DNP. The DNP can be a natural voice for the underserved, for the etiology of health disparities, and for his or her own scope of practice with legislators. In following bills, both local and national, DNPs can provide important background information for their legislators and their profession. Laws are complex and legislators increasingly rely on important sources for information; DNPs can provide important counsel on issues related to finance and health care outcomes.

ESSENTIAL VI: INTERPROFESSIONAL COLLABORATION FOR IMPROVING PATIENT AND POPULATION HEALTH OUTCOMES

The dedication of multiple professionals is required to answer important ethical, legal, and legal policy questions. If outcomes of health interventions are related to pure access-to-care principles, then collaborative efforts on the part of the DNP leader should take place on boards and in professional organizations. At the point of being doctorally prepared, the "right" to sit at the table with other professionals requires a sense of one's own discipline and the fundamental assumptions that underlie that discipline. The discipline of nursing has moved through much iteration since it was first recognized as having its own philosophical posture. Yet, the reluctance of nursing professionals to engage in higher level decisions has dampened its voice.

New models of payment for health care services have been provided in recent health care reform initiatives in which providers and hospitals are given financial incentives to provide good quality at cost-lowering rates. Although this may seem paradoxical, it is one way to encourage investment in systems that provide efficient and quality care to patients.

The legal and ethical considerations for this domain include the performance in a wide range of activities that can and should direct issues of social justice. The 2008 "financial meltdown" that resulted in a global recession revealed the issues of leaving business practices to "business experts." This author takes the position that DNPs should consider offering their skills, knowledge, and talents in collaboration *outside* of the health care system as much as they consider operating within that structure. Outside influences on the ways in which money flows to support the health care of individuals include both governmental and private organizations that direct programs and fund research grants. Issues of "big picture" proportion have often been neglected by nurses in the face of more pressing, individual patient or system needs. The importance of engaging in collaborative efforts has been particularly underscored by the length of time it has taken to gain traction on a cogent health care bill that began in President Clinton's term and continues in the present-day administration.

Why leave the voice only to politicians and pundits? The DNP is uniquely situated to provide that voice.

▪ ESSENTIAL VII: CLINICAL PREVENTION AND POPULATION HEALTH FOR IMPROVING THE NATION'S HEALTH

The financial cost of prevention is relatively low in comparison to the cost of treatment, yet prevention is uniquely underfunded. For any given outbreak, whether an aggressive influenza or a food-borne illness, the public outcry, especially driven by the media, is loud and emphatic. Yet, when the disease is no longer in the headlines, the tendency to move away from the notion of public health is strong.

There are many reasons for this, including the federal cut to public health funding included in the ACA (Rapaport, 2015). The responsibility of the DNP lies in the ethics of distribution of justice in the context of fairness of resource management. In addition to dealing with insurance company lobbyists, political campaigns, and the sometimes ill-informed vox populi, the DNP is charged with standing for the needs of an entire population as needs arise. Using the early AIDS epidemic as an example, the history of which is carefully constructed in both scholarly and lay publications, the lack of response by the political forces at the time led to a delay of funding to study, and indeed control, the epidemic. This is in no doubt partly due to the fact that the initial, infected population was from a "marginalized" population. Many lessons were learned from this bleak episode in our nation's recent history, but the charge for the DNP is to argue for a financial remedy irrespective of *who* is affected by any given disease, both to provide humane treatment *and* to protect the public.

ESSENTIAL VIII: ADVANCED NURSING PRACTICE

Perhaps nowhere is the field more in need for the DNP than the translation of solid, important evidence into direct practice. Whether the DNP is in direct patient care, such as an NP, or in direct administrative responsibility within organizations or as an independent consultant and teacher, the most important role that can be engaged is that of advancing the discipline of nursing.

Issues of trust in the U.S. financial system emerged strongly in the beginning of the collapse of the "housing bubble," the existence of packaged home loans to those with little ability to pay, "credit default swaps" sold to global partners, and the various "Ponzi" schemes such as those perpetrated by Madoff. Medicare fraud and inappropriate billing are among those practices that have displaced the public trust.

Nurses are well positioned to change that low level of trust to a higher one. Nurses continue to enjoy high positions in the public trust ratings; DNPs can—and indeed should—continue to manage the financial and ethical obligations placed before them.

The notion of "nursing practice" must include the ethics and legal complexity associated with the management of financial obligations and regulatory efforts on behalf of those most in need. That would include not only the individual patient, but also the system in which those patients find themselves.

In a broader interpretation, DNPs who can integrate within the political and legislative system can provide important information to guide lawmaking and public health policy directives. Milstead (2012) suggests that nurses are "articulate experts" who can address the rational shaping of policy. This may mean working directly with lobbyists, who can (and do) work toward special interests. In 2009, the American Nurses Association (ANA) reported spending $1,197,342 on its lobbying efforts, whereas the American Hospital Association (AHA) spent $13,585,000. This level of disparity often speaks to the "attention" each legislator gives to the issues that are raised.

The area where APRNs could support the financing of a just public health care policy might be in "grassroots" initiatives. DNPs can form powerful coalitions and address issues of cost, how money is spent and on whom. Any initiative can receive attention if the volume of letters, emails, and telephone calls reach the attention of legislators (or their health aides).

CONCLUSION

The cost of health care continues to outpace other industries. The cost of research, particularly for the design and implementation of new medications or invasive devices, is necessarily high, as is the investment by corporations into this type of discovery. Issues related to the recruitment and protection of human subjects, the number of phases and trials, and the management of large data sets are expensive. To fail to acknowledge that corporations that invest large resources and time to discovery should be compensated is to deny the very basis of American capitalism. The issue should not be that corporations should not receive just compensation, but rather what is the definition of just compensation.

Political pressure, certainly by lobbyists, is designed to maintain the status quo for large benefits to executives and to shareholders. What is required of the DNP is to assist in the notion of what is "fair" to charge for innovation and who should be able to receive novel therapies. It is a discussion that occurs with great difficulty in the United States. The dialogue that emerged during the debates around health care reform, rather than assisting the creation of a "social contract," resulted in polarizing positions that continue to divide the country as "pro" or "con." Is it possible to reach a compromise between profit, cost, and delivery?

One of the most important documents to be written, the Declaration of Independence, took approximately 17 days to complete. This treatise served (and continues to serve) as a foundation for the important notions of freedom and fair representation. Could such an accomplishment occur in today's world of special interests, divisive politics, and large amounts of money spent by corporations interested not in public health, or ethics, but in bottom-line profit for their shareholders?

Yet, in counterargument, the shareholders are not some vague entity, they are us. The shareholders of large corporations include tens of thousands of average workers whose 401(K) plans are invested on their behalf; undoubtedly, some of those investments include large pharmaceutical and medical equipment companies. Is it fair to ask single individual workers to withhold their investments in such potentially profitable companies as a counterbalance to the rising costs of health care?

Important in this discussion of financial management is the notion that Americans have some responsibility to decide where their money is spent and on whom. The questions related to "financial triage" are theoretically possible to answer, but in each individual case, decisions become more difficult to make. Conflicts of conscience, respect for persons versus the greater good, intervene in the immediacy of decisions required by life and death events.

A critical framework that can serve as a foundation for an ethical, lawful, and cost-effective health care policy relies on three important pillars: (a) quality and safety of care, (b) access to care, and (c) cost. Can all three be justified under one social contract? Interestingly, studies continue to demonstrate that simply increasing spending does not influence population mortality. Rather, infrastructure that includes environmental health, vaccinations, and clean air and water has more greatly impacted population health. Life expectancy models reflect this notion, as reported by the Organisation for Economic Co-operation and Development (OECD, 2011), and compare the United States and the United Kingdom at 78 years at $7,538 per capita versus 79.9 years at $3,129.

What explains this significant difference? One could speculate that the United Kingdom has more sophisticated public health access, or better genetic pools, but the notion that the United States spends twice the amount for less years of life requires deeper exploration. Certainly the notion of private versus public health care is a comparison that should be explored, perhaps as one mechanism to be included in subsequent political discussions about health care reform.

The quality and safety issues can and should fall under the ethical practices of the DNP as the notion of "first, do no harm" is foundational to the responsibilities and promise to the patient (or organization). In addition to the ethical perspective, mistakes cost money. That money must necessarily be diverted from one area to another, or it is simply lost to the organization. None of those alternatives offers a reasonable choice.

Access issues are important to discuss in light of the notion of "personal responsibility." Economists use two terms to defend insurance company practices. *Adverse selection* is defined as a person who seeks coverage solely on the likelihood that he or she intends to experience higher costs (e.g., early cancer symptoms). *Moral hazard* describes the use of insurance for purposes other than health (e.g., cosmetic surgery). From an ethical perspective, do these actions constitute a "distributive justice" approach, where all individuals are accorded equal shares? Justice involves the fair treatment of all humans and should not favor one group of individuals based on the ability to be resourceful over another who may not have the means to accomplish the same benefits.

The patient (or consumer of health care) must also be educated to understand the individual responsibility to share the burden and to not take more than one needs. These principles, although seemingly obvious, are necessary to reinforce as the DNP meets with the public.

The DNP is uniquely positioned to render a compromise among disparate perspectives, as the *DNP Essentials* offer an important roadmap to solution. When taken both as a single essential, or viewing them as a whole, no other doctorally prepared individual has such a recipe for potential success.

Coleman, Bouësseau, Reis, and Capron (2007) made this important statement:

The ethical obligations of those who work for health are as old as the health professions themselves; indeed, the commitment to place the interests of clients above all else is one of the hallmarks of professionalism. (p. 504)

This statement colors carefully the issue of how the individuals with the newest doctoral degree in nursing can influence one of the oldest notions of social justice and legal protections for the individuals, populations, and systems. It is a challenge for which the education prepares the student; it is the moral conscience that sustains that student throughout his or her career.

CRITICAL THINKING EXERCISES

1. You are the chief nurse executive at an organization that provides clinic services to Medicare patients; there are seven clinics located in underserved areas. While visiting one of the clinics, you perform a routine audit. You notice that one physician, who has been excluded from the Medicare program due to a prior felony conviction for accepting kickbacks for referrals, has submitted bills for $165,000 for services rendered. You contact the physician and she refers you to her attorney. Her attorney says she thought she was following the law when she submitted bills for services her employee performed. The patients received the services and there have been no reported complaints.

   The physician speaks three languages fluently, and the patients at this clinic have nothing but praise for his care. You have had a great deal of difficulty locating a qualified physician who is willing to work in this crime-ridden area.
   a. What is your first action?
   b. How do you justify this action based on legal and ethical guidelines?
   c. What is your second action?
   d. How do you justify this action based on legal and ethical guidelines?
   e. What is your final action?
   f. How do you justify this action based on legal and ethical guidelines?

2. You are an NP who sees mostly post-head trauma patients and refers many of these patients to physical and occupational services. On one routine follow-up visit, your patient claims that he has not had any of the services you suggested, even though you saw several bills from the consulting provider.

   You ask for an audit and discover that the owner of the service submitted $1.28 million in claims for occupational therapy services that were not provided. The owner used Medicaid provider numbers of licensed therapists without their consent to bill for the never-performed services.
   a. What is your first action?
   b. How do you justify this action based on legal and ethical guidelines?
   c. What is your second action?
   d. How do you justify this action based on legal and ethical guidelines?
   e. What is your final action?
   f. How do you justify this action based on legal and ethical guidelines?

3. You are the chief nursing executive for a small rural clinic that provides contraception services to low-income individuals. An insurer, providing care under the ACA, has rejected paying the claims, stating that they are a not-for-profit religious organization and are not obliged to

cover these services. You check your records and find that nonpayment for contraception places a significant financial burden on the clinic. These individuals do not have access to any other health care services in the region.

a. What is your first action?

b. How do you justify this action based on legal and ethical guidelines?

c. What is your second action?

d. How do you justify this action based on legal and ethical guidelines?

e. What is your final action?

f. How do you justify this action based on legal and ethical guidelines?

4. You are an NP in a small hospital and you are reviewing the chart of a patient who underwent a second abdominal surgery. Six months after his initial surgery, the patient had to return to surgery for removal of a retained surgical instrument, an 11-inch retractor. On his follow-up appointment, your review of his medical record reveals that the discharge diagnosis for his second surgery was abdominal adhesions and there is no mention of removing the retractor in the surgical report. As you review his chart, you question if the incident was reported as a "never event." You practice in a state that has mandatory reporting of never events.

a. What is your first action?

b. How do you justify this action based on legal and ethical guidelines?

c. What is your second action?

d. How do you justify this action based on legal and ethical guidelines?

e. What is your final action?

f. How do you justify this action based on legal and ethical guidelines?

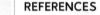

REFERENCES

Abelson, R., & Sanger-Katz, M. (2016, October 25). A quick-guide to rising Obamacare rates. *New York Times*. Retrieved from https://www.nytimes.com/2016/10/26/upshot/rising-obamacare-rates-what-you-need-to-know.html

American Association for Ambulatory Health Care. (2016). Accreditation handbook for ambulatory health care. Retrieved from https://www.aaahc.org/Global/Handbooks/2016/HB16_FNL-interactive_v2.pdf

Berlinger, N. (2008). Medical error. In C. Mary (Ed.), *From birth to death and bench to clinic: The Hastings Center bioethics briefing book for journalists, policymakers, and campaigns* (pp. 97–100). Garrison, NY: The Hastings Center.

Boyd, A. (2011). An analytics education. Retrieved from http://viewer.zmags.com/publication/03b6e869#/03b6e869/7

Cavaliere, F. J., Mulvaney, T. P., & Swerdlow, M. R. (2010). Teaching business ethics after the financial meltdown: Is it time for ethics with a sermon? *Education, 131*(1), 3–7.

Centers for Disease Control and Prevention. (2015). *Health insurance coverage: Early release of estimates from the National Health Interview Survey, January–June 2015*. Retrieved from http://www.cdc.gov

Coleman, C. H., Bouësseau, M. C., Reis, A., & Capron, A. M. (2007). How should ethics be incorporated into public health policy and practice? *Bulletin of the World Health Organization, 85*(7), 504.

Congressional Budget Office. (2017). American Health Care Act: Cost estimate. Retrieved from https://www.cbo.gov/publication/52486

Dall, T. M., Chen, Y. Z., Siefert, R. F., Maddox, P. J., & Hogan, P. F. (2009). The economic value of professional nursing. *Medical Care, 47*(1), 97–104.

Graf, M. M., Van Quaquebeke, N., & Van Dick, R. (2011). Two independent value orientations: Ideal and counter-ideal leader values and their impact on followers' respect for and identification with their leaders. *Journal of Business Ethics, 114*, 185–195. Retrieved from http://www.springerlink.com/content/g3127141361g6755

Institute of Medicine. (2000). *To err is human: Building a safer health system*. Washington, DC: National Academies Press.

Institute of Medicine. (2010). *The future of nursing: Leading change, advancing health*. Washington, DC: National Academies Press.

Institute of Medicine (U.S.) Committee on Understanding Premature Birth and Assuring Healthy Outcomes, Behrman, R. E., & Butler, A. S. (2007). *Preterm birth: Causes, consequences, and prevention*. Washington, DC: National Academies Press.

Kaiser Family Foundation. (2017). Health reform. Retrieved from http://kff.org/health-reform

Kereiakes, D. J., & Willerson, J. T. (2012). U.S. health care: Entitlement or privilege? Retrieved from http://www.circ.ahajournals.org

LaCorte, R. (2017, March 13). WA governor says health care analysis confirms worst fears. *U.S. News & World Report*. Retrieved from https://www.usnews.com/news/best-states/washington-dc/articles/2017-03-13/wa-governor-says-health-care-analysis-confirms-worst-fears

Lane, S. G., Longstreth, E., & Nixon, V. (2001). *A community leader's guide to hospital finance: The access project*. Boston, MA: Harvard School of Public Health.

Mello, M. M., Studdert, D. M., Thomas, E. J., Yoon, C. S., & Brennan, T. A. (2007). Who pays for medical errors? An analysis of adverse costs, the medical liability system and incentives for patient safety improvement. *Journal of Empirical Legal Studies, 4*(4), 835–860.

Milstead, J. A. (2012). Advanced practice nurses and public policy, naturally. In J. A. Milstread (Ed.), *Health policy and ethics* (4th ed.). Burlington, MA: Jones & Bartlett.

National Health Care Anti-Fraud Association. (2010). *Combating health care fraud in a post-reform world: Seven guiding principles for policymakers: A white paper*. Retrieved from http://www.nhcaa.org

Organisation for Economic Co-operation and Development. (2011). Retrieved from http://stats.oecd.org

Rapaport, L. (2015, November 18). U.S. public health funding on the decline. *Reuters Health News*. Retrieved from http://www.reuters.com/article/us-health-publichealth-funding-idUSKCN0T735R20151118

Raphael, C., & Fowler, N. (2001). Financing end-of-life care in the USA. *Journal of the Royal Society of Medicine, 94*(9), 458–461.

Saccoccio, L. (2011, March). *Improving efforts to combat health care fraud* (Report to U.S. House Committee on Ways and Means Subcommittee on Oversight), Washington, DC. Retrieved from https://waysandmeans.house.gov/UploadedFiles/Socc.pdf

Sakowski, J. A., Kahn, J. G., Kronick, R. D., Newman, J. M., & Luft, H. S. (2009). Peering into the black box: Billing and insurance activities in medical group. *Health Affairs Web Exclusive, 28*(4), w544–w554.

Society of Actuaries. (2008). Retrieved from http://www.soa.org

U.S. Census Bureau. (2010). Home page. Retrieved from https://www.census.gov/2010census

Velasquez, M., Andre, C., Shanks, T., & Meyer, M. J. (2010). What is ethics? Retrieved from https://www.scu.edu/ethics/practicing/decision/whatisethics.html

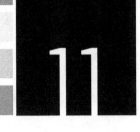

11 Evolution of a Project: The DNP as Project Manager

Elena Capella and Kathleen M. Nakfoor

We are what we repeatedly do. Excellence, then, is not an act; it is a habit.

(Aristotle, 384–322 BCE)

Peter Drucker (2001) has long called for "systematic abandonment," claiming a product is virtually obsolete at the time of its launch. He went on to state that knowledge workers who are in the process of continuous learning would replace blue-collar workers. Decentralized organizations with spontaneous, ad hoc, flexible teams are in a better position to innovate because they are at the microeconomic level and nearer to events (Drucker, 2001). Drucker's recommendations have been instilled in health care organizations, primarily through the Institute for Healthcare Improvement (IHI) and its focus on the diffusion of innovation through small tests of change. The reduction in product life cycles combined with the growing complexity of projects and need to integrate divergent sectors makes project management a standard rather than a unique way of doing business (Larson & Gray, 2011). The torrent of incessant change in organizations and the demand to remain flexible have led to the evolution of high-performing, cross-functional teams working on "projects." Although hierarchical, mechanistic health care oligopolies had a measure of success in the past, they now struggle to provide quick turnaround on projects in the rapidly changing, complex environment of the 21st century. To meet the changing demand, organizations turn to project teams that have developed into ubiquitous hybrid, flat, organic teams led by skilled project managers. In this new model, subject matter experts collaborate to complete projects that range from single-process improvements to complex projects. Organizational management teams are leaner, as project managers replace middle managers to oversee internal and outsourced projects. Service organizations have replaced manufacturing models, creating a need for strong interpersonal skills. Project management calls for a balance of task-oriented and relationship-oriented competencies to meet the demands of on-time, zero-error customer service.

DEFINITION OF A PROJECT

The Project Management Institute (PMI), in its *A Guide to the Project Management Body of Knowledge*, defines a project as, "a temporary endeavor undertaken to create a unique product, service or result" (PMI, 2004, p. 1). Ultimately, the goal of a project is to fulfill a need, usually an internal or external customer need (Larson & Gray, 2011). Larson and Gray describe how a project consists of a predetermined objective to be completed within a specified target date. In general, projects require the involvement of several departments and professionals coordinating on work that has never been done before and is due to be completed within specific time, cost, and performance parameters.

Larson and Gray (2011) describe the technical and sociocultural dimensions of the project management process. The technical side of project management refers to the preparation of a work breakdown structure (WBS), preparing schedules and budgets, resource allocation, project mapping, and control. The mechanical or precise skills side of project management is static, guided by rules that are straightforward, as opposed to the sociocultural side, which requires interpersonal skills to meet the demands of project management in today's organizational environments. Goleman (1998) describes these types of interpersonal skills, particularly when used in organizations, as emotional intelligence, or the management of feelings that support team processes and accomplish shared goals. Interpersonal skills are critical to building teams, negotiating, traversing the formal and informal politics of the organization with the needs of the customer always at the forefront. This chapter further explores the spectrum of technical and sociocultural skills of project management, as well as the doctor of nursing practice (DNP) preparation to meet such demands.

THE DNP AS PROJECT MANAGER

Key drivers in the demand for organizational change in health care delivery are current initiatives to redesign health care delivery through innovation, such as the accountable care organization (ACO). The DNP will play a critical role in change at this macrosystem level, as well as the mesosystem and microsystems level. The American Association of Colleges of Nursing (AACN), in *The Essentials of Doctoral Education for Advanced Nursing Practice* (2006), delineates the eight essential core competencies that will prepare the DNP as both a participant and leader in change and project management (AACN, 2006):

1. Scientific Underpinnings for Practice
2. Organizational and Systems Leadership for Quality Improvement and Systems Thinking
3. Clinical Scholarship and Analytical Methods for Evidence-Based Practice
4. Information Systems/Technology and Patient Care Technology for the Improvement and Transformation of Health Care
5. Health Care Policy for Advocacy in Health Care
6. Interprofessional Collaboration for Improving Patient and Population Health Outcomes
7. Clinical Prevention and Population Health for Improving the Nation's Health
8. Advanced Nursing Practice

Improvements in practice are neither sustainable nor measurable without corresponding changes in organizational structure, organizational and professional culture, and financial structures to support the changed practice (AACN, 2006). The DNP graduate is prepared with leadership, assessment, and communication skills to perform project management at every level of the health care organization. The DNP will be armed with the "essential" competencies to be an effective project manager: applying evidence-based research; collaborating at the micro-, meso-, and macrosystem level; contributing to the financial analyses; performing an organizational needs assessment; knowing when to utilize technology; and adding value through the balance of cost and quality at every phase of the project.

▦ THE PHASES OF PROJECT PLANNING

Projects have a finite progression span consisting of the analysis/design, planning, implementation, and concluding phases, with each phase overlapping the other at variable lengths. The four phases will be discussed in the following portions of this chapter to equip the DNP with the foundation for successful project planning and management.

The analysis/design phase explores the factors necessary to ensure the project goals and outcomes are aligned with the organization's strategic plan, delineates project specifications, performs financial analyses, and builds a team capable of completing tasks and accepting responsibilities. The next phase, the planning phase, is more extensive than the design phase. In the planning phase, schedules and budgets are prepared with accompanying resource allocations, including staffing. At this phase, risks are identified and mitigated when feasible. The implementation phase is typically the longest and most labor intensive of the four phases of project management. It is in this phase that the project is built, implemented, and monitored to verify costs and schedules meet baseline projections. The concluding phase consists of final testing and deployment, training the end user, sign-off by appropriate parties, and transfer of key documents related to the projects. For ease of discussion and clarity, the chapter is organized according to the four phases of a project.

THE ANALYSIS/DESIGN PHASE

The project charter is generated at the executive level and authorizes the DNP project manager to initiate the project and access the organization's resources to complete the project. Three principal documents used in project management are the project charter, project scope statement, and project plan. The project scope statement describes the work to be accomplished, including deliverables, and the project management plan states how the work is to be completed (PMI, 2004).

The DNP project manager begins a project by performing an organizational need and readiness assessment within the organization (Larson & Gray, 2011). Key indicators are analyzed, such as the alignment of the stakeholders' expectations and leadership support for the project, including the allocation of resources to meet the cost and personnel demands of the project. It is important to determine whether the project leader and team members have been given the appropriate amount of authority and are capable of completing the project. Evaluation of the mission, vision, and culture of the organization is critical to the potential success of a project, as well as verification that the project manager and team members are a good match for the project and the organization. How the project goals fit with the strategic goals of the organization is another key consideration. Ultimately, a determination is needed that the project adds value to the organization and key stakeholders agree with this financial analysis. Projects in health care organizations are held to a high level of accountability because the projects affect health outcomes. They are expected to be based on sound clinical evidence and measured against projected outcomes.

Early in the analysis/design phase, a review of organizational documents including committee minutes and decision-making records provides the DNP project manager with information to guide the planning process (Harris, Roussel, Walters, & Dearman, 2011). These records shed light on how decisions are made, identify the key decision makers, and signal potential pitfalls. If the DNP identifies troubling trends, such as a series of former projects that failed to be implemented, an opportunity exists to discuss these failures, identify the factors that led to the failures, and adjust the plan for the project.

Another way to gather more information about potential support is to discuss the project with a variety of leaders who will be involved in the project, as this will provide information on the leadership group's support as a whole. If the leaders in the organization have similar expectations and are consistent in their approval of the project, the DNP will be more confident and broad support will likely be sustained throughout the project planning and implementation phases. A particularly promising sign is when the leaders in the organization are skilled in articulating the goals of the project, defining its benefits, and inspiring others to accept the project's worth. These emotionally intelligent leaders stimulate enthusiasm and motivation in others and can be helpful in the project development phase. The DNP project manager builds continuing relationships with these individuals who are allies that give support when the project stalls or is in need of additional resources. Building collegial interprofessional partnerships is an essential element of DNP practice in advocating projects that lead to better clinical outcomes (AACN, 2006).

The methods that DNP project managers use to confirm alignment with the strategic mission will vary but often include interviews of top and middle management combined with a review of strategic planning documents. Developing a list of questions based on the DNP's expert understanding of the organization makes the interview discussion more productive. The DNP project manager uses advanced communication skills to explore the project's alignment with strategic plans such as the Five Whys questioning method. The Five Whys method was developed by Sakichi Toyoda to reduce the number of false assumptions made during service quality evaluation (Pojasek, 2000). This communication technique delves deeper into the interviewee's perspectives to uncover a richer understanding of the reasons for their point of view. During the interviews, the DNP project manager may uncover disagreement among members of top and middle management on the goals of the organization, which is called an implementation gap (Larson & Gray, 2011). Uncovering this gap early on in the project selection process can help the DNP project manager pick projects that are more likely to be successful. The interviews also provide the DNP with insight into the political environment and which leaders will be persuasive advocates for or against specific projects. This early exploration is an essential step in evaluating which projects have the greatest potential for completion and sustainability. Projects lay the foundation for the organization's development and are more likely to be successful when they add value, align with the overall strategic plan, and engender support from management.

Smart Goals and Aim Statements

Before committing to a project that will have a significant impact on the organization, the DNP project manager develops specific goals for the potential project. A clear goal statement that accurately represents the project is essential in the selection process to determine which projects are implemented by the organization. Goal clarification is the process of communicating desired results in a clear manner, which serves to guide and direct employees toward completion of the project. Developing goals using the SMART goals framework is an effective way to ensure goals are properly formulated. In the SMART goals method, goals are developed that are specific, measurable, attainable, realistic, and time bound. Early drafts of a goal statement are reviewed and revised to verify they meet SMART goal standards. It is particularly important that the goals be free of jargon and written in a manner understood by all stakeholders involved in the project. The strongest goal statements are succinct and explicit to such a degree that they do not require readers to read attachments or addendums to understand the goals. This concise clarity makes goal statements useful to team members who periodically need to review the goal statement and redirect their activities.

The IHI's Science of Improvement: Tips for Setting Aims (2017a) provides specific recommendations for the development of aim statements in health care organizations that are helpful for DNP project managers. The inclusion of numerical goals is recommended because projects that have a specific numerical aim are more likely to be completed. According to the IHI, numerical goals support change by directing measurement and creating an ongoing "tension" about the progress of the change. Another recommended practice is to develop stretch goals to indicate that maintaining the status quo is not good enough. DNP project managers discuss the aim statement with stakeholders and provide team members regular feedback to support the project's progress.

As outlined in *DNP Essential IV*, the DNP project manager uses information to provide a feedback mechanism on practice with the goal of improving patient care (AACN, 2006).

On occasion, the DNP may determine that the project team has experienced "aim drift," the unconscious or deliberate backing away from a stretch goal that requires team discussion and corrective action. In this type of situation, it may be necessary to redirect the aim statement, perhaps to a smaller part of the goal. The process of redirection must be carefully analyzed to represent a deliberate decision based on sound decision making. The DNP project manager has a significant body of knowledge to help some team members persuade others to practice in the direction of better clinical outcomes (AACN, 2006).

Integral to the DNP's success of project planning and management is a thorough understanding of systems theory and complexity science. Systems theory was first proposed in 1928 by biologist Ludwig von Bertalanffy (1950). He questioned the prevailing idea that a system could be disassembled into its parts and laid out linearly to explain the interworkings of the system. Von Bertalanffy proposed that the interworkings of the system could only be explained by looking at the *interrelationship* of its parts, particularly their cause-and-effect relationship. The DNP project manager applies systems theory to health care's predominately open systems. Open systems depend on external resources for survival and success, as opposed to a closed system, which is entirely dependent on internal resources to be self-sustaining. Health care systems are dependent on many external sources, such as regulatory agencies, third-party payers, and professional organizations that advance changes in protocols and standards. In general, organizations transform inputs to outputs, depending on feedback, to maintain homeostasis. Health care systems respond to change in the environment, such as the need for adoption of a new clinical protocol, with conflict between the organization's parts and subsystems. A DNP project manager who takes on the project of implementing an updated clinical protocol uses systems thinking to understand that the resistance to change is in conflict with the goals of the organization, nursing, and medical staff to provide quality care. This conflict results in the development of a state of entropy or disorganization, which threatens the balance or homeostasis of the organization (Marriner-Tomey & Alligood, 2006). The DNP project manager sees the goal of establishing the new clinical protocol as an effort to reestablish stability and guide the organization to regain functional integrity. To accomplish homeostasis, the DNP leads the project team through the analysis of clinical evidence, agreement on a best-practice protocol, and the development of a mutually agreed-upon protocol consistent with shared values of the stakeholders. Promoting mechanisms for communication, feedback, and agreement is essential in the DNP project manager's effort to establish homeostasis and equilibrium (AACN, 2006). The DNP project manager uses systems theory to guide projects through a health care system characterized by a multitude of conflicting interdependent parts. Systems theory is a suitable model for project management because it describes interdependencies within a system and how these interdependencies can be coordinated to act as a whole.

Project Selection

After clarifying project goals and conducting evaluations of potential projects, the DNP project manager begins the selection process. Selection may be made based on predetermined criteria using a checklist or weighted scoring model. A common criterion for selection of business projects is the payback model, a measurement of the time it takes for the project to recover its investment (Larson & Gray, 2011). Many projects in health care settings follow the payback model, particularly those that involve new services such as the development of a new cardiac surgery center. A central feature of the payback model is the analysis of return on investment (ROI), which quantifies the project's value by determining the ratio of dollars gained by completing the project divided by dollars invested. Not all projects conducted in health care organizations are primarily driven by the payback model; some are driven by other factors, such as compliance with regulation or updates in clinical practice standards. Although the ROI may not be an essential driving force in a project, there is still need for the DNP project manager to plan, monitor, and control expenses. Essential to the DNP role is the ability to analyze the cost-effectiveness of projects, particularly those that improve health care outcomes (AACN, 2006).

The selection of an appropriate project management structure is another key decision in project management planning (Larson & Gray, 2011). Although multidisciplinary, cross-functional, and matrix teams may reflect the nature of the project, they create some dilemmas related to authority, responsibility, and setting priorities. Functional structures reflect the organizational design, but there is an associated reduction in coordination and project ownership. In contrast, the dedicated team operating as a separate unit under the leadership of a full-time project manager works well in organizations that do a significant number of projects, but can be costly. Ultimately, the best structure for a project team is the one that meets the needs of the project within the culture of the organization.

THE PLANNING PHASE

In the planning phase, the DNP project manager maps the project to illustrate its direction and sequence of events. Two common mapping techniques used in project management are activity on node (AON) and activity on arrow (AOA), which are diagrams that show the arrangement of activities, how they are sequenced, and interrelationships and dependencies of these activities to the project (Larson & Gray, 2011). An activity is a process that consumes time and is an essential part of the project's sequence of events. Burst activity has more than one activity immediately following it and has influence on dependent activities. In contrast, merge activity has more than one activity immediately preceding it and is dependent on completion of the preceding items. Connecting these activities is a line, called the path, that clearly delineates the sequence of dependent activities.

After the project has been selected, aligned with organizational goals, and mapped, a project team is assembled, needs assessment is completed, and potential risks are identified. An essential part of this phase is to identify resources and estimate costs to avert schedule delays and cost overruns. Two common factors in project execution are budgeting and scheduling constraints. When a project is behind schedule, costs are incurred to add resources and make up for the lost time. In turn, when money is short and costs have exceeded expectation, an attempt is made to shorten the schedule and compensate for the shortages. Trade-offs are continually being made to offset quality, time, and cost while managing the scope of the project. The challenge in the health care sector is to implement projects that maintain clinical, ethical, regulatory, and social standards, in light of the available resources. In health care settings, DNP project managers are likely to lead projects that focus on improving access, cost, and quality of health care services consistent with the highest standards.

The Cost of Quality

In his book, *Thriving on Chaos*, Tom Peters (1987) states that poor quality costs (a) manufacturing firms 25% of their personnel and asset costs and (b) service organizations up to 40% of these costs. Health care organizations are primarily service organizations and are subject to the high cost overruns that result from poor quality. Poor quality health services, such as preventable nosocomial infections, are costly and particularly impactful due to the unnecessary harm they cause patients. Preventing service quality failure is a primary focus of health care organizations due to public, government, and payer concerns related to the prevalence of medical errors and high cost of care. Error prevention efforts focus on the 1-10-100 rule: $1 spent on prevention will save $10 on analysis and $100 on failure costs. Put another way, if a defect is caught in the design phase, it has a relative cost of $1; at beta test phase $10; and after the release phase, when the defective product goes to the customer, $100. Developing a well-designed prototype will save the exponential costs of a subsequent recall. Quality has become a key business differentiator in current times. It is no longer just desirable to keep regulatory and contractual relationships—it is required; this is why quality is continually measured, tracked, and managed (Gunawardena, 2011).

Value has a direct relationship to quality and indirect relationship to cost. The DNP will assume the role of good steward of limited resources in the direction of improving quality. Originally written from an ecological perspective, Garret Hardin's (1968) article "The Tragedy of the Commons" is a lesson in the impact of resource overutilization on subsequent generations. Making decisions out of self-interest is often detrimental to the overall long-term goals and sustainability of an organization. When resources are finite, members of an organization are more likely to act out of self-interest, demanding the DNP project manager diligently manage resources. In the highly competitive environment of automakers, Japanese automakers obtained a competitive advantage over American automakers by replacing four bolts with one interchangeable bolt (Ross, 1995). This example shows how diligent stewardship of resources, even on low-cost items, can have a significant overall impact on savings. In the health care setting, net savings from one project can be utilized for services that would otherwise be unfunded. A preoccupation with quick fixes and short-term solutions detracts from the organization's ability to find new solutions to resolve problems. Koloroutis (2004) proposes using reflection in combination with deep analytical and creative thinking skills to find new solutions and balance the cost–quality equation. DNP project managers, working in organizations challenged with limited resources, are prepared to develop innovative and creative solutions, particularly when working with project teams on solutions to health care service delivery problems.

Organizational Culture

A sound assessment of organizational culture is a method DNP project managers use to identify and mitigate risk stemming from the organization's culture and subcultures. Organizational culture is an abstract conception of an organization's values, beliefs, and assumptions. Although these basic values, beliefs, and assumptions are difficult to identify, they can have a strong effect on how a project is perceived and whether staff members are willing to collaborate on the project. Culture can be overtly apparent, such as in the case of the organization that displays a values statement in the entry, stating that the organization values employee input. However, culture is more subtly or tacitly manifested, such as the observation that an employee hesitates to offer a viewpoint that differs from upper management. It is the subtle aspects of culture that are difficult to understand, particularly when the overt and tacit cultures contradict each other. The DNP project manager has an essential understanding of the way culture influences projects and is prepared to intervene to guide projects within a variety of subcultures toward completion (AACN, 2006). The DNP project manager has expert understanding of how to use and develop organizational culture as he or she guides project implementation (AACN, 2006).

Project Readiness

Once the risk reduction plan is determined, additional work is performed on the project plan to define it further in terms of the scope, priorities, work plan, and way in which the work plan will be integrated in organizational operations (Larson & Gray, 2011). The aim statement developed in the early stages of the project provides some information on the end result of the project, but more definition is done at this stage to specify the deliverables, milestones, technical requirements, limits and exclusions, and evaluation. Deliverables are the major products or results that must be finished before a project can progress to the next step. Milestones are groups of deliverables that represent a significant event or accomplishment. Consider the project of a hospital goal to open a new stroke center by a given date. The project manager would be responsible for assigning the development of policy and procedures to individuals within the organization. Each of these policies and procedures would be listed on the project plan as a deliverable, along with the name of the person responsible for the policy and the date the policy is due to be completed. The project

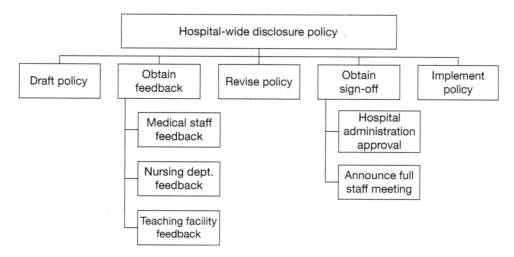

FIGURE 11.1 Work breakdown structure.

manager would also assign someone deliverables associated with collecting the policies, verifying the policies are complete, and sending them to the state for approval. Once these deliverables are completed and the organization receives notice from the state, the organization then reaches its milestone of obtaining state approval for the service.

Forecasting is the approximation of the time and cost it will take to complete project deliverables (Larson & Gray, 2011). Forecasting estimates are done to determine whether the project is worth doing, but also used to monitor the cash flow as the project progresses. When estimating costs, it is common practice to involve people familiar with the tasks, obtain estimates from several people, and base estimates on normal conditions. Determining the appropriate level of detail is important because too much detail may create a nonproductive accounting process, and too little detail may impair the monitoring process. In determining costs, there are direct costs that clearly connect to the project, such as labor, materials, and equipment, and there are indirect costs that are less clearly connected to the project but allocated as general administration and overhead costs.

A key element in this phase of the project is WBS, which is essentially an outline of the work elements and products for the project. The WBS, particularly if it is coded and entered into the information system, facilitates evaluation of the cost and time spent on a project. The document is arranged in a hierarchical order to provide management with feedback on performance at each organizational level. The WBS helps the DNP project manager manage the plan, schedule, and budget for the project, which relates to *DNP essentials* on cost-effective practices (AACN, 2006; see Figure 11.1). A companion document to the WBS is the responsibility chart, which summarizes the tasks to be accomplished during the project and assigns each task to a person within the organization. Members of the project team consult this document to view their responsibilities and assignments.

Managing Risks

Anticipating and mitigating risk, which is the potential loss, is an important task of the DNP project manager during the planning phase. Risk management is performed to identify potential loss and resolve issues before they have an impact on the organization. Although it is impossible for the DNP project manager to avert every risk, anticipating risk and assembling a team qualified to manage such risk is imperative to a successful project outcome. Open communication without the threat of reprisal is an approach DNP project managers use to allow for forthright communication. One of the techniques used to facilitate innovative problem solving is the brainstorming technique, in which ideas are encouraged, without judgment or censorship, to give team members an opportunity to express their unique notions.

Failure modes and effects analysis (FMEA) is used to anticipate and systemize risk. Through the FMEA process, a value is determined based on three variables: the probability of occurrence, impact should it occur, and likelihood the event would be detected (Larson & Gray, 2011). Risk severity is measured by calculating the risk value, which is a formula based on the impact, probability, and potential for detection. Determining a problem's risk value helps the DNP project manager prioritize projects based on a comparison of each potential project's risk values. Attention to every detail of the project with special attention to the problem-prone areas of budgeting, scheduling, and resource allocation is essential in project risk management.

The IHI encourages the use of plan–do–study–act (PDSA) and FMEA to mitigate risks that threaten projects designed to improve patient care (IHI, 2017b). Shewhart's model, which was subsequently modified by Deming, is called the PDSA cycle; it is, used to guide continual improvement processes by tracking the stages of the process. In the plan stage, data is gathered on the problem and its history. Experimentation begins in the do stage, when trial improvement projects are tested on a small scale. Results of the trials are evaluated in the study stage to determine whether they were effective. Successful improvements are adopted in the act stage. The PDSA process does not stop after the act stage, but begins again with focus on another promising improvement to test and evaluate. Following the PDSA ensures sustained focus on continual improvement activity.

FMEA is a method of proactively determining when and how a project is likely to undergo failure, understand the potential impact of the failure, and prioritize which parts of a process are in greatest need of solutions. The IHI process assigns a risk value, or risk priority number (RPN), based on a formula that includes the likelihood of occurrence, detection, and severity ($occ \times det \times sev = RPN$). A Likert scale is used to plot the elements of the formula for each project, and the projects with the highest scores are determined to be priorities because works on these projects are likely to have the most positive impact on the quality of care.

DNP project managers attend to the four steps in the risk management process: risk identification, risk assessment, risk response development, and risk response control (Larson & Gray, 2011). Through open communication and collaboration with key stakeholders, the DNP project manager identifies potential threats and analyzes threats in terms of severity, likelihood of occurrence, and whether or not the risk can be controlled. The DNP project manager prepares contingency plans and implements the plan in the event a threat occurs. A common risk to health care projects is a staffing shortage during a holiday season. The DNP project manager prepares a risk assessment based on the likelihood of occurrence and the severity of impact, and develops contingency plans that are ready in the event of its occurrence.

The ways DNP project managers mitigate the risks vary depending on the assessment of the situation. If the risk is associated with lack of sustained leadership support, the DNP project manager may elicit the support of board members and executive-level staff to shepherd the project to its completion. In addition, enlisting the support of stakeholders who are skilled in communication and collaboration is another way to increase support and mitigate risk. The DNP project manager will need to maintain communication and build trust with these individuals to sustain their support throughout the project. Monitoring capital allocations and requirements is another way to reduce risks that might have a negative impact on the project. During the project selection and team member appointment, the DNP uses project risk management techniques that reflect an awareness of risk as well as plans to mitigate risk.

THE IMPLEMENTATION PHASE

Establishment of a regular meeting that includes communication from project team members and leadership is commonly used during the implementation phase to disseminate status and milestone reports throughout the organization. In addition, these meetings can be used for communication aimed at solving problems with progress on deliverables and handling other action items (Larson & Gray, 2011). Communication between team members and leadership can be in written or electronic form, but generally includes several scheduled meetings. Depending on the scope of the project, communications may be handled in a previously existing operations meeting to ensure all members of the operations group are apprised on the project's progress. It is common for team members to report their progress on deliverables and ask team members for advice on resolving problems. The team discussion is focused on solving problems and moving the project toward completion. There is a high level of accountability when the meetings are regularly scheduled, and particularly when they include leadership in addition to members of the project team. The DNP project manager uses advanced communication skills during these meetings to ensure mutual understanding of progress on the project deliverables (AACN, 2006). Effective communication, in the form of clarifying the goals, deliverables, and responsibilities, facilitates collaboration and coordination to project completion.

Effective communication also depends on active listening to purposefully listen to others' perspectives (Salmon, 2011). Because people speak at a slower rate than listeners comprehend, it is natural for the listener to experience mind drift during conversations. To avoid mind drift, an effective project manager willfully concentrates on what is being said and offers verbal feedback to confirm what information was received.

Communication regarding the status of the project is also accomplished through diagrams and graphical displays. The DNP is prepared to use information technology to support and improve patient care and health care systems (AACN, 2006). Diagrams of the rich networks of individuals who will be affected by the project can be helpful in determining what input is needed to support a project. A map of dependencies can help the DNP project manager conceptualize the network of individuals who can potentially cooperate, approve, or oppose the project (Larson & Gray, 2011; see Figure 11.2). Using the brainstorming method to develop a map of dependencies is helpful because it is better to overestimate the number of individuals likely to be affected by the project than underestimate them. As the DNP project manager reviews the map of dependencies and considers the stakeholders and their perspectives, there is an opportunity to begin formulating strategies to build relationships to support the project.

A Gantt chart is a bar chart used as a project scheduling tool during the project monitoring phase (Larson & Gray, 2011; see Figure 11.3). It is basically a breakdown of the project into activities with start and finish times. Gantt charts are most effective when the name of the responsible party is clearly displayed and these members of the team report their progress with the deliverables. Although the Gantt chart is helpful in providing a visual display of time and scope, it is somewhat limited.

Additional tools are used for analysis in project management, including the project evaluation and review technique (PERT). PERT is a statistical analysis tool used to analyze and represent project tasks. It is designed to show the critical path, which is the longest possible continuous pathway from the initial event to the terminal event (Larson & Gray, 2011). A delay along the critical path will create a delay in reaching the project completion by the same amount. A series of delays along the critical path will have a cumulative effect on the delay. The PERT chart is helpful in showing the project team' progress along the critical path (see Figure 11.4). Essential elements of the PERT chart are projections for the optimistic time (OT), which is the minimum time required to accomplish the task; the pessimistic time (PT), which is the maximum possible time required if everything goes wrong; and the most likely time (MT), which is the normal estimate of the time required to accomplish a task. Projections of the optimistic, pessimistic, and

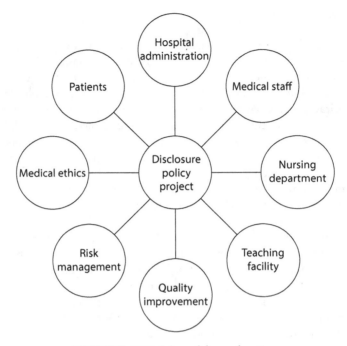

FIGURE 11.2 Map of dependencies.

most likely time frames help the DNP project manager model potential scenarios for project completion. The PERT chart gives the DNP project manager the ability to determine the float or slack, which is the amount of time that a project task can be delayed without causing a delay in subsequent tasks.

Larson and Gray (2011) recommend developing a risk breakdown structure (RBS) that is based on the WBS and the risk profile. An RBS not only identifies the general risk, such as personnel shortages, but answers "why" and when such shortages may occur for the development of contingency plans to adjust for the anticipated gaps. Structured questions are included in the risk profile that is designed to identify risk, actions to mitigate such risk, and the means of averting the subsequent costs. Risks are evaluated through the answers to questions such as: Are the customer and developer expectations aligned? Is the staff assigned just to this project or is their time divided among other work responsibilities? Are the financial resources allocated specifically for this project or contingent on other variables out of the project manager's control? Ultimately, the DNP project manager uses the risk severity matrix diagram to display the level of impact and likelihood of occurrence of risks related to the project.

Preparation for Changes in the Project Plan

Normal conditions are used in the forecasting process, but the project manager must be prepared for unusual conditions that require adjustment in the form of a contingency plan. One common change in project planning is a request to reduce the project's duration, to bring it in ahead of the normal schedule (Larson & Gray, 2011). Consider the situation of a DNP project manager who is working with a team to implement a new oncology drug protocol. The project has been scheduled to take 6 months, but the physicians in the oncology department have approved the protocol 2 months before the completion date and ask that it be implemented immediately. In this case, the DNP project manager would consider the need to compress the project schedule and its clinical and financial implications, including the cost of staff overtime. The project management

Deliverable	Responsible for deliverable	Jan 9	Jan 16	Jan 23	Jan 30	Feb 6	Feb 13	Feb 20	Feb 27	Mar 4	Mar 11	Mar 18	Mar 25	Apr 2	Apr 9	Apr 16	Apr 23	Completion date
Research best practices	Director of quality improvement	■	■															
Draft policy	Director of quality improvement			■														
Obtain medical staff feedback	Hospital chief medical officer					■	■	■	■									
Obtain nursing dept. feedback	Hospital chief nursing officer						■											
Obtain teaching facility feedback	Teaching facility medical officer						■											
Revise policy	Director of quality improvement									■	■							
Hospital admin. approval	Chief operating officer											■	■					
Announce in full staff meeting	Chief operating officer														■			
Implement policy	Chief operating officer																■	

FIGURE 11.3 Gantt chart.

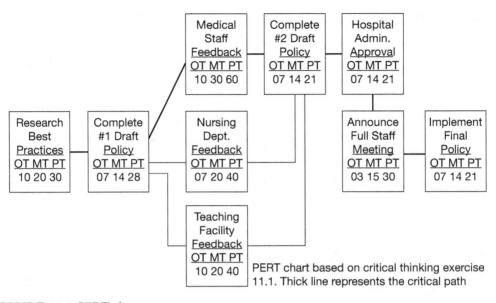

FIGURE 11.4 PERT chart.

MT, most likely time; OT, optimistic time; PERT, Project Evaluation and Review Technique; PT, pessimistic time.

term for the greatest time reduction possible under realistic conditions is called the project's crash time (Larson & Gray, 2011). DNP project managers prepare for contingencies, such as projecting crash times, by preparing the documentation in advance to demonstrate the implications of changing the project plan.

Team Dynamics

As stated earlier in this chapter, projects require a variety of individuals to come together and collaborate to bring a project to completion. These groups are essential to project management because the diverse experiences and backgrounds of the members foster optimal decision making. There is a synergistic effect in the group process in which the group produces more knowledge than each of the members working on his or her own (Lasker & Weiss, 2003). Using a group process also increases the likelihood that the project will gain acceptance throughout the organization because there is an increase in the general awareness of the value of the project and importance of the deliverables when more people are involved in the project.

The ability to work in teams is not a naturally acquired skill, but is essential for every member of the project management team and particularly for the project manager. Managing projects in a complex health care setting requires DNP the project managers to have a good understanding of how teams develop and function. Of particular importance is the ability to distinguish dysfunctional from functional conflict, to identify when to intervene and restore function. Functional conflict supports the goals of the group and is a productive part of the group process (Amason, 1996). In contrast, dysfunctional conflict hinders group performance and requires the DNP project manager to intervene and get the membership back on course. The DNP project manager may need to establish ground rules for the team and state that personal attacks are not allowed, and if they occur, they will be addressed immediately during the meeting. In this way, the DNP project manager is prepared to use sophisticated expertise in assessing the organization and facilitating changes in practice delivery (AACN, 2006).

The five-stage model of group development (Tuckman & Jensen, 1977) sheds light on the phases of group activity and how DNPs can manage the process. In the forming stage, group members are unclear or disagree on the purpose of the project. When group members are unclear on the purpose, the DNP can offer guidance and support and clarify project goals. In the next stage, the storming stage, members of the group struggle for power and experience conflict. Coaching members through the conflict is a way that DNPs keep the group moving toward the goals. Members experience role clarity in the norming stage, and the DNP project manager reinforces roles during this part of the group process. In the performing stage, group members focus on performing tasks associated with the goals, and the DNP project manager delegates tasks to group members. At the end of the group process, group members are satisfied with completing their tasks and meeting the goal. In this stage, the adjourning stage, the DNP project manager recognizes accomplishments and acknowledges member contributions.

There are problems for DNP project managers to solve as they work with the group on a project. Group work takes more time and not all the decisions and tasks benefit from group discussion. The DNP project manager monitors group interactions and tasks, and, when appropriate, asks group members to do work on their own or in subgroups and report their findings to the full project team to expedite project completion.

Among the threats to the group process, groupthink is particularly formidable because it is difficult to identify, much less address. Groupthink is a phenomenon in which members of a group strive to be in agreement with each other even though, in their private analysis of the problem, they do not agree (Janis, 1972). The team members experiencing groupthink appear to be in agreement, when in actuality they are not. Groupthink limits the adequacy of the decision made by the group and puts the project in jeopardy. The most common contributing factors that lead to groupthink are a strong sense of group cohesiveness in the presence of high stress or recent failures, which make group members afraid to make incorrect decisions. Groupthink can be detrimental to the completion of a project because members fail to solve problems or select the best alternatives. To avoid groupthink, the DNP project manager can appoint someone to criticize and test group recommendations, called a devil's advocate (Packer, 2009). If the DNP project manager is concerned that a leader's power-based presence is the source of the group's unwillingness to make decisions, the DNP can discuss the situation with the leader and suggest the leader not attend some of the critical decision-making meetings. The DNP project manager can also use nominal group technique and ask members to document their opinions anonymously (Andersen & Fagerhaug, 2000). The ideas are then listed on the white board for the group's discussion, free of influence due to judgments about the source of the comments. When working with groups, it is essential that the DNP project manager facilitate positive team dynamics and intervene when there is potential risk to keep the group performing at an optimal level as it solves problems and produces deliverables.

When working with teams, the understanding of organizational culture and subculture helps the DNP project manager anticipate potential conflict and take measures to minimize its impact on the project. Schein (1996) described culture as patterns of shared assumptions that inform actions and beliefs of members of a group. Culture may arise from organizational values, beliefs, and assumptions or from across the organization as in the case of occupational communities. Occupational communities have shared assumptions that come from outside the organization, based on common educational backgrounds, professional requirements, and interactions with colleagues from the same field. Nurses and physicians fall into the occupational communities of the operator culture, a culture that is composed of people who perform work, as in clinical work. The executive culture is composed of people who focus on efficiency and productivity, which has different values from those of the operator culture. When these occupational communities align and coordinate activities around shared goals, adoption of projects progresses. When environmental conditions change, such as in a budget crisis or with a shortage of staff, these occupational communities experience conflict and impaired coordination that can potentially inhibit progression on project goals. Schein's (1996) research suggests that when management and operator goals are aligned around a shared goal, projects and innovations progress in support of organizational goals. The DNP project manager monitors conflict within the group and determines when intervention is needed to realign members around a shared goal. If needed, realignment can be accomplished by reinforcing the team member's shared goals, communicating how these goals relate to the project, and emphasizing how the project will benefit from the team's collaboration and coordination.

Appreciative inquiry is another method that can be used to realign member goals to the project goals (Harris et al., 2011). This process of inquiry consists of four phases: discovery, dreaming, designing, and delivering the project. Because appreciative inquiry begins with a focus toward the mutual goals and potential benefits of the project, it tends to confirm team member collaboration and alignment on the goal. It differs from routine business planning, which focuses on specific activities and tasks, but does not emphasize shared goals. DNP project managers use appreciative inquiry to align staff to core values, as well as motivate team members to stretch to higher performance levels. Appreciative inquiry is an inspirational approach that is a good choice in health care settings in which staff members are professionals who share common goals for quality service delivery and patient safety. DNP project managers are well prepared to play a role in managing interprofessional teams and guiding them to complete projects to improve patient care and organizational outcomes (AACN, 2006).

Projects bring together a collection of people from divergent skills, organizations, and, perhaps, countries. The DNP project manager uses leadership, collaboration, and negotiating skills to bridge the differences among and between divergent groups. The sociocultural dimension of project management, discussed in the first part of this chapter, reflects the dynamic nature of collaborating on projects. When working with divergent groups, the DNP project manager may elect to use negotiating skills that promote the win–win approach. Successful negotiating rules encompass the technique of "principled negotiation," the product of the Harvard Mediation Project and three of its founders, Fisher, Ury, and Patton (1991). Their guiding premise is to separate the people from the problem and focus on interests, not positions. The DNP project manager is prepared to invent options for mutual gain and use the best alternative to negotiated agreement (BATNA) technique when dealing with individuals hesitant to compromise.

The Change Process

Understanding the dynamics of the change process and how to intervene to facilitate acceptance of the project is essential for the DNP project manager (AACN, 2006). Lewin (1948) explained that the change process is made up of three distinct phases: unfreezing, change, and refreezing. The first phase, unfreezing, is an essential precipitating factor for a change in established practice or status quo. Unfreezing an established practice requires a significant amount of disconfirming information delivered in an informed manner, particularly when working with health care professionals who are trained in evidence-based practice. In the planning phase of the project, the DNP project manager is prepared to do a thorough evaluation of evidence, both in favor of and against the project. The application of knowledge from diverse sources and multiple disciplines is essential to DNP practice (AACN, 2006). The DNP project manager discusses the evidence in a forthright, informed, and deliberate manner to establish trust, authority, and credibility with other members of the team.

An important element of the change process is to create a sense of psychological safety (Schein, 1992). Psychological safety occurs when individuals believe that change can be made without harm to their personal values or integrity. Individuals are more likely to participate in change if they feel that they personally will not experience failure. An individual's sense of psychological safety is increased when he or she is able to discuss his or her concerns with empathetic and supportive peers who serve as role models. DNP project managers understand how to guide, mentor, and support others through the change process (AACN, 2006). When others accept the need for change, they begin to incorporate the new attitudes or behaviors that align with their understandings of project expectations. Refreezing occurs when individuals involved in the change process have thoroughly incorporated new attitudes or behaviors into practice.

DNP project managers may elect to use force field and SWOT analysis (one considering strengths, weaknesses, opportunities, and threats) to evaluate the conflicting factors involved in the change process (Harris et al., 2011). This type of analysis identifies the driving forces that direct behavior away from the project's goals and restraining forces that prevent movement toward the project's goals. Force field analysis is a tool used for weighing pros and cons, whereas SWOT analysis focuses on the internal strengths and weaknesses, as well as the external opportunities and threats. Both methods provide the DNP project manager with insight into ways to reduce the impact of the opposing forces and strengthen supporting forces. In general, change is more acceptable when driving forces outweigh the negative impact of restraining forces. Clarification of the forces involved in a project helps the DNP project manager develop agreement on an effective project plan (AACN, 2006).

DNP project managers also keep the stages of innovation in mind as they interact with others to complete a project. Rogers's (2003) work on the decision innovation process describes how networks of individuals go through phases before adopting a change in practice. According to Rogers, there are five stages through which individuals pass during the innovation process: knowledge, persuasion, decision, implementation, and confirmation. The DNP project manager promotes adoption of the project by spreading knowledge on the needs, goals, strengths, and limitations of the project. As the DNP project manager discusses the project and its outcomes with others, the ideas are tested and evaluated. DNP project managers are in a good position to persuade others to accept the project and commit to the deliverables and time frames because they are skilled communicators (AACN, 2006). These skills of persuasion help others on the project team accept the project plan and agree to complete their assigned deliverables at the specified time. The stage in the change process called implementation occurs when the members of the team complete their deliverables in a timely manner. The last stage, the confirmation stage, is an important factor in sustaining the change. This stage in the change process begins when the DNP project manager confirms team members completed the deliverable on time, usually during a project team meeting, which serves to reinforce accountability to complete projects on time. The DNP project manager's understanding of the decision innovation process guides the project team to recognize the importance of the project's deliverables and milestones.

When needed to make progress on the project, the DNP project manager acts as a change agent to drive changes in behavior, attitudes, and, ultimately, practices. Change agents are individuals who influence others' decisions to accept change in the direction deemed desirable by the change agent (Rogers, 2003). There are eight functions that are typically performed by change agents: (a) developing the need for change in others, (b) establishing a relationship to exchange information, (c) assessing problems with the exchange of information, (d) creating the intent to change in others, (e) establishing similarity, (f) building credibility, (g) working with the influential, and (h) evaluating the change in practice. According to Hudak, Brooke, Finstuen, and Trounson (2002), organizations expedite the adoption of new projects by assigning skilled individuals, such as DNP project managers, to lead the change process on new initiatives.

Rogers (2003) formulated a model to show how change agents use effective communication skills during the change process. Change agents communicate by establishing meaningful dialogue with people who can influence select social networks within the organizations. Because they mediate others' understanding of the change throughout the project, change agents play an important role in the diffusion of a change throughout an organization. Research on change agents shows they use communication, debate, and negotiated understanding as major tools in promoting the adoption of a new project or practice (Sharma, 1997). Conversely, individuals who do not engage in negotiating understandings through communication and debate will not be effective in promoting adoption of innovation. Communication is an essential element of the change process, and DNP project managers use their communication and collaborative skills to advocate for projects that improve health care practice (AACN, 2006).

THE CONCLUDING PHASE

After all deliverables have been produced and milestones met, the project has been completed, but not finished. Concluding is the phase when the project team reflects on the project, performs an evaluation, and produces documentation that will inform future projects (Larson & Gray, 2011). To begin the process, the DNP project manager determines if the project delivered met the goal expectations of the project. A review of the aim statement and feedback in the form of interviews or surveys can help the project manager with this part of the project. Next, the project manager considers the efficacy of the management of the project. For this part of the process, the DNP project manager reviews deliverables and time frames to provide more information on how smoothly the management process went. Lastly, attention is given to how the project met customer expectations. Interviews or surveys can help the DNP project manager obtain feedback from stakeholders and customers. The goal of this part of the project is to reflect on the process and determine what worked well and what could have been done better.

To document the project evaluation, the DNP project manager develops an executive summary with the project's history, activities, and learning opportunities (Larson & Gray, 2011). Effective executive summaries are succinct, clear, and forthright in their discussion of the strengths and weaknesses of the project. Included in the executive summary is a statement of the project goals, how the goals were met, and quality and satisfaction with deliverables. A summary of the procedures and systems used, recommendations, and lessons learned is also included. Appendices are attached to the executive summary for those who want to review supportive information in a more thorough manner. The documentation in the executive summary provides a historical record of the project that is used by others who lead future projects. Future project leaders will likely value the section that addresses lessons learned and use these lessons to inform their own projects.

Agile Project Management

Chris Argyris's (1993) conceptualization of double-loop learning, in which organizations shift paradigms by questioning the norm associated with linear thinking, provides the basis for many of the techniques organizations use, including project management. In contrast to the traditional model, agile project management does not progress in a linear direction (Larson & Gray, 2011). There are times when there is a need for a design with incremental phases in which the end-product evolves over time through multiple iterations. Agile project management is ideal for phased testing of new ideas at the microsystem level. To better understand agile project management, let us take a moment to compare traditional project management to agile project management. Traditional project management is premised on the initial development of a perfect prototype during the analysis and design phase. The project has a finite scope, with little or no change after the design phase, and minimizes stakeholder feedback during the course of the project life cycle. Traditional project management relies on fixed deliverables and milestones during the course of the project, with evaluations performed postimplementation. In the traditional method, the project is designed once and completed, but in agile project management, multiple iterations are designed and implemented as new information about the project evolves. Agile project management embraces flexibility, responds to feedback from stakeholders, and encourages development during the iteration phases of the project. The DNP project manager uses agile project management when the project would benefit from a short design phase, broad scope, or rotating stakeholders who are often the end user in this dynamic process.

The design phase of a traditional project is often several months, as opposed to weeks in agile project management for each iterative cycle's own analysis and design, testing, and evaluation. The iterative cycles are analogous to the "small tests of change" promulgated by IHI as a process to stimulate innovation (www.ihi.org). In 1986, Hirotaka Takeuchi and Ikujiro Nonaka coined the term *scrum* when describing commercial product development, using the analogy of a rugby team holding onto the ball while ever changing its placement among team members (Larson & Gray, 2011). To demonstrate the concept of scrum, consider a hospital setting with a cross-functional team representing each hospital department. They meet to brainstorm the development of a portable cart that can quickly be converted into an isolation bed anywhere in the hospital. The cart would be the first of its kind. An inexpensive prototype is developed based on the input of team members and placed on a randomly chosen unit for 2 weeks. Each week the team convenes to evaluate the cart, encouraging input from the end user. Every week a new iteration of the product is developed and moved to a new department for its use. Several iterations are created until every department has given feedback on its design. The finished design is successfully developed for less cost and with specifications that meet the needs of each department.

SUSTAINABILITY

Project implementation can take a significantly long period of time, perhaps months to a year, before roles are defined; staff, including administrative staff, is trained; technology is put in place; or other resources are acquired. It is a natural for the team to experience implementation fatigue and lose interest in supporting the project. Once a project is implemented, members of the organization have a sense that the project is completed and there is no longer any need for continued support. However, projects require ongoing care and maintenance even after they are implemented, so any sense of complacency is a threat to the ongoing sustainability of the project. To control this threat, DNPs design projects with sustainability in mind.

A useful framework for understanding sustainability was developed by Shediac-Rizkallah and Bone (1998). They describe sustainability as a project's ongoing viability once the development is done. It is essentially the process of locking the project into routine operations. In their model, there are three aspects of the project to be considered for sustainability: project design, factors within the organization, and factors outside the organization.

PROJECT DESIGN

In the project design phase, DNPs promote project sustainability by involving stakeholders to secure their commitment to the value and success of the project, which ultimately lays the foundation for lasting support for the project. Ensuring that project designs allow for modification makes those projects more likely to have lasting viability than those that cannot be adjusted for changing needs and conditions. Another design feature that supports sustainability is the development of a monitoring plan to demonstrate the continued value of the project. The DNP's attention to these design elements during the early phases of the project will have a positive effect on the long-term viability after the project.

FACTORS WITHIN THE ORGANIZATIONAL SETTING

DNPs also assess factors within the organizational setting to determine the potential sustainability of the project. One important task DNPs do is to identify program champions early in the development phase because they can make adjustments to ensure the project is effective and foster continuation. In addition, DNPs verify the project is aligned with the goals and changing operating procedures of the organization to ensure that projects have ongoing relevance. It is also critical that the DNP understand the organization's underlying capacity and its willingness and ability to standardize operations, because these factors will support a project's sustainability.

FACTORS OUTSIDE THE ORGANIZATION

External factors are outside the control of the organization, but it is worthwhile for DNPs to do an analysis of external factors likely to affect the project's viability. These external factors include the favorability of external economic factors, the effect of market forces, the constraints of legislation, and the availability of reimbursement that might influence the project.

The DNP has a strong commitment to the sustainability of the project, and this is a consideration from the beginning of the project. It is important for the DNP to select programs that are (a) strongly related to the organization's mission and culture and (b) have the support of upper management. The task workload should be reasonable and fit within staff members' responsibilities. Thoughtful modifications may be necessary to make the project more effective, and the modifications should not impair the project's core components that contribute to its effectiveness. It is important to (a) identify and support a program champion and (b) to take a leadership role in both initial program development and planning for sustainability. When designing and implementing the project, it is critical to emphasize the project's benefits for involved stakeholders. The goal is for the DNP to "routinize" the project and make it part of the core operations of the organization.

▥ SPREAD

The IHI defines spread as the dissemination of a successful project, practice, or knowledge to a different care setting (www.ihi.org). DNPs seek out opportunities to implement best practices and disseminate knowledge within their organizations, including the knowledge gained from the implementation of projects. The following information on spread is useful in guiding the DNP on how to disseminate projects throughout the organization.

Developing a plan for spread starts at the beginning of the initial project and continues throughout the project (Massoud, Nielsen, Nolan, Schall, & Sevin, 2006). Many of the design features previously discussed in this chapter have already set the groundwork for the spread plan. This section of the chapter highlights those elements to show how developing a plan for spread can help the DNP project reach additional units or departments. If the organization has made great strides in testing and implementing a project, it may be time to replicate the gains from the initial work and implement a spread plan. The goal of the spread plan is to ensure that the project interventions can be implemented in a similar organization.

The IHI describes a three-part plan for spread that includes the following steps: laying the foundation for spread, developing an initial plan for spread, and refining the plan. This section of the chapter explains how the DNP develops a plan and a course of action for spreading a project across the organization.

LAYING THE FOUNDATION FOR SPREAD

The spread plan will be most successful with the support of leadership in the form of an executive sponsor accountable to the CEO and board of directors. As in the design for the original project, it is important to involve the stakeholders who will be affected by the implementation. The appointment of a day-to-day spread leader is useful to act as coach, coordinator, motivator, and connector for the spread work. It is very important that the day-to-day leader be someone who has project management expertise and who can effectively communicate, motivate, and coordinate resources to support the spread effort. This individual is responsible for ensuring that there is a clear message about the importance of moving the project from a single department to other units within the facility.

Sharing the results of the successful project is important in the initial spread plan. Discussing the results will attract attention to the value of the interventions and the positive impact on patient care outcomes. Sharing the experience of a successful project helps make the case for a wider implementation, particularly when it is a first-hand example from the organization. This is an opportunity to take advantage of the experience and expertise of the project team and provide learning from their successes and challenges. It is beneficial for experts to provide examples from other departments in the organization to help new teams implement the interventions because they have credibility.

DEVELOPING THE INITIAL PLAN FOR SPREAD

In developing the plan for spread, the team works with senior leadership to put together the spread plan and monitor the progress toward the goal. The first step in developing the spread plan is formulating an aim statement. The aim statement may be a modification of the one used in the original project and should address the intent, target level of performance, target population, and time period for the project. It serves as the guiding document to direct the deliberate actions of the spread team.

Spread occurs more rapidly when the pilot project is linked to the other units in a direct way. The plan should account for opportunities to use unit or department reporting relationships, medical staff committees, and other structures to engage clinicians and staff in the spread process. It is helpful to determine whether there are differences in the new unit that might impact how the intervention is implemented.

Some attention should be given to information system changes, such as data collection methods, information system templates, and phone or pager enhancements, that would facilitate spread from one unit to another. It is important to make the process as easy as possible to facilitate adoption. The goal is to have the project perceived as part of routine operations, rather than a special project. It is necessary to focus on the value the project has already added and the ways in which this value is to be expanded across the system.

The plan for communication is an important part of the spread plan. The communication channels used in the initial project are a starting point to increase awareness about the project. Hospital-wide meetings, newsletters, media coverage, and special events can build interest and motivation. The use of stories and results from prior successes will educate staff and promote collaboration. In any communication plan, it is important to identify the target audience and the messages that will be most effective for the audience. It can be helpful to incorporate what was learned during the initial project by those who were involved because their stories are authentic and have credibility.

Feedback is a critical element of the communication plan because it establishes accountability for results and provides encouragement and support from leaders. This can be done in regular meetings with staff and leaders, review of results at staff meetings, and linking results to leadership and management performance reviews. The executive sponsor plays an important role in the communication plan by conveying the importance of the interventions and listening for issues, stories, and success from those involved in the implementation.

A measurement system to track the adoption of the project over time is critical to success. For this to be beneficial, it is important to identify how to measure the rate of adoption. It is helpful to provide regular feedback on progress in reaching target goals and in the rate of adoption of each element of the project to the senior leadership and units making the change. This focuses attention on the work and can be an important source of information about emerging issues that need to be addressed by either the leadership or the frontline teams to accelerate spread.

REFINING THE PLAN

Adjustments in the spread plan may be necessary to accelerate adoption of the project. By monitoring reports, the spread team can identify the need for adjustments. Additional data can be obtained from the frontline units and departments through formal reports, regular surveys, informal conversations, or other methods.

Many of the evidence-based projects developed in health care settings are implemented in just one location (Berwick, 2003). Although a project may be successful, it is uncommon for a project to be disseminated to relevant units, often because staff have limited knowledge and skill in diffusion of innovation and spread. The DNP who is knowledgeable about project management and spread is in an ideal position to provide additional value and improvement in patient care outcomes by replicating projects to relevant locations within the organization.

■ CONCLUSION

As DNP project managers lead projects through the analysis and design, planning, implementation, and concluding phases, they evaluate problems for cause-and-effect relationships, explore interrelationships across systems, and advance the projects in collaboration with others. In the analysis and design phase, the DNP project manager ensures that the project is aligned with the organization's strategic plan, project specifications are defined, and the project team is assembled with responsibilities assigned. The WBS is built by defining the project schedule, budget, and associated staff during the planning phase. Risks are identified and mitigated when feasible. The implementation phase includes ongoing risk aversion and identification through the FMEA or PERT process, as well as monitoring and adjusting resources, staff, and costs. Training, final testing, exchange of documentation, and sign-off are completed during the concluding phase. The testament of the DNP project manager's commitment and expertise is the executive summary, which documents an evaluation of the goals and performance, as well as lessons from the project to add to the organization's body of knowledge and set the stage for future projects.

Project management is no longer delegated to one or two departments in an organization; rather, it is now integrated into every important aspect of organizational operations. The need for innovation, continuous learning, rapid response to change, and the complexities of operations require the expertise and discipline of a skilled project manager. Agile project management, with its demands for innovation through small tests of change, is managed through feedback and multiple design iterations toward the desired outcome. The DNP project manager is prepared with the "essentials" defined by the AACN (2006): a practitioner, skilled in leadership, financial and organizational analyses, collaboration, communication, critical and creative thinking, team building, evidence-based research, negotiating, and informatics skills. To meet the challenge of advocating for best clinical practice, the DNP gains project management skills, including the development of product specifications, network maps, deliverables, milestones, budgets, schedules, and tasks that match the skills of personnel and resource allocation. Ultimately, it is through the expert application of organizational theories, including group, systems, complexity, and change theories, that the DNP project manager effectively manages projects in collaboration with others at the microsystem, mesosystem, and macrosystem level.

CRITICAL THINKING EXERCISES

1. SCENARIO-BASED DISCUSSION OF AIM STATEMENT

The scenario: You are a DNP clinical coordinator in an urban teaching hospital that includes medical school students as well as a physician residency program. A medical resident inadvertently injected air into a patient's central line, after an unexpected interruption, which resulted in the patient experiencing an air embolism. The patient was subsequently treated in the ICU and has made a full recovery. After much discussion between nursing staff, medical residents, and supervising physicians, the resident and supervising physician disclosed the error and apologized to the patient.

You are troubled by the delay in the disclosure and the lack of coordination between the nurses, supervising physician, and residents. You discuss your concern with the chief nursing officer (CNO) and ask to lead a project to develop a hospital-wide disclosure policy that includes the medical staff and teaching facilities, and also places more emphasis on appropriate elements of the apology. The CNO supports your plan and announces her support during a nursing leadership meeting. You review hospital policies and find that the hospital has a nursing policy for disclosing medical errors, but the policy does not address medical students, residents, or supervising or attending physicians. You conduct interviews with key members of the hospital and medical staff to reveal that there has been no collaborative discussion regarding medical error disclosure between the hospital and medical staff, much less with the affiliated teaching facilities.

Working with the CNO, you have selected a project team that includes administration; staff nurses; medical staff members; faculty and students from the medical school; and members of the medical ethics, quality improvement, and risk management committees; as well as a former patient. Initially, you begin by drafting an aim statement to present to team members at the first meeting. Patterned on the SMART goals method, the aim statement is to reflect specific, measurable, attainable, realistic, and time-bound goals, but you also review IHI recommendations for aim statements for guidance. The IHI information regarding aim statements can be found from the following website:

www.ihi.org/knowledge/Pages/HowtoImprove/ScienceofImprovementTipsforSettingAims.aspx.

Exercise: Develop an aim statement that reflects both SMART goals and IHI recommendations that you plan to present to the project team. What are some of the most important considerations in writing the aim statement? What type of comments do you anticipate from the various team members? How will you respond to their comments?

2. SCENARIO-BASED DISCUSSION OF SWOT ANALYSIS

Members of the team agree on the aim statement that you, as the DNP project manager, developed in Exercise 1 and they are ready to start developing the hospital-wide policy. Before starting on the policy, you ask team members to participate in a SWOT analysis to explore potential risks and drivers for the project.

SWOT analysis is used in the planning stage of project management to identify the internal strengths and weaknesses, as well as the external opportunities and threats related to a project. In a SWOT analysis, the first step is to clarify the goal of the project and to verify that all members of the team understand the goal. The next step is to systematically evaluate favorable and unfavorable factors related to the goal of the project. Using SWOT analysis provides the project team with an organized framework for analyzing factors that will most likely contribute or detract from the project.

Project managers often do a SWOT analysis with project teams by documenting it on a white board as group members generate their comments and ideas. For this exercise, draw a line on a blank piece of paper in half lengthwise and then in half crosswise, so there are four quadrants marked on the page. Then place an S (for internal strengths) in the left upper quadrant, a W (for internal weaknesses) in the right upper quadrant, an O (for external opportunities) in the left lower quadrant, and a T (for external threats) in the right lower quadrant. Consider the different perspectives of your team members and generate the comments that you anticipate from team members as they complete the SWOT analysis. Make sure to document anticipated comments on the corresponding SWOT analysis quadrant. What comments do you expect team members to offer during the SWOT analysis? Once you have completed documenting the four quadrants of the SWOT analysis, review the document. How has the SWOT analysis changed your impression of the project and its driving and restraining forces?

3. **SCENARIO-BASED DISCUSSION OF CHANGE IN LEADERSHIP**

The team is halfway through the project when you receive word that the chief medical officer (CMO) is planning to retire in a month. You are concerned about the project because the CMO was a strong supporter of the hospital-wide disclosure policy and, according to your Gantt chart, it will be 2 months before it is ready for presentation to the full medical staff. The CMO was a trusted member of the medical staff who had a high level of authority and credibility with her colleagues. What steps will you take to ensure that the project continues to progress toward completion? How will you identify additional individuals who can help guide this project toward completion?

4. **SCENARIO-BASED DISCUSSION OF CONCLUDING PROCESS**

The procedure was presented to the full medical staff and approved after a lively discussion regarding the risks and benefits of having a hospital-wide disclosure policy. You worked with several key physicians who voiced their support and presented evidence from medical journals to reduce the physicians' concerns that disclosing medical errors would increase lawsuits. A few suggestions were made to make some minor changes in wording. The wording changes have been completed and you are ready to call the project to a close. What are your next steps? How will you ensure that an effective evaluation is performed? Provide a description of the important elements of the project conclusion process and explain why these elements are important.

REFERENCES

Amason, A. C. (1996). Distinguishing the effects of functional and dysfunctional conflict on strategic decision making: Resolving a paradox for top management teams. *Academy of Management Journal*, 39(1), 123–148.

American Association of Colleges of Nursing. (2006). *The essentials of doctoral education for advanced nursing practice*. Washington, DC: Author. Retrieved from http://www.aacnnursing.org/Portals/42/Publications/DNPEssentials.pdf

Andersen, B., & Fagerhaug, T. (2000). Nominal group technique: Generating possible causes and reaching consensus. *Quality Progress*, 33(22), 144.

Argyris, C. (1993). *Knowledge for action: A guide to overcoming barriers to organizational change*. San Francisco, CA: Jossey-Bass.

Bertalanffy, L. (1950). An outline of general system theory. *British Journal for the Philosophy of Science*, 1(2), 134–165.

Berwick, D. M. (2003). Disseminating innovations in health care. *Journal of the American Medical Association*, 289(15), 1969–1975.

Drucker, P. F. (2001). *The essential Drucker: Selections from the management works of Peter F. Drucker*. New York, NY: HarperCollins.

Fisher, R., Ury, W., & Patton, B. (1991). *Getting to yes: Negotiating agreement without giving in* (2nd ed.). Boston, MA: Houghton Mifflin.

Goleman, D. (1998). *Working with emotional intelligence*. New York, NY: Bantam.

Gunawardena, I. (2011). Organisational learning: Where professions rule. *British Journal of Health Care Management, 17*(10), 470–476.

Hardin, G. (1968). The tragedy of the commons. *Science, 162,* 1242–1248.

Harris, J. L., Roussel, L., Walters, S. E., & Dearman, C. (2011). *Project planning and management: A guide for CNLS, DNPs, and nurse executives.* Sudbury, MA: Jones & Bartlett.

Hudak, R. P., Brooke, P. P., Finstuen, K., & Trounson, J. (2002). Physician executives share insights on ways to influence people. *Physician Executive, 28*(5), 29–32.

Institute for Healthcare Improvement. (2017a). Science of improvement: Tips for setting aims. Retrieved from http://www.ihi.org/resources/Pages/HowtoImprove/ScienceofImprovementSettingAims.aspx

Institute for Healthcare Improvement. (2017b). Science of improvement: How to improve. Retrieved from http://www.ihi.org/resources/Pages/HowtoImprove/ScienceofImprovementHowtoImprove.aspx

Janis, I. L. (1972). *Victims of groupthink.* Boston, MA: Houghton Mifflin.

Koloroutis, M. (2004). *Relationship based care: A model for transforming practice.* Minneapolis, MN: Creative Health Care Management.

Larson, E. W., & Gray, C. F. (2011). *Project management: The managerial process* (5th ed.). Boston, MA: McGraw-Hill.

Lasker, R. D., & Weiss, E. S. (2003). Creating partnership synergy: The critical role of community stakeholders. *Journal of Health and Human Services Administration, 26*(1), 119–139.

Lewin, K. (1948). *Resolving social conflicts: Selected papers on group dynamics.* New York, NY: Harper & Row.

Marriner-Tomey, A. M., & Alligood, M. A. (2006). *Nursing theorists and their work* (6th ed.). St. Louis, MO: Mosby.

Massoud, M. R., Nielsen, G. A., Nolan, K., Schall, M. W., & Sevin, C. A. (2006). *Framework for spread.* Cambridge, MA: Institute for Healthcare Improvement.

Packer, D. J. (2009). Avoiding groupthink: Whereas weakly identified members remain silent, strongly identified members dissent about collective problems. *Psychological Science, 20*(1), 546–548.

Peters, T. (1987). *Thriving on chaos: Handbook for a management revolution.* New York, NY: Knopf.

Pojasek, R. B. (2000). Asking "why?" five times. *Environmental Quality Management, 10*(1), 79–84.

Project Management Institute. (2004). *A guide to the project management body of knowledge* (3rd ed.). Newton Square, PA: PMI Publishing.

Rogers, E. M. (2003). *Diffusion of innovations* (5th ed.). New York, NY: Free Press.

Ross, J. (1995). *Total quality management: Text, cases, readings.* Delray Beach, FL: St. Lucie Press.

Salmon, B. M. (2011). Resolve conflicts through active listening. *Washington Informer, 46*(9), 56–59.

Schein, E. H. (1992). *Organizational culture and leadership* (2nd ed.). San Francisco, CA: Jossey-Bass.

Schein, E. H. (1996). Three cultures of management: The key to organizational learning. *Sloan Management Review, 38*(1), 9–20.

Sharma, A. (1997). Professional as agent: Knowledge asymmetry in agency exchange. *Academy of Management Review, 22*(3), 758–799.

Shediac-Rizkallah, M. C., & Bone, L. R. (1998). Planning for the sustainability of community-based health programs: Conceptual frameworks and future directions for research, practice and policy. *Health Education Research, 13,* 87–108.

Tuckman, B. W., & Jensen, M. A. (1977). Stages of small group development revisited. *Group and Organizational Studies, 2*(2), 419–427.

12 Health Care Grant Writing in Acute, Ambulatory, and Community Care

Mary Lynne Knighten

KEY TERMS

DNP grant seeker

DNPs and grant writing

grant seeking

grant writing

grant writing for community
  care

grant writing for DNP-led
  projects

grant writing for health care
  programs

grant-writing skills

health care grant writing

novice grant writers

nurses and grant writing

proposal writing

As health care evolves in the United States, nurses play a unique and valuable role in meeting growing demand. The aging nursing workforce, implementing the changing face of the Affordable Care Act, and nursing and physician shortages contribute to the forecasted need for more health care professionals. The number of nurse practitioners (NPs) is projected to increase by 30% to 72,100 by 2020, according to a report by the U.S. Health Resources and Services Administration (HRSA, 2016), which is expected to ease some of the physician shortage in primary care. The face of advanced practice nursing has experienced sweeping changes related, in large part, to several landmark reports and position statements in the last decade. In *Health Professions Education: A Bridge to Quality* (Institute of Medicine [IOM], 2003)—a follow-up report to the IOM Committee report, *Crossing the Quality Chasm*, published in 2001—the IOM Committee on the Health Professions Education states, "All health professionals should be educated to deliver patient-centered care as members of an interdisciplinary team, emphasizing evidence-based practice (EBP), quality improvement approaches, and informatics" (IOM, 2003). The American Association of Colleges of Nursing (AACN) 2004 *Position Statement* articulated a target date by which advanced practice registered nurses (APRNs) would be required to enter the field with a doctoral degree rather than the previously accepted master's degree.

According to the AACN (2004), several factors influenced the migration to a clinical or practice doctorate, including ". . . the rapid expansion of knowledge underlying practice; increased complexity of patient care; national concerns about the quality of care and patient safety; shortages of nursing personnel; demands for a higher level of preparation for nurses who can design and assess care and lead; shortages of prepared nursing faculty, leaders in practice, and nurse researchers; and increasing educational expectations for the preparation of other health professionals." The 2004 AACN *Position Statement* clearly outlined the need for administrative and advanced practice leaders with stronger preparation in systems-based practice improvement and translational research (AACN, 2004). These goals are consistent with the IOM's *Future of Nursing: Leading Change, Advancing Health* report released in October 2010, with recommendations to "prepare and enable nurses to lead change to advance health" and to "double the number of nurses with a doctorate by 2020" (IOM, 2010).

In 2007, the American Organization of Nurse Executives (AONE) published a position paper that supports the doctor of nursing practice (DNP) as a terminal degree option for practice-focused nursing, while not eliminating nursing master's degree programs in both specialty and generalist courses of study (AONE, 2007). Likewise, the American Association of Nurse Anesthetists (AANA) supports doctoral education as the entry level for nurse anesthesia practice by 2025 (AANA, 2017) and the National Association of Clinical Nurse Specialists (NACNS) endorses the DNP degree for entry level of practice for clinical nurse specialists (CNSs) by 2030 (NACNS, 2015).

According to Cronenwett and colleagues, studies evaluating impact and effectiveness demonstrate that APRNs make important contributions to access, quality, and cost of health services. The DNP was developed with the intent to prepare nurses with the core competencies required to improve health care systems through administrative leadership and advanced practice roles (Cronenwett et al., 2011, p. 10). It is imperative that DNPs, whether they practice in hospitals or communities or work as APRNs or in the boardroom as chief nursing executives, be prepared educationally, intellectually, economically, and clinically to effect the types of broad system changes needed for nursing practice and health care to survive in an era of radical health care reform.

Cronenwett et al.'s work further proposes that nursing is a public good, and at this particular time, the public good is defined with respect to health in the context of health care reform (Cronenwett et al., 2011, p. 10). For this reason, nurses with a DNP degree possess the specific skills needed to address the issues and achieve the goals related to better access, reduced health disparities, balanced quality and cost, improved health literacy, enhanced practice, and sustainability of health care and health care systems.

ESSENTIALS OF DOCTORAL EDUCATION FOR ADVANCED NURSING PRACTICE

The AACN *Essentials of Doctoral Education for Advanced Nursing Practice* guidelines (AACN, 2006) set the playing field for preparation of nurses to undertake the enormous task of health care system improvement along with managing the economic impact of such a task. DNP graduates must be skilled in working with organizational, advocacy, and policy issues while actually providing or paving the way for the provision of safe, efficient, high-quality patient care. The DNP curriculum defines eight *Essentials* that are the foundational outcome competencies deemed essential for all graduates of a DNP program regardless of specialty or functional focus (AACN, 2006). Distinguishing abilities and proficiencies of DNP graduates related to systems improvement and management of organizational, financial, political, cultural, and economic perspectives are depicted in Exhibit 12.1. The focus on DNP abilities and proficiencies for the purposes of this chapter is on financial and business management, applying EBPs to build systems of care, and evaluating outcomes, and it will be concentrated specifically on grant writing for health care programs.

GRANT WRITING FOR HEALTH CARE PROGRAMS

Nurses in general choose the nursing profession based on numerous personal variables: They had a role model who was a nurse that influenced their choice, they wanted to help people, they wanted to influence health, or they had a first career that was not fulfilling or ended and nursing looked like a stable and/or financially rewarding second career. Nurses do not generally enter the profession so they can focus on numbers, budgets, economics, funding sources, or health care dollars.

So why in the world do DNP students and subsequently DNP graduates need grant-writing knowledge and skills, and how do they go about building this toolkit? This question is fundamental to understanding the full scope and role of the DNP regardless of the practice setting,

EXHIBIT 12.1 DNP **A**bilities and **P**roficiencies **R**elated to **S**ystems **I**mprovement and **E**conomics

Essential I: Scientific Underpinnings for Practice

Conceptualizing new care delivery models based on contemporary nursing science; develop and evaluate new practice approaches based on theories from nursing and other disciplines

Essential II: Organizational and Systems Leadership for Quality Improvement and Systems Thinking

Employing principles of business, finance, economics, and health policy to:

- Incorporate quality improvement strategies in creating and sustaining changes at the organizational and policy levels
- Develop and implement effective plans for practice-level and/or system-wide practice initiatives
- Develop and implement strategies and tactics that will improve the quality of care delivery

Analyzing the quality and cost-effectiveness of care delivery and practice initiatives, accounting for risk and improvement of health care outcomes

Essential IV: Information Systems/Technology and Patient Care Technology for the Improvement and Transformation of Health Care

Using principles of economics and finance to redesign effective and realistic care delivery strategies

- Developing and/or monitoring budgets for practice initiatives

Designing, selecting, and using information systems/technology to apply budget, productivity, and decision support tools to evaluate programs of care, outcomes of care, and care systems

Essential V: Health Care Policy for Advocacy in Health Care

Equipping DNPs to design, influence, and implement health care policies that frame health care financing, practice regulation, access, safety, quality, and efficacy, as outlined in the IOM 2001 report

Supporting practice by creating, optimizing, and sustaining organizational and policy-level changes with corresponding changes in:

- Organizational arrangements
- Organizational and professional culture
- Financial structures

IOM, Institute of Medicine.

Adapted from *The Essentials of Doctoral Education for Advanced Nursing Practice* [Educational Standards], AACN, 2006.

and goes back to the abilities and proficiencies needed to effect systemic change. As health care moves toward more EBP, nurses and health care practitioners are faced with the challenge of validating current therapies and implementing EBP without the organizational, personnel, or financial resources to do so (Hess & Steffes, 2011, p. 12).

Many nurses may be intimidated by the thought of grant writing, feel inadequate to pursue grant funding, and perceive the process as overwhelming. Compounding this, the review of literature has revealed a dearth of information published on how a nurse would first begin and complete the process of writing for a grant, with a significant gap and few resources for nurses who are novice grant writers (Hess & Steffes, 2011, pp. 12, 13).

Still, nurses in many different settings are expected to write grants and obtain funding. *The Nurse's Grant Writing Advantage: How Grant Writing Can Advance Your Nursing Career* by Rebecca Bowers-Lanier explains the process and gives practical advice on how to be successful. The book has 10 chapters explaining how to view grants from the eyes of a philanthropist, write the proposal, create a budget, go for the "ask," and excel at a site visit (Bowers-Lanier, 2012). Another book, *Grant Writing Handbook* (second edition), by Holtzclaw, Kenner, and Walden (2009), is a reader-friendly primer that follows a logical path and recognizes that grant writing is an essential skill for today's nurse. Of particular importance are the topics that address ethical dilemmas related to grants and life after grants.

A national research study was conducted that surveyed health education faculty about their grant-writing activities. Two barriers were identified among faculty for grant writing: heavy teaching loads and administrative or committee assignments. The study concluded that most faculties do not feel prepared to write grants; however, many faculties were of the opinion that grant writing should be a formal part of graduate student learning (Kleinfelder, Price, & Drake, 2003). DNP programs should include exercises to develop grant-writing skills, and some programs may require submission of a grant to a funding agency as part of the qualifications to progress to doctoral candidacy.

DNPs are in a unique position to use principles of economics and finance to redesign effective and realistic care delivery strategies in order to conceptualize and implement new care delivery models based on contemporary nursing science. The development and monitoring of budgets and finances are key subsets of financial skills. Generally, contemporary operating budgets in the acute hospital, ambulatory, or community settings are based on historic operating expenses and revenues, or increasingly are zero based. This leaves the DNP with little to no margin for increases related to redesigning care delivery models, implementing quality initiatives, initiating performance improvement strategies, or creating new service lines—except, of course, to become leaner. With keen eyes on financial stewardship, productivity, and budget variances, it is likely unbudgeted initiatives would be difficult to implement, regardless of their merit, unless funding is found. Obtaining funding through philanthropic and grant sources in a tight financial and economic situation could be the answer to the difference between system improvement and organizational inertia.

DNPs should develop grant-writing skills for several reasons:

- Resources for grant writing may not be immediately available to them.
- Professional grant writers, while experts at format and fund mining, usually need content experts to identify appropriate practice tactics, develop the clinical portions of the grant, and define meaningful metrics.
- The DNPs' educational process prepares them for all aspects of grant writing, based on the AACN *The essentials of doctoral education for advanced nursing practice (DNP)*, including the scientific foundation and analytic methods for EBP, organizational leadership skills for quality improvement and systems thinking, epidemiological principles of population health, knowledge of health care policy and advocacy, interprofessional collaboration, economics, informational technology systems, and risk assessment/mitigation skills (AACN, 2006).
- Critical thinking skills possessed by DNPs can ensure that the scientific quality, practice relevance, and value for return on investment (ROI) are infused onto the grant proposal.
- Personal experience can ensure the DNPs' time is carved or "bought" out in the grant to leverage additional resources and/or focus on implementing practice initiatives within the context of grant deliverables above and beyond the everyday role.

According to an interview with Darlene Curley, MS, RN, "People who are philanthropists, who want to support their community and do good work, are interested in nursing. The nursing profession needs to tell the important story of their impact on patient care, and improving health in our country" (Curley, 2011, p. 335). Who better than DNPs to tell the story of the nursing profession, precisely because of their knowledge, expertise, and role in redesigning health care delivery, improving population health outcomes, and shaping public policy.

FINDING FUNDING SOURCES FOR HEALTH CARE GRANTS

To get started, The Grantsmanship Center recommends thinking about the problems or issues your organization is addressing and brainstorming key words and phrases to use in the research for grant funding (Hasselbring & Wiberg, 2016). For example, if you are looking to fund a new diabetes program, you might use *diabetes, diabetes treatment, diabetes prevention,* or *diabetes self-management* as key search words.

One of the most critical tactics in seeking grants is to know as much as possible about the grantor or funding agency before approaching them. Important characteristics with which to evaluate funding agencies are (Bauer, 2007, p. 198):

- Alignment of mission, vision, values, and goals
- Area(s) of interest, including areas in which they will not fund
- Previous activities funded
- Geographical funding preferences
- Process for and people involved in the funding decision process
- Requirements for metrics and reporting

As you explore information on grantmakers, ask yourself these additional questions:

- What is the typical grant award amount for an organization such as yours?
- Does the granting agency accept unsolicited applications? (If the answer is "no," do you have a relationship you can leverage?)
- Does the foundation have staff? (If so, this creates a level of approachability; Hasselbring & Wiberg, 2016)

If the characteristics of the funding agency do not match those of the project for which funding is being sought, it is advisable to keep on looking. Or, if the grant criteria force the DNP to design projects or programs that do not reflect the primary purpose of the work or exceed the capacity of the organization, this grant would not be a good "fit." It may be helpful to create a spreadsheet to list potential funding sources, as this will help focus the search, not just for the immediate project needs but also for the future. Often, one funding source may not fund an entire project; it is helpful to break down the project and seek funding from multiple sources, especially if a large amount of funding is needed.

Numerous resources may be used to find the appropriate grant funding for DNP-led projects. Grant search engines require little to moderate effort to yield potentially large funding opportunities. Such resources include the Foundation Center's *Foundation Directory* (www.foundationcenter.org), the National Institutes of Health (NIH) RePORT or Research Portfolio OnLine Reporting Tools (http://projectreporter.nih/gov/reporter.cfm), and the *Federal Register* National Archives and Records Administration (NARA; www.gpoaccess.gov/fr/index.html; Berger & Moore, 2011, pp. 168–169), as well as Grant Watch.com, Grant Vine (grantvine.net), and GrantForward (www.grantforward.com), to name a few.

Grant listservs require little effort beyond initial sign-up to have potential grant-funding opportunities delivered to your email inbox daily. Some prominent listservs that target health care initiatives include Grants.gov, RWJF Funding Alerts (fundingalert@rwjfmail.org) from the Robert Wood Johnson Foundation, and the California Health Care Foundation (info@chcf.org).

Many grant providers will provide funding for organizations but not individuals. According to the Gates Foundation website, some grant-seeking resources for individuals are:

- United Way (www.unitedway.org), which serves individuals and organizations through training, resources, and technical assistance
- Idealist.org (www.idealist.org), an interactive site where people and organizations can exchange resources and ideas and locate opportunities and supporters
- GuideStar (www.guidestar.org/Home.aspx), an online database of nonprofit organizations that includes their mission, programs, leaders, goals, accomplishments, and needs (Bill and Melinda Gates Foundation, 2017a). GuideStar also provides access to the Form 990s of foundations and other nonprofits

The NonProfit Times, the leading business publication for nonprofit management, provides a classic article on "Finding Grants in Online Databases" by Waddy Thompson (2007). It is also a source of "breaking news" on the nonprofit front.

TYPES OF GRANTS

There are numerous types of grants available from private, public, personal/family, and government (federal, state, and county) funders. Grants may be programmatic, project oriented, pilots for replication, research oriented, or educational (for training or fellowship) in nature. Rarely do grantors provide funding for overhead or usual and customary operating expenses. In DNP practice, grants will most likely be sought for purposes of translational research, application of EBPs to improve population health, or implementing strategies to effect system change. Since the premise for the DNP role is practice oriented and not research oriented, DNPs may pursue research grants, not so much as to perform original research, but to replicate studies or perform outcomes research. It is helpful to understand how to find the right funding source and the types of grants in order to determine the purpose for which DNPs will apply for grants.

Private Foundation Grants

Foundations will often fund projects and proposals that other funders will not. The application process is generally easier and shorter than the process required for research or government-funded grants; and the funding is usually more flexible. Private foundations generally were formed by wealthy benefactors who wished to reduce their tax burden and fund projects and organizations that further the interests, values, beliefs, and life works of those individuals. This is an important concept for grant seekers to understand, and the mission, vision, and values of the proposal should be synched with the mission, vision, and values of the funder. Within the private foundation genre, there are four subsets of private foundations that may further focus your fund-seeking proposal. These are *national general-purpose, special-purpose, community,* or *family foundations* (Bauer, 2007, p. 189).

- *National general-purpose grants* generally are made on the basis of a broad scope and impact across the nation and even the world. These foundations may use professional consultants as reviewers; like to create change; and generally prefer creative, innovative, or model projects that others can replicate. There are fewer than 200 national general foundations in the United States, and they include well-known foundations such as the Rockefeller and Ford Foundations.
- *Special-purpose foundations* are generally very large, are usually funded by large asset bases, and define their area of concern quite specifically. The Robert Wood Johnson Foundation, for example, is a special-purpose foundation associated with health care funding; the Bill and Melinda Gates Foundation provides domestic and international funding through its four primary divisions—Global Health, Global Development, U.S. Division, and Global Policy and Advocacy (Bill and Melinda Gates Foundation, 2017b); and the California Endowment's new

focus is building healthy communities in California. Although the funding results may be quite large, grant seekers should be aware that emphasis is placed on breakthrough contributions.

- *Community foundations* represent approximately 700 of the total private foundations (2,004). Their names usually allude to the area they serve (e.g., Glendale Community Foundation), and they wish to see their community members somehow served in the scope of the grants funded. Community foundation grants generally support replication projects rather than ground-breaking research or experimental approaches.
- *Family foundation grants* reflect the values of the family members whose interests have been memorialized by the creation of the foundation. This creates significant variability in funding purposes, criteria, and patterns among family foundations. Although family foundations represent the largest subset of private foundations, their asset base and subsequent funding amounts are generally quite small, and they typically fund on a local level (Bauer, 2007, pp. 189–191).

Private community or family foundations make good choices for DNPs to submit requests for proposals (RFPs) and applications. EBP application may be appealing to the general nature of the funders' focus on local or regional model, replication, and outcomes-oriented projects. Bauer (2007) also identifies a grant-funding resource in health care foundations created from the conversion or sale of nonprofit hospitals and health maintenance organizations to for-profit entities or which resulted from health care system mergers and acquisitions. Two such health care foundations, located in Los Angeles, are focused on funding community and organizational health-related projects.

- The Unihealth Foundation (created from the sale of eight hospitals, home health services, and senior citizen care services) is committed to being a pace-setter in health philanthropy and identifying and supporting innovative activities, while provoking and sustaining changes that positively impact health outcomes (Unihealth Foundation, n.d.).
- QueensCare (a health care foundation formed from the sale of a local hospital) supports several health care programs, including a Health and Faith Partnership, Pastoral Care, Hospitalization and Specialty Care, Grants and Scholarships, and QueensCare Health Centers. It strives to provide, directly and with others, accessible health care for uninsured and low-income individuals and families residing in Los Angeles County (QueensCare, 2014).

In addition to the aforementioned types of private foundation grants, some professional or membership organizations may provide funding in the form of grants or scholarships. These are usually in the area of professional interest; for example, the Association of California Nurse Leaders (ACNL) offers scholarships annually to nurses enrolled in advanced educational programs; the AONE, the American Psychiatric Nurses Association (APNA), Sigma Theta Tau International (STTI), and the Daisy Foundation, Inc. [U.S.] offer small research grants or scholarships. The Oncology Nursing Society (ONS) not only funds grants to its members, but also provides a mentorship program for grant writing (ACNL, 2014; APNA, 2017; Daisy Foundation, 2017; ONS, 2016; STTI, 2016). These are just a few names of organizations to which DNPs belong and may access grant resources.

An excellent resource to organize the ideas DNPs have about funding sources and pinpoint potential grantors is Bauer's grant seekers' private foundation decision matrix (see Table 12.1). The table summarizes the principal types of private foundation funding sources, as well as their major funding characteristics and preferences, similarities, and differences (Bauer, 2015, Kindle location 4028 of 5856).

Government Grants

Government grants may be funded as federal, state, or local (county or city) grants. In the 1970s, a movement grew to allocate federal dollars, based on federalism or the belief that the federal government should give funds back to the state and local governments to set their own agendas

TABLE 12.1 Grant Seekers' Private Foundation Decision Matrix

Type of Foundation	Geographical Need	Type of Project	Grant Award Size for Field of Interest	Image	Credentials of PI/PD	Pre-Proposal Contact	Application	Review System	Grants Admin. (Rules)
National General Purpose	National need—local regional population	Model Innovative	Large Medium	National image	National	Write, phone, email	Short concept paper—longer form if interested	Staff and peer review	Few audits and rules
Special Purpose	Need in area of interest	Model Innovative Research	Large to small	Image not as critical as solution	Strong image in field of interest	Write, phone, email	Short concept paper—longer form if interested	Board review (some staff)	Few audits and rules
Family	Varies—but geographic concern for need	Innovative Replication Building/Equipment Some Research	Medium Small	Regional image	Local, regional	Write, phone, email	Short letter proposal	Board review	Very few audits and rules
Nonprofits, Service Clubs, and others	Local	Replication Building/Equipment Scholarship	Small	Local image and member involvement	Local	Write, phone, email, present to committee or member	Short letter proposal	Committee review and/or member vote	Few audits and rules

Reprinted from Bauer (2015).

PI/PD, principle investigator/project director

(Bauer, 2007, p. 76). This concept is still seen borne out today, except in the arenas of research or demonstration grants, where tighter control is needed. Government grants are probably among the toughest funding sources to pursue and achieve a successful award for a variety of reasons.

• The applications are long, complicated, and both time- and resource-intensive.
• Requirements vary from agency to agency and program to program within the government.
• There is usually a short (45- to 60-day) response turnaround time frame, but a longer (3- to 6-month) review process.
• Grantees are required to submit frequent reports, keep accurate project records, and agree to audits and site visits by government personnel (Bauer, 2007, p. 77).
• Applicants run the risk of writing proposals that require more than the person or organization can support in order to meet rigorous grant requirements.
• Funding is often very competitive, requiring with little provocation for grants to be dismissed.

Government grant opportunities can be found in the Catalog of Federal Domestic Assistance and on Grants.gov, whereas contracts are advertised in Federal Business Opportunities (Bauer, 2015, Kindle location 1945).

DNPs who are sharp and perspicacious or have relationships with local government entities may recognize when the federal government creates a funding "pass-through" to state agencies or programs, and then the state can fund projects or programs its constituents or elected officials find valuable. Examples of monies that may pass through from the federal government to the states are Centers for Medicare and Medicaid Services (CMS) or Department of Homeland Security funds. Examples of state-appropriated funds are dollars from the tobacco company settlement and funding created for the Department of Mental Health to develop mental health services.

Ultimately, government grants are awarded to the person or organization whose proposal most clearly aligns with the publicized grant guidelines. Helpful tips from astute foundation directors are:

• Know what is coming and be "proposal-ready."
• Network to develop relationships with key agencies, such as local Workforce Investment Boards (WIBs) and program offices in the state or nation's capital.
• Look for demonstration projects to package creative ideas that will result in a large impact; assume a project management approach to successfully write and execute government grants.
• Ask for lots of feedback and be prepared to accept criticism from experts; "it is better to hear it from an expert now, rather than a review later" (Schilling, 2003, p. 150).
• Utilize an advocate or lobbyist.
• Sign up for regular notifications from grant listservs and use search engines.
• Consider using private foundations or community funding for small parts of a project, and use the results of that project to leverage a government grant application for the larger project.

Research Grants

Conducting health research that is of good quality can be extremely costly. Securing funds for research can be time-consuming, with numerous individuals and groups competing for a limited amount of funding. The competition for these funds is only likely to increase. The process of converting a good idea into a research project with potential for funding requires time and expertise. It is important that the research project provides relevance, scientific quality, and value for the money awarded (Bogg, Flynn, & Prescott, 2010, p. 549) and includes scalability.

Some practical considerations in applying for research funds are recommended by Bogg et al. (2010). The preparatory work to be completed prior to writing and submitting a research grant application requires a significant amount of intellectual, methodological, and practical work, which may not be sequential (Flynn, Watmough, Wright, & Fry, 2010). At the same time as research ideas are beginning to evolve, the current state of knowledge and evidence is being appraised, and a methodological plan is being formed, a suitable grant-awarding body should also be identified (Bogg et al., 2010, p. 550). At the point a funding agency is identified, it is imperative that the goals of the research are well matched with the purpose and mission of the grantor.

Anthony H. Mann (1998), professor of epidemiological psychiatry at De Crespigny Park's Institute of Psychiatry in London, recommends in his classic seminal 1998 article, "Preparing a Grant Proposal: Some Points for Guidance," a fundamental recipe or general layout for biomedical research grants. Table 12.2 depicts and describes the six sections of a typical research grant, which are often weighted.

Most research funding agencies use a structured application form, employ a method of electronic submission, and require clear concise writing by imposing word and/or page limits. A simple checklist can make a difference in the quality of the research grant proposal (Bogg et al., 2010, p. 551), such as the checklist in Exhibit 12.2.

Some contemporary funding sources for nursing or patient care research grants, in addition to those previously mentioned, are Patient-Centered Outcomes Research Institute (PCORI) and NIH. The NIH is known for scoring promising research grant applications and returning them to the author for revision and resubmission.

TABLE 12.2 Six Sections of a Typical Research Grant

Section	Description
Aims and objectives	• Brief and focused • Covers the intent of the study • Consistent with the conclusions of the literature review • Indicates the need for the proposed research
Hypothesis	• Follows the general aims • Lists topic the research will examine and hope to prove • Accurately written • Accompanied by an appropriate sample size calculation
Introduction/ background	• Makes the case for the proposed research • Brief, comprising no more than 25% of the overall proposal • Terminology used is clarified • May include a "lay" summary, which explains methods and ideas made accessible to all readers • Literature review cannot be exhaustive; include more recent research, with controversial or relevant findings
Methodology	• Most important section of the grant proposal • Provides detailed description of research method, study design, setting, sampling strategy, sample size, measures, and methods for analyzing the data • Subheadings are suggested: General Strategy, Setting, Sample, Assessment Measures, Procedures/Protocol, Time Scale, and Analysis • Comprises 50% to 70% of a successful application
Justification of support requested	• Justifies resources required, including staff and equipment • Identifies a lead researcher • Includes research team, disciplines, training, expertise, qualifications, roles, and previous research experience
Budget	• Itemized costs and descriptions of all resources • Collaboration with finance department is recommended • Careful planning to prevent underfunding; it is rare for grantors to provide supplementary money for poor planning or salary increases

Source: Adapted from Mann (1998).

EXHIBIT 12.2 Checklist for Research Grant Application

- Is the research question clearly stated?
- Have you identified why this work is important and relevant and what it will add to our knowledge of health?
- Does it demonstrate that you have knowledge of previous research in this area?
- Are your study aims and objectives clearly stated?
- Is the method of investigation relevant to what you want to find out?
- Will your method of investigation enable you to deliver the research aims?
- Does the proposal show how you have conceptualized the whole project?
- Is the study well planned with no obvious omissions?
- Does it explain how the results will be evaluated or how you will measure project success?
- Is the proposed length of the study realistic in terms of what you plan to achieve?
- Have you identified key dates or milestones in the life of the project?
- Have you identified any ethical considerations and outlined the mechanisms in place to ensure good research governance?
- Have you clarified any patient and public involvement in the research?
- Have you provided a clear and comprehensible lay summary of your project?
- Is the knowledge and experience of your research team appropriate and relevant for delivering the project?
- Have you clarified what each team member will contribute to the project?
- Have the estimated project finances been realistically costed out?
- Are the funds requested within any financial limits set by the fund awarding body?
- Have you included your reference list?
- Have you completed the monitoring information required by government or regulatory agencies (if applicable)?
- Have you had your proposal peer reviewed?
- Have you followed any instructions and/or guidelines for application?

Source: Reprinted from Bogg et al. (2010).

Private Industry Grants

Another type of funding that may be very attractive to DNPs comes from private industry. The thing to remember is that the guiding principle of corporate philanthropy is the concept of self-interest; however, the basis for corporate giving is the Internal Revenue Act of 1935. This made it legal for corporations to deduct up to 5% of pretax revenues for charitable contributions. Furthermore, in 1953, in *A.P Smith Manufacturing Co. v. Barlow et al.*, the New Jersey Supreme Court ruled that corporate contributions for purposes other than a direct benefit to the business are legal (Bauer, 2007, p. 239).

Pharmaceutical companies and other industries may support investigations that test or evaluate their products (Berger & Moore, 2011, p. 168). These companies have a long history of partnering with private or public agencies to support community health initiatives and further the health of the community. In one such partnership, Pfizer, Inc. partnered with the Union for International Cancer Control (UICC) and funded the Seeding Progress and Resources for the Cancer Community (SPARC): Metastatic Breast Cancer (MBC) Challenge, designed to support the implementation of projects that address the specific needs of women with metastatic breast cancer globally in 2015. Pfizer accepted proposals again for 2017 to expand the program

(Pfizer, 2017). In another such collaborative, Pfizer Independent Grants for Learning and Change (IGLC) partnered with the Smoking Cessation Leadership Center (SCLC) at the University of California, San Francisco, to provide $4.3 million in funding for community outreach projects to increase education to clinicians and physicians so these health care professionals could then better educate their patients about smoking cessation (Jensen et al., 2017; SCLC, 2016). Supply chain collaboratives, such as CardinalHealth, offer grant opportunities not related to their products or vendors but that create impact to improve health. The CardinalHealth E3 Grant Program commits $1 million annually to initiatives that improve the effectiveness, efficiency, and excellence of health care, as well as identifying grant resources on their website (Cardinal-Health, 2017).

A creative twist in the private industry grant-funding genre is "social media grant giving," which weighs heavily in favor of communities and organizations that are digitally sophisticated, but which do not necessarily create accountability for outcomes as much as they create popularity and mass advertising goodwill. Two such social media funding opportunities emerged in 2010 and 2011. Pepsi's Refresh Campaign commenced, in which Pepsi gave away $15 million during a daily vote program. Kohl's retail chain conducted a similar popularity-based grant program, called Kohl's Cares, dispensing $500,000 to 20 private and public schools (Wahtera, 2010, para. 4).

Although not a grant resource from a purist standpoint, it would be remiss to not mention crowdfunding, otherwise known as peer-to-peer fundraising campaigns, as an "out-of-the-box" funding mechanism. According to Chance Barrett, CEO of Crowdfunder (Barrett, 2013), crowdfunding, or collaborative funding via the web, is one of the standouts for exponential growth in this evolving collaborative economy.

Many grantors provide tutorials, webinars to discuss RFP processes, proposal writing courses, or guides for grant applications. DNPs would be wise to partake in these helpful tactics, especially as novice grant writers. Two organizations whose helpful tactics are of excellent quality are the NIH *Quick Guide for Grant Applications* (NIH, 2010), which gives step-by-step instructions on how to successfully complete major sections of the SF 424, or PHS398 Grant Application, and the Foundation Center's *Proposal Writing Short Course*—in person or online (Foundation Center, 2017), which may not only improve the potential for success in grants submitted to the Foundation Center, but will also help develop grant- or proposal-writing skills in general.

THE GRANT-WRITING PROCESS

The grant-writing process involves the execution of several tactics, including locating funding sources (discussed previously), understanding project guidelines, establishing an action plan, addressing grant components, soliciting letters of support, building credibility, justifying budget requests, and "wrapping the package" (Hester, 2000, p. 22). The Writing Center at the University of North Carolina, Chapel Hill, has a good schematic, depicted in Figure 12.1, which demonstrates the circular sequence of the grant-writing process.

The Writing Center offers ten simple but compelling tips:

1. Begin early.
2. Apply early and often.
3. Do not forget to include a cover letter with your application.
4. Answer all questions and preempt all unstated questions.
5. If rejected, revise your proposal and apply again.
6. Give them what they want. Follow the application guidelines exactly.
7. Be explicit and specific.
8. Be realistic in designing the project.

9. Make explicit the connections between your research questions and objectives, your objectives and methods, your methods and results, and your results and dissemination plan.

10. Follow the application guidelines exactly. (We have repeated this tip because it is very, very important.)

Many other universities have grant-writing resources for their students, so if the university the DNP student attends does not, do a little exploring. Some universities with grant-writing resources include California State University, Los Angeles (http://web.calstatela.edu); University of Tennessee (www.utc.edu); California State University, Dominguez Hills (www.csudh .edu); San Diego State University (www.sandiego.edu/soles/gateways/faculty-and-staff/resources -for-researchers), and Harvard University School of Public Health (hsph.harvard.edu), to name a few.

The Texas Higher Education Control Board (THECB) has sponsored a competitive process for a number of nursing grants, including Hospital-Based Nursing Education Partnership Grant

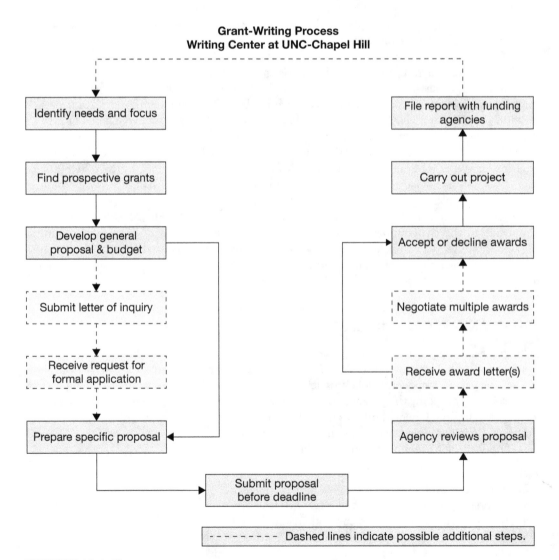

FIGURE 12.1 Grant-writing process.

Source: The Writing Center (n.d.).

(HNEP) and the Nursing Innovation Grants, for over a decade. In addition to a grant application format, their nursing innovations proposal outline includes some sensible grant-writing tips (THECB, 2017):

- Solicit matching funds from stakeholders.
- Identify partners that have the capacity and expertise to lend credibility to the proposed project.
- Remain client focused throughout your application.
- Include both data and individual narratives throughout the application because some reviewers respond better to hard statistics and percentages, whereas others relate more easily to a narrative that focuses more on the individual benefactor.
- Avoid passive voice and unsupported assumptions.

GRANT STYLE AND FORMAT

There appear to be numerous styles and formats for grant applications and proposals, and many grantors now have easy to follow online application processes. Ideally, the DNP grant seeker should rigorously follow the format and style required by the grantor; failure to do so could result in the proposal or application not making it past the initial screening. However, sometimes the format is left open, or a letter of request or intent followed by a proposal narrative or proposal letter is requested. In these cases, Table 12.3 depicts several acceptable formats suggested by some notable funders.

In reality, every successful grant began with a really good idea. And, even if the grant was not funded, it does not mean that the idea was not a good one; it may mean that it was not the right timing or the right funder. Turning a really good practice, research, or project idea into a well-written grant proposal takes planning and commitment, may be long and daunting, and—yes—can even be fun. Projects that significantly advance science, match the interests of the funding source, and provide rapid transitions from research to practice are projects that are attractive to funding organizations (Gitlin & Lyons, 2008). Writing an effective grant application combines scientific and scholarly rigor with innovation and creativity (Berger & Moore, 2011, p. 170). The writing should be clear, organized, parsimonious, and flow well throughout the document. Berger and Moore (2011) further identify characteristics of well-written grants, including:

- Avoid use of redundant phrases, words that are too big, and long, rambling sentences.
- Avert misunderstanding by leaving out jargon, trendy phrases, acronyms, and abbreviations.
- Keep sentences to fewer than 12 words and paragraphs to fewer than six sentences in length.
- Be truthful; do not exaggerate, inflate ideas, or use excessive adjectives.
- Use an active voice, and check grammar, punctuation, and spelling; consider using a style manual.
- Define key terms when first introduced in the grant.
- Deliver a clear and precise message.
- Ensure sources are credited properly, prepare a reference list, and include key evidence supporting your proposal.

GRANT PROJECT PLANNING AND EXECUTION

Once you have decided to submit an application, you should establish a work plan to develop the project design, write the proposal, and construct the final application. Critical tasks during this planning phase include completing a thorough review and scrutiny of the RFP; confirming the ability and availability of staff to participate in writing and producing the application; announcing to higher organizational leadership, staff, and potential stakeholders outside the program your intent to submit an application; and holding a meeting with team members and partners to discuss the feasibility of the project (THECB, 2017).

TABLE 12.3 Components of a Proposal

Foundation Center (Foundation Center, 2017)	Minnesota Council on Foundations (Davis, 2005)	Writing Center at University of North Carolina, Chapel Hill (The Writing Center, n.d.)
		Title Page: Brief, yet explicit title of the project, names of grant team/principal investigators, institutional affiliation, name and address of granting agency, project dates, amount of funding requested, and signatures of personnel authorizing the proposal
Executive Summary: Umbrella statement of your case and summary of the entire proposal (1 page)	*Summary:* Summary of the proposal; purpose is to assist the reader to follow your argument in the proposal itself (2–3 sentences)	*Abstract:* In some situations, this is required in addition to an executive summary; should give the first impression of the project. Most abstracts state the general purpose, specific goals, research design, methods, and significance (contribution and rationale)
	Organization Information: Tells the funder about your organization and why it should be trusted to use funds effectively (2–3 paragraphs)	
Statement of Need: Why the project is necessary (2 pages)	*Problem/Need/Situation Description:* This is where the convincing argument occurs to demonstrate the importance of the project and your organization's expertise to handle it. Do not assume the funder knows much about your subject area	*Introduction:* Covers the key elements of the proposal, including problem statement, purpose, goals or objectives, and significance of the project
		Literature Review: Reviewers want to know whether the preliminary research has been done to undertake the project; seen more often in research grants; literature reviews included should be selective and critical, not exhaustive

(continued)

TABLE 12.3 Components of a Proposal (*continued*)

Foundation Center (Foundation Center, 2017)	Minnesota Council on Foundations (Davis, 2005)	Writing Center at University of North Carolina, Chapel Hill (The Writing Center, n.d.)
Project Description: Details of how the project will be implemented and evaluated; includes objectives and goals. Methods, staffing/administration, evaluation, and sustainability (3 pages)	*Work Plan/Specific Activities:* Organizational overall goals of the project and plan to solve the problem	*Project Narrative:* The "meat" of the proposal; includes a detailed statement of the problem, objectives or goals, hypotheses, methods, procedures, outcomes or deliverables, evaluation, and results dissemination; should preempt and/or answer all reviewer questions
	Outcomes/Impact of Activities: Describe the impact and what will change as a result of the project. Impact is difficult but necessary to define	
		Personnel: Explains staffing requirements in detail, including current staff (include CVs) and recruitment of additional staff
Budget: Financial description of the project plus explanatory notes (1 page)	*Budget:* Shows expenses and income for the project, including other funding and future funding (1–2 pages); divide the expense side into three sections: personnel expenses, direct project expenses, administrative or overhead expenses	*Budget:* Itemizes project costs; generally includes a spreadsheet and narrative (or justification); suggests including narrative even when one is not specifically requested to explain the budget
Organization Information: History and governing structure of the nonprofit; its primary activities, audiences, and services (1 page)		
	Evaluation: Tells how you will know you have achieved the desired impact(s)	
Conclusion: Summary of the proposal's main points (2 paragraphs)		
		Time Frame: Explain in detail and include a visual version

(*continued*)

TABLE 12.3 Components of a Proposal (*continued*)

Foundation Center (Foundation Center, 2017)	Minnesota Council on Foundations (Davis, 2005)	Writing Center at University of North Carolina, Chapel Hill (The Writing Center, n.d.)
	Supplementary Materials: May include such materials as IRS tax-exempt letter, list of board members and affiliations, financial statements, organization's budget for current and next fiscal year	
Letter Proposal: Format requested occasionally instead of full scope of proposal; includes the "ask," description of need, what you propose to do, agency data, budget data, the "close," and any additional information		

CVs, curricula vitaes; IRS, Internal Revenue Service.

Project Planning Tools

Once the idea takes root and the proper funding source has been identified, it is advisable to create a timeline and/or use a project planning tool. An excellent project planning tool can be found in *The "How To" Grants Manual: Successful Grantseeking Techniques for Obtaining Public and Private Grants* (Eighth Edition), which is downloadable from the David G. Bauer Associates, Inc. website (see Figure 12.2). The Project Planner (Bauer, 2015, Kindle location 3108 and 3111 of 5856) includes categories for key grant project objectives and methods, outcomes, times, personnel, resources, costs, activities, and milestones.

Figure 12.3 shows an example of a simple timeline created by this author using an Excel spreadsheet to create a Gantt-type chart for project milestones. Obviously, any abbreviations would be explained in the grant narrative.

A number of technical resources are available for project planning and Gantt chart development. One of the prominent products is Tom's Planner (www.tomsplanner.com), created by a former project manager in the Netherlands who was frustrated with making a Gantt chart in a spreadsheet. Thomas Ummels, the CEO and founder of Tom's Planner, provides an easy-to-use-and-share web-based Gantt chart and project management product with drag-and-drop simplicity. It is free for individuals, with price points at professional and unlimited levels (see Figure 12.4), and can be easily exported to a spreadsheet. Project Plan 365 Online (www.projectplan365.com/projectplan/projectplanfree.html) in a purchased version or a free version (copyright, Housatonic Inc. 2002–2017) opens and creates files up to 2MB, and it includes templates for Gantt charts, task management, resource sheets, and graphs and usage monitoring tools. Another useful product is Mavenlink (http://start.mavenlink.com/project-management-software-premier), a cloud-based application that was voted the most popular project management software in 2016. Others are QuickBase.com and SmartSheet.com. And there are always the various print versions of project planning tools available at Amazon.com or Staples.

Grant writing may require a team effort, and while grant writing can be a successful team-building exercise (Siemens, 2010), DNPs need the right people with the right expertise

PROJECT PLANNER

PROJECT TITLE: _____

Project Director: _____

Proposed Start Date _____

Proposal Year _____

A. List project objectives or outcomes A. B.

B. List methods to accomplish each objective as A-1, A-2, ... B-1, B-2, ...

	MONTH		TIME	PROJECT PERSONNEL	PERSONNEL COSTS				CONSULTANTS CONTRACT SERVICES				NON-PERSONNEL RESOURCES NEEDED SUPPLIES - EQUIPMENT - MATERIALS					SUB-TOT ACTIVITY COST	MILESTONES PROGRESS INDICATORS		
	Begin	End			Salaries & Wages	Fringe Benefits	Total		Time	Cost/Week	Total		Item	Cost/Item	Quantity	Tot cost		Total I,L,P	Item	Date
	C/D		E	F	G	H	I		J	K	L		M	N	O	P		Q	R	S

Total Direct Costs or Costs Requested From Funder

Matching Funds, In-Kind Contributions, or Donated Costs

Total Costs

% of Total

FIGURE 12.2 The project planner.

Source: Reprinted from Bauer (2015).

	Q1CY11	Q2CY12	Q2CY12	Q2CY12	Q2CY12	Q2CY13
	Dec-11	Mar-12 Apr-12 May-12	Jun-12 Jul-12 Aug-12	Sep-12 Oct-12 Nov-12	Dec-12 Jan-13 Feb-13	Mar-13
Cardinal E3 Grant submission 12/2/11						
IRB approval (12/2/11 anticipated date)						
Grant awards announced						
Design HF curriculum and Teach-Back Protocol						
Curriculum/protocol approval (PFAC, PCT, ED Council)						
Curriculum/protocol approval (QACIB, QPS, PFAC)						
Train initial cohort of nurses, pharmacists, & PFA						
Implement Teach-Back: HF/ med management						
Implement Pharmacist Post Disch Phone Calls						
Governing Board approval curriculum/protocol						
Develop monitoring forms						
Train second cohort of nurses, pharmacists, & PFA						
Data collection/data analysis						
Data reporting at QACIB/QPS (quarterly)						
Incorporate Teach-Back in new hire orientation						
Final grant progress report						

FIGURE 12.3 Sample chart for project milestones.

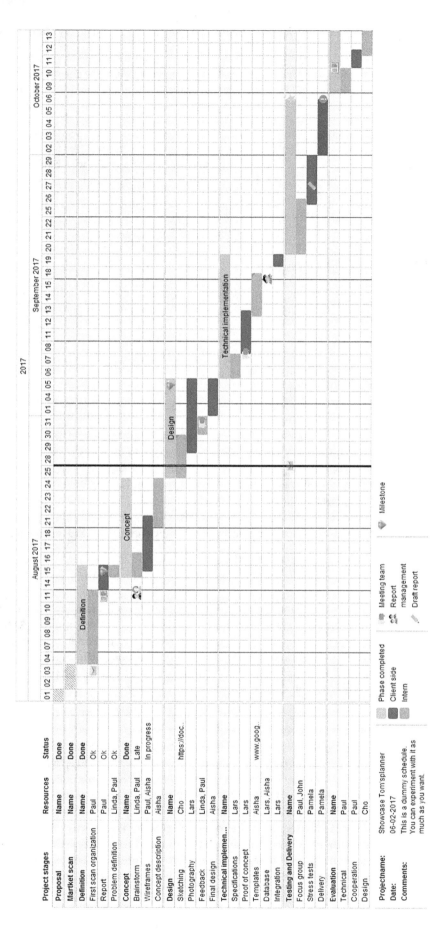

FIGURE 12.4 Tom's Planner.

Source: Reprinted with permission from Tom's Planner N.V.

and credibility on the team for planning, writing, executing, and evaluating the grant project. According to Berger and Moore (2011), some critical grant-writing roles to include on your team include:

- *Principal investigator (PI):* is responsible for all aspects of grants involving research projects
- *Co-investigator (Co-I):* works with the PI to identify and prepare drafts; provides formative and summative reviews in specific sections; and does the footwork of the grant, which may include preparing for Institutional Review Board (IRB) presentation, designing tools to be used in the project, troubleshooting problems, and so forth
- *Statistician:* works with the PI and Co-I to develop the specific aims and metrics, determines the plan of analysis, assists in developing the database, and supervises the analysis
- *Consultant:* provides expertise and experience in one or more focus areas. This is a role that can add credibility to the project
- *Coordinator:* assists with the grant application and coordinates all required sections and materials to be included in the application. The coordinator manages and coordinates personnel and procedures of the funded grant and may be synonymous with the position of grant manager
- *Budget coordinator:* identifies all costs related to the project, determines what funding mechanism will provide the right resources, and tracks responsible spending of the funds. This may also be a member of the organization's foundation
- *Editor/proofreader:* is an expert in the use of the English language and effective grantsmanship, who polishes the application before submission (Berger & Moore, 2011, p. 170)
- *Research assistant:* assists the PI and Co-I
- *Project manager:* writes and submits the grant, manages the execution and deliverables, and submits final reports. This may be a member of the organization's foundation
- *Professional grant writer:* serves as the technical writer in situations where the project manager plays more of a clinical expert role or has little grant-writing experience. Often, the cost of a professional grant writer can be included in the funding request
- *Executive sponsor:* lends administrative support, expertise, or credibility to the project. For example, some funders will not accept a project application without the CEO writing a letter of support

The most important step, which is mentioned exhaustively in the literature, is to follow the instructions and guidelines as presented by the funding agency. It is a good idea to write the proposal and then put it aside, review it later to ensure the directions have been followed, and then review it again at the eleventh hour before submission. Schilling (2003) recommends getting input from others and then giving your "finished" grant to a designated person in your organization who assembles the whole package a full week before it is due (although this may well be you; foundation staff who are good at this are most willing to help). They look at the proposal with fresh eyes and can catch subtle and glaring errors or identify omissions.

Executing the Grant-Funded Project

Once funded, the real work begins in executing the project and achieving the aims, outcomes, and/or deliverables. Again, the timeline or project planning tool is helpful to keep the project on track. In most cases, DNPs cannot and should not add the project and grant deliverables onto already full professional plates; however, sometimes the funding augments projects and programs that already exist. Requesting resources during the course of the budget planning to assist the DNP in executing the project is advised. It is wise to try and plan for unexpected circumstances such as staff attrition and/or changes in organizational priorities, which can broadside the grant project quickly. For example, in one organization, when a department was closed and the project manager resigned, the executive sponsor, who was also the PI, had to assume the project manager's functions. If the targeted outcomes or deliverables are not achieved, most grantors will request that the funding be returned, although some are willing to work with the grantee if unanticipated events occur that interfere with the execution. It is wise to determine up front how the grantor will respond if funds are not used or if there is interference in the execution of the project as designed.

The aspiring grant seeker will necessarily deal with failure along the way. Not all grant letters result in requests for proposal, and not all proposals or applications are funded. Savvy grant writers are always looking for the next funding opportunity, and many sections of the grant may be "recycled" and used in a new grant. While submitting the same proposal to multiple funders is not ethical, DNPs can, based on education and practice, realistically identify opportunities in systems of care that may be rewritten and submitted to different funders. Alternatively, the proposal can be revised and resubmitted in another funding cycle.

▪ CONCLUSION

DNP education and practice lends itself to the ability and need to write grants to obtain funding for EBP changes, to redesign care delivery systems or programs of care, and to positively influence population health. With the economic environment in the face of health care reform today, grant-writing skills are not just nice; they are imperative DNP skills.

CRITICAL THINKING EXERCISES

1. "Smoke-Free SFMC" Project, St. Francis Medical Center, Lynwood, CA

Established in 1945, St. Francis Medical Center (SFMC, 2013) is the only comprehensive, nonprofit health care institution serving Southeast Los Angeles. The medical center operates a 384-bed acute care hospital, one of the busiest private emergency and Level II trauma centers, a family life center with state-of-the-art neonatal intensive care, a health benefits resource center, and a children's counseling center. Additionally, SFMC sponsors a behavioral health service line with a 40-bed locked acute behavioral health unit (BHU), outpatient psych services (OPS), and a psychiatric evaluation team (PET) for psychiatric crises. Over $10,000 per year was spent by the medical center to purchase cigarettes for psychiatric inpatients.

SFMC provides quality medical care, educational programs, school-linked health services, and support services to the 1,000,000 residents of communities in Southeast Los Angeles County including Lynwood, South Gate, Downey, Huntington Park, Bell, Cudahy, Bell Gardens, Maywood Compton, and the Watts and Florence-Firestone sections of Los Angeles. Within service planning areas (SPAs) 6, 7, and 8, which encompass the major communities within SFMC's service area, Hispanics are the largest [growing] ethnic group at 56.8%, followed by Whites at 16.3% and African Americans at 13.0%. This is according to U.S. Census Bureau and American Community Survey 2010 statistics.

Based on the most recent data from the Los Angeles County Department of Public Health, from 2000 to 2009, the leading causes of mortality in Los Angeles County were coronary heart disease, stroke, lung cancer, emphysema, and Alzheimer's. In SPAs 6, 7, and 8, coronary heart disease was also the leading cause of death. Compared to the other SPAs and the county, SPA 6 has the highest percentages of adults living with one or more chronic health conditions. Overall, Southeast Los Angeles residents suffer from significant risk factors associated with cardiovascular disease, such as hypertension, diabetes, high cholesterol, and smoking.

Smoking is a controllable risk factor, and EBP shows that smoking cessation is effective in lowering risk, reducing complications of chronic illness, and improving quality of life. According to the Cigarette Smoking in Los Angeles County: Local Data to Inform Tobacco Policy (Los Angeles County Department of Public Health, Office of Health Assessment and Epidemiology, 2010) report produced by the Office of Health Assessment and Epidemiology at the County of Los Angeles Public Health Department, all the communities served by SFMC are at the third or fourth quartile for prevalence of smokers (Los Angeles County Department of Public Health, Office of Health Assessment and Epidemiology, 2009). This equates to nearly 115,000 estimated smokers in the communities located in SFMC's primary service area. According to the Los Angeles County Department of Public Health, Office of Health Assessment and Epidemiology (2015), 13% of adults smoke cigarettes. Tobacco use in the county is lower than the national average of 19%, but remains slightly above the *Healthy People 2020* target of 12% or fewer adults using tobacco.

- Approximately 8,600 lives and $4.3 billion are lost due to medical care and lost productivity costs associated with smoking and smoking-related diseases in Los Angeles County each year.
- The leading causes of smoking-related death are lung cancer, coronary heart disease, and chronic obstructive airway disease (COPD).
- 17% of households with children report tobacco smoke exposure in their homes (Los Angeles County Department of Public Health, Office of Health Assessment and Epidemiology, 2015).

A decision was made to have the medical center, situated on a 121-acre campus, including the medical office building, progressive care unit (housing the behavioral health service line), and children's counseling center (two sites), completely smoke-free for patients, visitors, employees, medical staff, and volunteers within 6 months of starting a health and wellness journey. This was an unbudgeted initiative to improve the health outcomes of the community requiring massive culture and systems change. A grant was available from Los Angeles County for $5,000 per site to implement smoke-free policies and practices. The deliverables specified by the grantor were:

- Develop a smoke-free policy and achieve a smoke-free campus
- Develop and implement smoking cessation protocols
- Purchase signage
- Participate in educational webinars and monthly conference calls (two people per site)
- Consent to technical site visits by government officials

The SFMC Foundation did not have a grant writer available for a small grant; however, a DNP student working at the medical center needed to write a grant project for class. The grant application was due 30 days from the time the DNP student became aware of its existence.

A. What steps does the DNP student need to take to leverage this grant opportunity in a short submission time frame?
B. What grant components should be included in the grant framework?
C. What resources may exist from the grantor, medical center, community, state, and/or nation to maximize the economics for the unbudgeted "Smoke-Free SFMC" initiative?
D. How can the numerous departments and service lines on the campus be leveraged to increase the grant award?
E. Who (if anyone) does the DNP student need on the grant planning, writing, and executing team?
F. How will outcomes be measured for the various populations impacted (patients, visitors, associates, medical staff, and community) by the grant tactics?

2. A local Southern California hospital serving 5.5% of Los Angeles County's population recently conducted a triennial community needs assessment and some of the significant community health needs identified were:

- Obesity/overweight
- Diabetes
- Cardiovascular disease
- Hypertension
- Cholesterol

Hospital leadership identified an opportunity to better serve the community, particularly patients with chronic illnesses, and prevent medical readmissions. A private foundation was approached about funding a project to improve patient and family decision making about health issues and medical crises. The primary grant deliverable was to increase the number of patients completing advance care planning (over baseline). The ultimate goal was to reduce unnecessary readmissions for persons with chronic illness by leveraging 24-hour community support for them at home.

The DNP on the team, who is an NP, is having success with the advance care planning conversations he is having with patients about their chronic conditions, goals for overall wellness, and how to manage a declining chronic disease trajectory. The patients and families are responsive and express gratitude that someone is talking with them about quality of life. However, he is worried that he may not be able to meet the grant deliverables.

After the multiyear grant was awarded, some unanticipated issues arose during the project execution phase, including turnover of key hospital personnel who were grant team members, delays in onboarding additional NPs, difficulty obtaining patient-level and aggregate data from the hospital's data systems, conflict over patient care goals between attending physicians and the project medical staff, and lack of willing/able 24-hour response community resources, such as home health agencies that will respond to the patient's home rather than an on call phone triage service.

The first-year grant report is due in a few months, and the DNP is unable to tell if efforts have been successful in reducing readmissions; he is concerned about the resistance of the medical staff and lack of 24-hour response community resources. He cannot do it all! He makes an appointment to discuss this with the grant project manager and hospital administrator, who is the project's executive sponsor.

A. In your opinion as a DNP, is this grant-funded project salvageable?
B. What steps should the DNP take to get the project on track?
C. Who are the key stakeholders that the DNP needs to engage and what should be expected of the stakeholders?
D. What other resources at the hospital can he employ to assist with this project?
E. What does the DNP need from his executive sponsor and the project manager?

3. A university professor who has conducted research for many years of his career submitted a grant to the NIH to request funding to integrate a Spanish-Language Hospice video in the discharge planning processes for a number of hospitals surrounding the university. The grant application, which was very prescriptive, detailed, and time-consuming, was scored and returned.

The professor, who is the principal investigator, saw the value of conducting a small-scale feasibility study in one hospital with the intent to use those results to leverage another NIH grant application. The Spanish-Language Hospice video would be incorporated into the palliative care process, whereby Latino patients with palliative care and end-of-life needs would be triaged to watch the video with their family before discharge and prior to an order being written for hospice services. Data would be gathered before and after the video is watched, the results analyzed, and a feasibility index calculated. He engages a DNP as Co-I who will assist with the feasibility project design and execution, prepare the project for presentation to the IRB, guide the palliative care NP, and, in general, act as liaison to the hospital.

A. What types of data should be gathered before and after the video intervention?

B. What types of considerations should be given to the patient and/or family regarding participation in the study?

C. As the Co-I, you have never participated in a feasibility study; how does this align with the DNP scope of practice focus being on applying EBP?

D. You are asked as the Co-I to calculate the feasibility index. What do you need in order to complete this task?

E. What quantitative and qualitative data will be important to take away from this study to assist the professor in rewriting the NIH grant application?

4. The health ministry in your faith community provides ongoing health promotion and disease prevention outreach to congregants within the context of their faith tradition, and to the community. As the director of health ministry, you are a DNP with many years of experience in acute care, faith community nursing, and community health.

The DNP also participates in a regional health ministry organization that often collaborates on projects. The other faith community nurses feel there is not enough being done to prevent bacterial pneumonia, and the mortality associated with pneumonia and influenza, and want to pursue a grant to provide vaccinations in each of their faith communities.

The DNP educational program instilled rigor for the *DNP Essentials . . .* so the DNP knows there must be more than a "feeling" before embarking on a journey to address influenza and pneumonia prevention using EBP with the goal to reduce mortality.

A. Which of the eight *DNP Essentials* play a role in utilizing the DNP's skills to advance this project?

B. What databases or resources would the DNP need to investigate to validate the incidence and prevalence of bacterial pneumonia in the local community?

C. What type(s) of grantors should be considered for this project?

D. What project planning tactics would the DNP need to apply and when should this start?

E. What would the DNP need to include in the budget for this annual multiorganization project?

F. What considerations need to be accounted for when operating vaccination clinics in the community?

REFERENCES

American Association of Colleges of Nursing. (2004). AACN position statement on the practice doctorate in nursing [Position paper]. Retrieved from http://www.aacnnursing.org/Portals/42/News/Position-Statements/DNP.pdf?ver=2017-08-02-103159-760

American Association of Colleges of Nursing. (2006). *The essentials of doctoral education for advanced nursing practice* [Educational Standards]. Retrieved from http://www.aacnnursing.org/Portals/42/Publications/DNPEssentials.pdf

American Association of Nurse Anesthetists. (2017, March 23). AANA announces support of doctorate for entry into nurse anesthesia practice by 2025 [Press Release]. Retrieved from http://www.aana.com/newsandjournal/News/Pages/092007-AANA-Announces-Support-of-Doctorate-for-Entry-into-Nurse-Anesthesia-Practice-by-2025.aspx

American Organization of Nurse Executives. (2007). Consideration of the doctorate of nursing practice. Retrieved from http://www.aone.org/resources/doctorate-nursing-practice.pdf

American Psychiatric Nurses Association. (2017). American Psychiatric Association research grants. Retrieved from https://www.apna.org/i4a/pages/index.cfm?pageid=3741

Association of California Nurse Leaders. (2014). Scholarship Opportunities from ACNL. Retrieved from http://www.acnl.org/index.php?option=com_content&view=article&id=134:scholarships&catid=20 :site-content&Itemid=204

Barrett, C. (2013, May 3). Top 10 crowdfunding sites for fundraising. *Forbes*. Retrieved from https://www .forbes.com/sites/chancebarnett/2013/05/08/top-10-crowdfunding-sites-for-fundraising/#e8dfa3e38506

Bauer, D. G. (2007). *The "how to" grants manual* (6th ed.). Lanham, MD: Rowman & Littlefield.

Bauer, D. G. (2015). *The "how to" grants manual: Successful grantseeking techniques for obtaining public and private grants* (8th ed.). Lanham, MD: Rowman & Littlefield. (Kindle version)

Berger, A. M., & Moore, T. A. (2011). Effective grant writing. *Journal of Infusion Nursing, 34*, 167–171.

Bill and Melinda Gates Foundation. (2017a). How we work: Grant seeking resources. Retrieved from http:// www.gatesfoundation.org/How-We-Work/General-Information/Grant-Seeking-Resources

Bill and Melinda Gates Foundation. (2017b). What we do. Retrieved from http://www.gatesfoundation.org/ What-We-Do

Bogg, J., Flynn, M., & Prescott, J. (2010). Applying for research funds. *British Journal of Cardiac Nursing, 5*, 549–553.

Bowers-Lanier, R. (2012). *The nurse's grant writing advantage: How grant writing can advance your nursing career*. Indianapolis, IN: Sigma Theta Tau International.

CardinalHealth. (2017). E3 Grant Program. Retrieved from http://www.cardinalhealth.com/en/about-us/ corporate-citizenship/community-relations/healthcare/e3-patient-safety-grant-program.html

Cronenwett, L., Dracup, K., Grey, M., McCauley, L., Meleis, A., & Salmon, M. (2011). The doctor of nursing practice: A national workforce perspective. *Nursing Outlook, 59*, 9–17. doi:10.1016/j.outlook.2010 .11.003

Curley, D. (2011). The importance of philanthropy in nursing: An interview with Darlene Curley, MS, RN/ Interviewer: Donna M. Nickitas. *Nursing Economic$, 29*, 335–338.

Daisy Foundation. (2017). Research and EBP grants. Retrieved from https://www.daisyfoundation.org

Davis, B. (2005). Writing a successful grant proposal. In *Guide to Minnesota grantmakers* (pp. 1–6). Minneapolis: Minnesota Council of Foundations. Retrieved from http://www.mcf.org

Flynn, M., Watmough, S., Wright, A., & Fry, K. (2010). Health research in context: Defining the research question and designing the study. *British Journal of Cardiac Nursing, 5*, 346–349.

Foundation Center. (2017). Proposal writing short course [Educational Standards]. Retrieved from http:// www.foundationcenter.ngo/getstarted/tutorials/shortcourse/index.html

Gitlin, L. N., & Lyons, K. J. (2008). *Successful grant writing* (3rd ed.). New York, NY: Springer Publishing.

Hasselbring, P., & Wiberg, K. (2016). Finding the right funders. Retrieved from https://www.tgci.com/articles/ finding-right-funders

Hess, K., & Steffes, A. (2011). What one takes for "granted" about grant writing. *The Kansas Nurse, 86*(3), 12–15. Retrieved from http://www.ksnurses.com

Hester, S. H. (2000). Strategies for successful grant acquisition. *Journal of the New York State Nurses Association, 31*(1), 22–26.

Holtzclaw, B., Kenner, C., & Walden, M. (2009). *Grant writing handbook* (2nd ed.). Burlington, MA: Jones & Bartlett. Retrieved from http://www.jblearning.com/catalog/9780763756024

Institute of Medicine. (2003). *Health professions education: A bridge to quality*. Washington, DC: National Academies Press.

Institute of Medicine. (2010). *The future of nursing: Leading change, advancing health* (White Paper). Retrieved from https://www.nap.edu/read/12956/chapter/1

Jensen, T., Hennein, R., Saucedo, C., Clark, B., Waldrop, J., & Schroeder, S. (2017). An industry/academia collaborative to support smoking-cessation grants. *American Journal of Preventative Medicine, 52*(2), 232–236. doi:10.1016/j.amepre.2016.09.013

Kleinfelder, J., Price, J., & Drake, J. (2003). Grant writing practice and preparation of university health educators. *American Journal of Health Education, 34*(1), 47–53.

Los Angeles County Department of Public Health, Office of Health Assessment and Epidemiology. (2009). *Key indicators of health by service planning area* [Epidemiological Report]. Retrieved from http://www .publichealth.lacounty.gov/ha

Los Angeles County Department of Public Health, Office of Health Assessment and Epidemiology. (2010). Cigarette smoking in Los Angeles County: Local data to inform tobacco policy. Retrieved from http:// www.publichealth.lacounty.gov/ha/reports/habriefs/2007/Cigarette_Smoking_Cities_finalS.pdf

Los Angeles County Department of Public Health, Office of Health Assessment and Epidemiology. (2015). *Community needs assessment.* Retrieved from http://www.publichealth.lacounty.gov/plan/docs/CHA_CHIP/LACDPHCommunityHealthAssessment2015.pdf

Mann, A. H. (1998). Preparing a grant proposal: Some points for guidance. *International Review of Psychiatry, 10,* 338–343.

National Association of Clinical Nurse Specialists. (2015). *NACNS position statement on the doctor of nursing practice.* Retrieved from http://www.nacns.org/wp-content/uploads/2016/12/DNP-Statement1507.pdf

National Institutes of Health. (2010). Quick guide for grant applications [Instructional Brochure]. Retrieved from http://www.nih.gov

Oncology Nursing Society. (2016). Grants and scholarships. Retrieved from https://www.ons.org/education/grants-scholarships

Pfizer. (2017, March 8). The Union for International Cancer Control and Pfizer announce next phase of global grants initiative supporting metastatic breast cancer patients [Press Release]. Retrieved from http://www.pfizer.com/news/press-release/press-release-detail/the_union_for_international_cancer_control_and_pfizer_announce_next_phase_of_global_grants_initiative_supporting_metastatic_breast_cancer_patients

QueensCare. (2014). QueensCare history. Retrieved from https://www.queenscare.org/about/history

Schilling, L. S. (2003). Ten things I learned while writing my last research grant. *Pediatric Nursing, 29,* 150–151.

Siemens, L. (2010). The potential of grant applications as team building exercises: A case study. *Journal of Research Administration, 41*(1), 75–91.

Sigma Theta Tau International. (2016). Nursing research grants. Retrieved from http://www.nursingsociety.org/advance-elevate/research/research-grants

Smoking Cessation Leadership Center. University of California, San Francisco. (2016). Retrieved from http://smokingcessationleadership.ucsf.edu/partnerships/pfizer-iglc

St. Francis Medical Center. (2013). *SFMC Community Benefit Programs: FY 2013 update* [Annual Report]. Lynwood, CA: Linda Woo, Community Affairs Director.

Texas Higher Education Control Board. (2017). Research and project grants. Retrieved from http://www.thecb.state.tx.us/index.cfm?objectid=B85D3933-C8DB-F8A6-3E2C2992B67B1058

The Writing Center. (n.d.). Grant proposals (or give me the money!) [Technical guidelines]. Retrieved from http://writingcenter.unc.edu

Thompson, W. (2007). Finding grants through online databases. *The Nonprofit Times.* Retrieved from http://www.thenonprofittimes.com/news-articles/finding-grants-through-online-databases

UniHealth Foundation. (n.d.). History. Retrieved from http://www.unihealthfoundation.org/history

U.S. Health Resources and Services Administration Health Workforce. (2016). Projecting the supply and demand for primary care practitioners through 2020. Retrieved from https://bhw.hrsa.gov/health-workforce-analysis/primary-care-2020

Wahtera, R. (2010, September 9). Conflicting trends in grant making: What do you think? [Online forum comment]. Retrieved from http://grant-writing-resources.blogspot.com

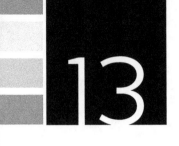

13 The Efficient Hospital of the Future

Lisa J. Massarweh

KEY TERMS		
contingent workforce	human capital	roster
efficiency	productivity	value

Now more than ever, it is essential to gain clarity about what it takes to execute in increasingly complex hospital operations. Tighter regulations, a focus on value-based purchasing (VBP), the challenges of adhering to multiple union contracts, and a dwindling supply of caregivers can make it difficult to understand what it takes to lead safe and efficient hospital operations today and in the future. This chapter focuses on providing a better understanding of the cost drivers in hospital operations as well as a review of four essential strategies that result in more efficient care delivery. Priorities for tactical execution across the value-driven equation lie in the areas of leadership alignment, quality care delivery as a business strategy, data analytics, human capital management, and the integration of technology for clinical decision support.

THE PERFECT STORM

In 2010, the Affordable Care Act (ACA) legislation passed, providing health care access to an additional 32 million Americans (Institute of Medicine [IOM], 2011). Provisions in this act converged with those available through the Centers for Medicare and Medicaid Services (CMS) to move more closely toward rewarding those hospitals that delivered quality care delivery while penalizing those that failed to meet defined thresholds and shifted traditional care delivery models from volume to value. Although the current political environment and the future of the ACA remain uncertain, the fundamental need to provide health care to those in need remains. Health care projections include a rising demand for nursing care overlaid atop a growing utilization of services by an aging population and diminishing supply of nurses. The supply–demand mismatch predicts an estimated void of approximately 36% of nursing jobs, representing vacancies of up to 260,000 positions by 2025 (IOM, 2011). The nurse executive will need to strategically think in light of the graying of America, changes in financial incentives as a result of VBP, and the uncertainty of future health policy in order to achieve efficient hospital operations. Nursing shortages may lead to unfilled shifts in the hospital setting. As a result of these unfilled shifts, operational leadership may turn to the use of extra shifts or overtime shifts to meet care demands. An abundance of research exists (Bae, 2013; Blouin, Smith-Miller, Harden, & Li, 2016; Ellis, 2008; Lerman et al., 2012; Martin, 2015; Reese, 2011; Smith-Miller, Shaw-Kokot, Curro, & Jones, 2014; Steege & Pinekenstein, 2016; Stimpfel & Aiken, 2013; The Joint Commission [TJC], 2011; Trinkoff, Le, Geiger-Brown, Lipscomb, & Lang, 2006) citing the impact of patient care outcomes and cost to the organization when nursing shifts or work weeks are extended. These factors converge to produce an urgency to assess and evaluate strategies necessary to meet future care delivery demands.

Strategic hospital leadership requires astute business and operational knowledge. This chapter makes the argument that the nurse executive is perhaps the single most qualified professional to address the care needs of the future. This leader holds the keys, wielding knowledge of hospital operations as well as an understanding of key data points to strategically identify and execute strategies against principal cost drivers. The practice essentials of the doctor of nursing practice (DNP) preparation (American Association of Colleges of Nursing [AACN], 2006) uniquely prepare this executive to affect practice change. Areas of curricula preparation include systems thinking for quality improvement, analytical methods of application of evidence, use of information systems to transform care, collaboration among professions, and policy application.

SHIFTING OUR MENTAL MODELS

Hospital financial measures have historically been grounded in models associated with illness care, fee-for-service reimbursement, and accounting mechanisms focused on official "12 midnight census" for workforce planning. Nursing units are often seen as cost centers as opposed to areas that positively impact quality care delivery, thus affecting overall cost avoidance. These perspectives become important as hospital staffing typically accounts for more than half of the cost equation (Schouten, 2013). A strong case can be made to better understand hospital operations with regard to matching supply and demand efficiently. In order to accomplish this, thinking must shift to a future of care delivery that values patient- and family-centered care and leverages the core business of health promotion with robust data analytics. Strategic positioning requires alignment between executive "C-suite" leaders including the chief executive officer (CEO), chief financial officer (CFO), and chief nursing officer (CNO). This alignment begins with an understanding of the core business and the ability to distill that essence into a unique strategic value position upon which decision making is based. This is neither a quick exercise nor a laundry list of operational initiatives to tick off the "to-do" list; rather, it is a strategic intent that will provide a bellwether upon which choices can be made (Porter, 2011). These choices include what to do as well as what not to do. Partnering with C-suite colleagues in dialogue to define evidence-based clinical quality initiatives is a unique responsibility of the nurse executive. Gaining clarity and alignment, in and of itself, will assist in eliminating wasted hospital resources (MacLeod, 2016). This is the first essential step necessary to gain operational efficiencies.

ESSENTIALS THAT IMPACT HOSPITAL EFFICIENCY

ESSENTIAL 1: ORGANIZATIONAL VISION AND CULTURAL ALIGNMENT

Although much has been written about the importance of aligned leadership, it is the role of the C-suite executive leaders to clearly articulate the organization's vision. The team must be able to express to all levels of the organization how value-based care delivery fits the care priorities and future vision of the organization. Collins and Porras (2011) identify three requirements for articulating a vision: identification of the (a) organization's core purpose, (b) few fundamental values held as sacred, and (c) desired long-term future state of the organization. These concepts are important and must be adequately identified and clearly expressed. It is this strategic vision aligned to values and behaviors that will speak to the entire team. Once these foundational elements are identified, the broader vision can be put into practical application of actionable strategic priorities that are supported and tracked to the articulated vision. The American Organization of Nurse Executives (AONE, 2015) provides a framework for nurse manager development upon which to build.

ESSENTIAL 2: QUALITY CARE AS A COST-EFFECTIVE STRATEGY

The hallmark of an efficient hospital is one in continual pursuit of excellence. Focusing well on a few key clinical initiatives can make significant initial improvements in reducing hospital length of stay, improving patient outcomes, and affecting the overall cost of care. The DNP stays abreast of scholarly works that inform contemporary nursing practice. He or she is charged with facilitation, application, and evaluation of innovative care delivery. In addition, he or she commands a fluency in process improvement, quality management principles, and human capital development. Data provided at the individual nursing unit level and aggregate medical center level can identify populations associated with higher cost of care, readmission rates, and variation in practices; these all lend opportunities for improvement. This leader understands that community and hospital macrosystem priorities affect care delivery at the nursing unit or microsystem level. The use of these data to understand specific care improvement opportunities, while applying quality improvement techniques, can inform the DNP on value-added priorities upon which to focus. Addressing nurse-sensitive hospital-associated complications may have immediate and meaningful impact on the value equation of hospital care delivery. In a 5-year longitudinal study, Yankovsky, Gajewski, and Dunton (2016) looked at falls and pressure ulcer outcome rates compared to direct productive hours per patient day to understand efficiency trends over time in 1,217 hospitals. Overall, findings revealed that acute care nursing units are becoming more efficient. Inclusion of evidence-based practices as well as cultivating academic–clinical partnerships can engage frontline caregivers as well as inform policy and practice of care delivery protocols.

A simple use-case example of the benefits of early ambulation of hospitalized patients provides an illustration upon which to build. Morris (2007) was a pioneer who published findings about the impact of muscle wasting from immobility in hospitalized patients and its contribution to complications. Morris was an early advocate of patient mobility as a therapeutic treatment to care. Subsequent studies (Fleming et al., 2016; Hoyer et al., 2016; Wahab et al., 2016) across inpatient hospital care settings have demonstrated the impact of patient mobility affecting measurable reductions in hospital length of stay.

Value-based models take into consideration outcome measures rather than traditional methods of managing labor expenses. The DNP must have a solid understanding of current evidence-based literature, the acumen to produce a solid business case, and the political weight to influence other executives. A well-structured strategy focusing on safe quality care can translate to efficient care delivery that can be understood by all.

ESSENTIAL 3: ADVANCED ANALYTICS IN THE HUMAN CAPITAL EQUATION

Health care has a data problem. There is too much data in disparate systems that do not talk to each other, resulting in a deluge of information that is often not actionable. More than 90% of hospitals in the United States are now using electronic medical records (Ivory, 2015), yet there is a lack of interoperability for data systems to talk to one another. It is not atypical for a hospital's scheduling and staffing system to exist as a stand-alone system that is not interfaced or integrated to the electronic medical record, admission, discharge, and transfer systems, or patient classification systems. According to an IOM report focused on improving care at a lower cost (Smith, Saunders, Stuckhardt, & McGinnis, 2013), antiquated staffing practices create system stressors that result in emergency department overcrowding, delays in admissions, and adverse care outcomes. As technological growth outpaces the dissemination of new evidence, tools such as clinical decision support and data marts may improve the understanding of data for application of evidence into practice.

The Robust Roster

The IOM (2011), in its seminal work on the future of nursing, challenged governmental agencies and the nursing profession to better collect data and to build an infrastructure for workforce data analysis. Since this initial publication, a national workforce commission to collect and synthesize workforce needs has not materialized. Instead, many state nursing workforce centers are independently working to collect information on supply, demand, and education (Altman, Butler, & Shern, 2016). On both a local and national level, accurate forecasting provides the foundation for effectively addressing the supply–demand challenges ahead.

Hospital nurse scheduling and staffing are dynamic complex processes. When the planned resource roster does not adequately address actual bedded census, day-to-day adjustments in staffing occur; the staffing office aims to fill vacant shifts while simultaneously satisfying regulatory and union requirements as well as staff preferences. When hospital nurse staffing demands stretch beyond capacity, typical responses are to fill the void with extra shifts, overtime, and use of contingent workforce. A measure to address expanding capacity is the ability to provide for extra shifts in a manner that does not unduly tax the nursing workforce by working them beyond 40 hours per week or beyond the scheduled shift length. The literature is rich in the adverse impact that fatigue plays to both the nurse and patient (Collins Sharp & Clancy, 2008; Rogers, Hwang, Scott, Aiken, & Dinges, 2004; Stimpfel & Aiken, 2013; Trinkoff et al., 2011). It is thus imperative that the DNP advocate and direct adequate resource planning.

Traditional planning for hospital nursing staff has started with inputs from official midnight census and/or historic average daily census volumes. These inputs are used to model future resource allocation across individual nursing units. Neither of these methods provides the necessary flexibility to address changing care delivery environments nor do they offer an adequate starting point to forecast the needs of the unit. Official census numbers often lack data capture of all the patients present on a nursing unit (e.g., those under observation or in procedural recovery) and, as such, underestimate the nursing resources required. The use of census averaging does not address the ebb and flow of inpatient census fluctuations and thus does not adequately match supply with demand across the shifts during the day. These antiquated models understate volume, resulting in a failure to allocate adequate staffing at the unit level (Hughes, Bobay, Jolly, & Suby, 2015). This may contribute to overextending staff in overtime shifts, adding unnecessary expense and introducing the unintended consequences of fatigue.

The ability to use analytics assists in matching supply and demand, along with informing a target for recruitment in areas of predicted risk. Leveraging technology to pull actual hourly census at the nursing unit level provides better initial inputs for rostering and allows the capture of seasonality of census distribution, thus allowing for better matching of needs by shift and day of week. Demand-based staffing at the unit, shift, and day of week level is informed by ratio or unit of service indicators; nonproductive allocation of sick, training, vacation, and holiday needs; as well as any additional unit specialty allocation. Data inputs from vacancy rates along with predictive analytics of retirement and attrition rates, changes in services, and membership demographics provide a greater specificity of inputs to create a more robust roster. This precision, in turn, lessens the burden of daily staffing and the unintended consequences of staff fatigue. Effective scheduling and staffing practices are tied to patient safety, employee satisfaction, and, if deployed correctly, can result in cost savings.

Performance Metrics

Key performance indicators for the human capital equation include understanding the impact of planned census on the resulting full-time equivalent (FTE) demand as well as realized actual census and actual FTE utilization. This assists the DNP in further understanding the drivers of labor expense. With this knowledge, the leader can evaluate if the plan was accurate and if the execution was efficient or if there was variance to either the plan or the operational execution. Other key human capital performance indicators include monitoring attrition rates, nonholiday overtime rates as a percentage of productive hours, nurse sensitive indicators, and employee injury rates. These key performance indicators are displayed in Exhibit 13.1.

EXHIBIT 13.1 Key Performance Indicators

Census (planned to actual)
FTE (planned to actual)
Nurse attrition (planned to actual)
Overtime (nonholiday) as a percentage of productive hours
Harm index (nurse-sensitive indicators)
Employee injury rate trends

FTE, full-time equivalent.

Once an informed roster has been established, it is imperative to develop defined strategies involving workforce planning and display a dashboard to effectively monitor the human capital equation. At a glance, key indicators should be visible that speak to the planned census and resulting planned resource need. An illustrative example is shown in Figure 13.1. The ability to quickly see the variance in both planned to actual census as well as the resulting planned to actual FTE utilization, including contingent workforce, provides a visual base to aid in understanding the human capital equation. Figure 13.2 further illustrates a driver diagram of the leading contributors to the human capital cost equation. This level of detail should be reviewed by the responsible leader at the nursing unit level as well as the DNP leader for the hospital as a whole. Once the principal cost drivers are identified, a specific corrective action plan can be developed.

ESSENTIAL 4: EMBRACE TECHNOLOGY

As staffing and scheduling technology advance, new opportunities unfold in the area of workforce flexibility. Leveraging technology is one strategy to aid in expanding capacity in light of a looming nurse shortage. Whether looking at an individual hospital or across a hospital system, research into hospital workforce flexibility shows the use of technology has demonstrated superior performance in staffing to demand at a favorable cost when compared to traditional hospital staffing practices (Drake, 2014; Wright & Bretthauer, 2010; Wright & Mahar, 2013). Typically hospital staffing relies on antiquated processes that often depend on individuals making their best decisions possible in the moment to cover unfilled shifts. The application of technology could facilitate complex computational analyses and confirm qualified nonovertime extra shifts within an individual hospital or across multihospital systems using a "sharing economy" much like processes used by Uber and Airbnb. Additionally, scheduling and staffing systems that are integrated with admission, discharge, and transfer (ADT) data as well as the patient classification system could further positively influence data-driven decision making at the front line. These systems allow a platform to affect operational efficiencies before the shift is deployed and thus get in front of value proposition incrementally, several times a day, before shift change occurs and resources are committed. Technology that applies predictive analytics and machine learning with regard to patient volume and patient condition could adjust for seasonal staffing, identify specific volume trends at a medical center level, and alert medical staff of either improving or deteriorating patient condition. These triggers might facilitate amending the patient's level of care placement or prompting the provider to evaluate the patient's readiness for discharge.

Use of Clinical Decision Support Tools to Support Efficiencies: Patient Placement

Bed management and patient placement are additional key drivers of resource utilization. Patients are admitted to nursing units throughout the day. The skill set of staff assigning bed status to the

	Planned Roster Need FTE	Hired FTE	Open Posted Vacant FTE	Contingent RNs (Non-LOA)	Var to Total Need FTE (Over/Under)	Forecasted Retirement & Departure	Per-Diem Headcount	Per-Diem % of Productive Hrs	Planned Total Census	Total Census PP 01	Total Census PP 02	Total Census PP 03	Staffed Patient Capacity	3 Pay Period Census Trend
ICU	42.00	36.55	2.40	5.40	3.05	2.18	9	5.55%	10.50	9.21	14.93	12.85	14	
6 South - MS overflow	0.00	17.00	0.00	0.00	-17.00	1.61	4	1.01%	0.00	0.17	6.25	0.57	15	
L&D	24.44	28.55	2.20	0.90	-6.31	1.63	10	12.56%	5.00	5.04	4.99	4.60	6	
5 South - OB&WB	18.00	16.80	0.00	0.00	1.20	0.43	8	11.85%	10.00	11.86	11.43	10.14	12	
IMN - NICU II	12.60	12.00	0.60	0.00	0.00	0.67	8	8.94%	2.00	2.16	1.86	2.00	4	
6 North - Tele	29.40	22.60	0.00	0.00	6.80	1.34	2	4.36%	16.52	18.62	21.43	20.59	16	
7 South - MS	25.80	14.80	0.00	2.70	11.00	0.76	4	9.54%	16.51	20.79	23.34	23.36	15	
5 North - Neuro Obs	45.00	39.60	2.60	0.90	2.80	1.70	6	5.16%	19.00	15.87	21.31	19.81	21	
	197.24	**187.90**	**7.80**	**9.90**	**1.54**	**10.32**	**51**	**7.41%**	**79.53**	**83.72**	**105.53**	**93.92**	**103**	

FIGURE 13.1 Executive dashboard.

FTE, full-time equivalent; L&D, labor & delivery; IMN-NICU II, intermediate nursery, level II; LOA, leave of absence; MS, medical–surgical; PP, postpartum.

Level of Care	YTD OT % of Prod (Exc. Holiday)	OT FTE (YTD)	Planned Annual Avg Total Census	Total Census Last 3 PP	Staffed Patient Capacity (Hired + Contingent)	Hired FTE	Current Contingent RN (Non-LOA)	Actual Productive FTE (YTD)	Actual Total FTE (YTD) (Prod + Non-prod)	Drivers					
										More Patients Than Plan?	Under Hired to the Plan?	Is Sick Leave an Issue?	Need Temp to Cover LOA?	Need Temp to Cover Open Postings?	Need more Hour Utilization from Per-Diem?
ICU	11.20%	4.3	10.50	12.33	14.00	36.55	5.40	38.40	46.63	Yes	Yes				
TELE	9.68%	3.0	16.52	20.21	16.00	22.60	0.00	30.57	36.76	Yes	Yes	Yes	Yes		
MEDSURG	18.52%	5.6	16.51	24.82	30.00	31.80	2.70	30.02	38.34	Yes		Yes	Yes		
NOU	5.65%	2.1	19.00	19.00	21.00	39.60	0.90	37.84	48.73		Yes	Yes		Yes	
L&D	11.14%	2.7	5.00	4.88	6.00	28.55	0.90	24.10	32.54		Yes	Yes	Yes	Yes	
OB	9.25%	1.6	10.00	11.14	12.00	16.80	0.00	17.11	21.72	Yes	Yes	Yes	Yes		
NICU	11.94%	1.5	2.00	2.01	4.00	12.00	0.00	12.80	16.28	Yes		Yes	Yes		Yes
	10.88%	20.8	79.53	94.39	103.00	187.90	9.90	190.84	241.00	Yes	Yes	Yes			

FIGURE 13.2 Detailed-drivers facility level.

FTE, full-time equivalent; L&D, labor & delivery; LOA, leave of absence; NOU, neurosurgical observation unit; PP, postpartum; YTD, year to date.

patient being admitted can be variable. As bed assignment typically occurs on an as needed basis, the ability to capture and data-mine the thought process of bed placement by experienced leaders is lost. This multivariate complex decision-making process is an environment ripe for data-mining. Often the opportunity is lost, as is the case when these processes reside in our heads and leverage pencil and paper.

A multihospital system set about a quality improvement project with the aims of (a) decreasing boarding time in the postanesthesia care unit and emergency department, (b) maximizing clinical grouping to enhance geographic patient distribution, (c) smoothing admissions and discharge volumes, (d) determining the need to utilize overflow units, and (e) maximizing distributed staffing efficiencies using known and expected admissions and discharges. A clinical decision support tool was developed to take inputs from hospital census and staffed beds, and specific patient care requirements (e.g., isolation room, telemetry, chemotherapy unit) using mathematical modeling suggest the admission unit maximizes efficiency of staff. Hourly census by type of service or level of care ordered was extracted from the electronic medical record for a year. This assisted the build team's understanding of specific peak bed need by time and day of week. Once the demand was confirmed, the CNO applied knowledge at both the micro and macro level to map the types of service with the number of beds designated for each service to the individual nursing units. The result created a clinical decision support tool that could ensure the CNO's plan was consistently acted upon with each patient admission, 24 hours per day, 7 days per week.

Human capital makes up over half of hospital operating costs. Staffing effectiveness provides the DNP with a solid platform upon which to exert influence and execute standardized processes to improve efficiencies and reduce variation and cost. An illustration of a strategic alignment of policies, workflows, and tools is provided in Figure 13.3.

Use of Clinical Decision Support Tools to Support Efficiencies: Nurse-to-Patient Assignment

The reoccurring act of assigning nurses to individual patients occurs several times per day in almost every hospital nursing unit across the nation with the start of each shift. This often under-scrutinized activity of workload distribution can have direct impact on the quality and safety of care delivery, nurse satisfaction, burnout, and cost (Cathro, 2013; Ellis, 2008; Quadra Med, 2013). Moving from paper-based systems to electronic versions can leverage heuristic rule-based logic to facilitate the nurse-to-patient assignment pairing that occurs across nursing units several times per day. Technology in this use-case application, as demonstrated by a multihospital system, provided a framework to support patient safety and patient care needs as well as address nursing factors while adhering to legal and contractual parameters. When clinical decision support tools that add value are embedded into existing workflows, cost and workforce optimization follow.

▨ CONCLUSION

Acute care delivery systems are the epitome of complexity theory in action where individual inputs affect the overarching performance of the whole. A confluence of factors including an impending shortage of nurses, the exponential growth of medical technology, and unknown political variables make the present time the right time to boldly act and affect change. Four essentials to address hospital efficiency have been explored.

The clinical experience, the ethos of the nursing profession steeped in its interaction and obligation to society, along with the academic preparation of the DNP place this leader in a unique transformational position to change the future of acute care delivery. Rather than relying on traditional retrospective reviews of missed opportunities, this leader possesses the knowledge

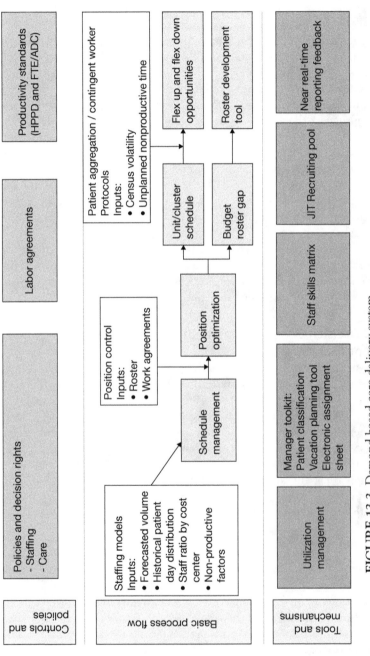

FIGURE 13.3 Demand-based care delivery system.

ADC, average daily census; FTE, full-time equivalent; HPPD, hours per patient day; JIT, just in time.

and skill set to get in front of the curve by utilizing data and evidence proactively to inform decision-making processes. In this role, the DNP is the health delivery advocate for patients and staff obligated to ensure the right resource in the right place at the right time; they are key to creating the efficient hospital of the future.

CRITICAL THINKING EXERCISES

1. In groups of three, with each person acting as one of the C-suite leadership roles, identify and share with the class your hospital's core values, core purpose, and what the future of the organization vividly looks like in 30 years.
    a. What do you personally value? What guides decision making and forms the foundation upon which you act? List three to five personal values and then compare and collectively identify your hospital's values.
    b. Identify the purpose of why your hospital exists today and for the next 100 years. Distill the essence of your presence by using the performance improvement techniques, asking the five whys, or using a fishbone diagram to get to the root. This purpose should have inspirational meaning to those working within your hospital.
    c. With clarity of your collective purpose and value system, envision and describe with strong conviction and in vivid detail your hospital 30 years from today. This should include a goal that aligns both purpose and values; when spoken, others say "wow" and understand it right away.
2a. Focus on a quality campaign of aggressive early ambulation. How will you differently consider and articulate patient and family engagement?
2b. What is the value proposition of adding one unlicensed nursing assistive personnel (UAP) for every eight patients planned in a 24-bed medical–surgical nursing unit?

> Assumptions: average wage rate of the UAP is $31/hour; tax and benefit burden is 36.5%; nonproductive add of 21%; average hospital cost is $3,200/patient/day. This initiative was able to yield an average reduction in length of stay by 0.4 days.
>
> *24 patients × 365 days × 0.4 length of stay reduction × $3,200 cost/patient day represents an $11.2 million cost reduction for an expense of $1.3 million in labor costs, resulting in a net cost avoidance of $9.9 million.*

2c. Consider the C-suite as your audience. How will you make the business case for this campaign?
2d. Now consider the nursing unit and patients as your audience. What elements of the delivery change? What stay the same and why?
3. Review the data presented in Figures 13.1 and 13.2. Based on this information, consider the following questions and provide an action plan that is aligned to the hospital's core purpose, vision, and values.
    a. Which units are running a census higher than the planned census?
    b. Which units are under hired to the plan?
    c. Which unit(s), when considering permanently hired nurses plus contingent nursing workforce, may be at risk for running overtime? Are these units experiencing high overtime?
    d. What considerations, other than census, are driving the costs in overtime utilization?
4a. In your original C-suite grouping, explore other examples ripe for technology advancement in the area of human capital management.
4b. Look to industry outside of health care to expand your thinking.
4c. Present your thoughts to the group with rationale that ties back to your strategic vision, and provide a sound business case for the improved efficiencies.

REFERENCES

Altman, S. H., Butler, A. S., & Shern, L. (Eds.). (2016). *Assessing progress on the Institute of Medicine report the future of nursing.* doi:10.17226/21838

American Association of Colleges of Nursing. (2006). *The essentials of doctoral education for advanced nursing practice.* Washington, DC: Author. Retrieved from http://www.aacnnursing.org/Portals/42/Publications/DNPEssentials.pdf

American Organization of Nurse Executives. (2015). Nurse manager competencies. Retrieved from http://www.aone.org/resources/nurse-leader-competencies.shtml

Bae, S. (2013). Presence of nurse mandatory overtime regulations and nurse and patient outcomes. *Nursing Economic$, 31*(2), 59–68, 89.

Blouin, A. S., Smith-Miller, C. A., Harden, J., & Li, Y. (2016). Caregiver fatigue: Implications for patient and staff safety, part 1. *Journal of Nursing Administration, 46*(6), 329–335.

Cathro, H. (2013). A practical guide to making patient assignments in acute care. *Journal of Nursing Administration, 43*(1), 6–9.

Collins, J. C., & Porras, J. I. (2011). Building your company's vision. In *On strategy* (pp. 77–102). Boston, MA: Harvard Business Review Press.

Collins Sharp, B. A., & Clancy, C. M. (2008). Limiting nurse overtime, and promoting other good working conditions, influences patient safety. *Journal of Nursing Care Quality, 23*(2), 97–100.

Drake, R. G. (2014). The "robust" roster: Exploring the nurse rostering process. *Journal of Advanced Nursing, 70*(9), 2095–2106. doi:10.1111/jan.12367

Ellis, J. R. (2008). *Quality of care, nurses' work schedules, and fatigue* [White paper]. Retrieved from http://www.wsna.org/assets/entry-assets/Nursing-Practice/2015/fatigue/Fatigue-White-Paper.pdf

Fleming, L. M., Zhao, X., Devore, A. D., Heidenreich, P. A., Yancy, C. W., Fonarow, G. C., . . . Kociol, R. D. (2016). Abstract 16757: Early ambulation among hospitalized heart failure patients is associated with decreased length of stay and higher rates of discharge to home. *Circulation, 134* (A16757, originally published November 11, 2016). Retrieved from http://circ.ahajournals.org/content/134/Suppl_1/A16757

Hoyer, E. H., Friedman, M., Lavezza, A., Wagner-Kosmakos, K., Lewis-Cherry, R., Skolnik, J. L., . . . Needham, D. M. (2016). Promoting mobility and reducing length of stay in hospitalized general medicine patients: A quality-improvement project. *Journal of Hospital Medicine, 11*(5), 341–347. doi:10.1002/jhm.2546

Hughes, R. G., Bobay, K. L., Jolly, N. A., & Suby, C. (2015). Comparison of nurse staffing based on changes in unit-level workload associated with patient churn. *Journal of Nursing Management, 23*, 390–400. doi:10.1111/jonm.12147

Institute of Medicine. (2011). *The future of nursing: Leading change, advancing health.* Washington, DC: National Academies Press. Retrieved from http://www.nap.edu/catalog/12956.html

Ivory, C. H. (2015). The role of health care technology in support of perinatal nurse staffing. *Journal of Obstetric, Gynecologic and Neonatal Nursing, 44*(2), 309–316. doi:10.1111/1552-6909.12546

The Joint Commission. (2011). Sentinel event alert: Health care worker fatigue and patient safety. Retrieved from https://www.jointcommission.org

Lerman, S. E., Eskin, E., Flower, D. J., George, E. C., Gerson, B., Hartenbaum, N., . . . Moore-Ede, M. (2012). Fatigue risk management in the workplace. *Journal of Occupational and Environmental Medicine, 54*(2), 231–258.

MacLeod, L. (2016). Aligning mission, vision, and values: The nurse leader's role. *Nurse Leader, 14*(6), 438–441. doi:10.1016/j.mnl.2016.09.005

Martin, D. M. (2015). Nurse fatigue and shift length: A pilot study. *Nursing Economic$, 33*(2), 81–87.

Morris, P. E. (2007). Moving our critically ill patients: Mobility barriers and benefits. *Critical Care Clinics, 23*, 1–20. doi:10.1016/j.ccc.2006.11.003

Porter, M. E. (2011). *HBR's 10 must reads: On strategy.* Boston, MA: Harvard Business School.

Quadra Med. (2013). *Five reasons why CFOs should care about staffing and acuity* [White paper]. Retrieved from http://www.quadramed.com/en/solutions_services/nursing/why_acuity_based_staffing

Reese, S. M. (2011). 10 ways to practice evidence-based staffing and scheduling. *Nursing Management, 42*(10), 20–24. doi:10.1097/01.NUMA.0000403286.72991.4c

Rogers, A. E., Hwang, W., Scott, L. D., Aiken, L. H., & Dinges, D. F. (2004). The working hours of hospital staff nurses and patient safety. *Health Affairs, 23*(4), 202–212. doi:10.1377/hlthaff.23.4.202

Schouten, P. (2013, October 2). Better patient forecasts and schedule optimization improve patient care and curb staffing costs [Newsgroup comment]. Retrieved from http://www.beckershospitalreview.com/hospital-management-administration/better-patient-forecasts-and-schedule-optimization-improve-patient-care-and-curb-staffing-costs.html

Smith, M., Saunders, R., Stuckhardt, L., & McGinnis, J. M. (Eds.). (2013). Best care at lower cost: The path to continuously learning health care in America. Washington, DC: National Academies Press. Retrieved from https://www.nap.edu/download/13444

Smith-Miller, C. A., Shaw-Kokot, J., Curro, B., & Jones, C. B. (2014). An integrative review: Fatigue among nurses in acute care settings. *Journal of Nursing Administration, 44*(9), 487–494.

Steege, L. M., & Pinekenstein, B. (2016). Addressing occupational fatigue in nurses. *Journal of Nursing Administration, 46*(4), 193–200. doi:10.1097/NNA.0000000000000325

Stimpfel, A. W., & Aiken, L. H. (2013). Hospital staff nurses' shift length associated with safety and quality of care. *Journal of Nursing Care Quality, 28*(2), 122–129. doi:10.1097/NCQ.0b013e3182725f09

Trinkoff, A. M., Johantgen, M., Storr, C. L., Gurses, A. P., Liang, Y., & Han, K. (2011). Nurses' work schedule characteristics, nurse staffing, and patient mortality. *Nursing Research, 60*(1), 1–8.

Trinkoff, A. M., Le, R., Geiger-Brown, J., Lipscomb, J., & Lang, G. (2006). Longitudinal relationship of work hours, mandatory overtime, and on-call to musculoskeletal problems in nurses. *American Journal of Industrial Medicine, 49*, 964–971. doi:10.1002/ajim.20330

Wahab, R., Yip, N. H., Chandra, S., Nguyen, M., Pavlovich, K. H., Benson, T., . . . Brodie, D. (2016). The implementation of an early rehabilitation program is associated with reduced length of stay: A multi-ICU study. *Journal of Intensive Care Society, 17*(1), 2–11. doi:10.1177/1751143715605118

Wright, P. D., & Bretthauer, K. M. (2010). Strategies for addressing the nursing shortage: Coordinated decision making and workforce flexibility. *Decision Sciences, 41*, 373–401.

Wright, P. D., & Mahar, S. (2013). Centralized nurse scheduling to simultaneously improve schedule cost and nurse satisfaction. *Omega, 41*, 1042–1052. doi:10.1016/j.omega.2012.08.004

Yankovsky, A., Gajewski, B. J., & Dunton, N. (2016). Trends in nursing care efficiency from 2007 to 2011 on acute nursing units. *Nursing Economic$, 34*(6), 266–276.

14

Entrepreneurial Leadership: Innovation and Business Acumen

KT Waxman and Marjorie Barter

KEY TERMS

business plan
entreleadership
entrepreneur
executive summary

intrapreneur
marketing mix
risk
strategic messaging

SWOT
venture

This chapter focuses on leadership knowledge and skills to navigate the health care macrosystem. The future will require innovative approaches and business applications designed by nurse leaders. *The Essentials of Doctoral Education for Advanced Nursing Practice* (American Association of Colleges of Nursing [AACN], 2006) provides an interesting roadmap for doctorally prepared nurses wishing to engage in entrepreneurial activity. The leadership and management skills needed to lead these redesign efforts are embedded in the doctor of nursing practice (DNP) standards. DNPs not only need to be able to speak the language of finance and business, but also need to market themselves both internally and externally. The *DNP Essentials* discussed in this chapter are *Essential II:* Organizational and Systems Leadership for Quality Improvement and Systems Thinking, and *Essential VI:* Interprofessional Collaboration for Improving Patient and Population Health Outcomes. This chapter also presents some key issues that have socialized nurse leaders and discusses roles for DNPs in the future health care organization. The first part of the chapter focuses on innovation and entrepreneurship; the second focuses on business acumen, planning, and building a solid business case.

▓ INNOVATION AND ENTREPRENEURSHIP

ENTREPRENEURSHIP

The concept of entrepreneurship is not a new one. A leader is someone who rules, guides, and inspires others. An entrepreneur is someone who organizes, operates, and assumes risk for a venture. The root of the word *entrepreneur* is a French word *entreprendre*, meaning, "one who takes a risk."

For centuries, enterprising people have developed new inventions and better ways to deliver goods and services. Entrepreneurial skills can be learned, and with mindful practice will promote creative ways of thinking about your organization. The pace of innovation has increased, creating a need for faster response time from nursing leaders who must evaluate and implement new technology and care delivery models. Every business, and health care is a business, requires leadership that can be entrepreneurial and innovative. The rising cost of health care and the many issues related to access and reimbursement for performance create an opportunity for nurses to design innovative products and services.

A term that has emerged in recent years is *entreleadership* (Ramsey, 2011). This is defined as "the process of leading to cause a venture to grow and prosper." Qualities of an entreleader include (a) passionately serving, (b) mavericks who have integrity, (c) disciplined risk takers, (d) courageous while humble, (e) motivated visionaries, (f) driven while loyal, and (g) influential learners (Ramsey, 2011).

INTRAPRENEURS AND ENTREPRENEURS

Intrapreneurs are employees within an established system that champion, manage, and embed new products and services within an organization. They have similar characteristics to entrepreneurs: commitment, motivation, and skills to take a risk and develop something new. Nurse leaders have an exceptional vantage point into the health care delivery system and are positioned to be successful intrapreneurs.

The practice of systematic and purposeful innovation creates successful change in economic or social endeavors. Entrepreneurs who learn the principles and understand the sources for innovative opportunity can create a new product or service of value. The foremost characteristic required is leadership. Successful entrepreneurs must have the ability to lead productive teams and inspire others to take a risk in developing new things (Meyer & Crane, 2015). Organizational structures can be developed through the strategic acquisition of people, processes, and technology that support innovation (Healthcare Financial Management Association, Fall, 2016).

Drucker (1985) identified information and events (Exhibit 14.1) that are reliable indicators of innovative opportunity. Analysis of these items can yield new insight that will lead to purposeful innovation. Examine the reasons for unexpected success or failure of a program or process improvement; then determine what caused the result. Could a different, more innovative approach have created another result? Is there incongruity between what you know should be and what actually happened? Why? Can you identify demographic changes or new knowledge that creates an opportunity to innovate?

The Centers for Medicare and Medicaid Services (CMS) has developed a Center for Medicare and Medicaid Innovation (The CMS Innovation Center, 2017) to encourage the rapid testing and implementation of best-practice models to deliver health care. This creates a perfect opportunity for entrepreneurial nurses to design and implement creative changes to improve patient care. Nurses are providing telehealth virtual home visits, teaching and mentoring lay health coaches using web-based tools, and virtually coaching new nurses in inpatient settings to improve retention (Sanford, 2011). The opportunity for nurses to be innovative and develop new programs or systems has never been greater.

EXHIBIT 14.1 Indicators for Innovative Opportunity

- Unexpected success or failure
- Incongruity between what is and what should be
- Innovation based on process need
- Changes that catch everyone unaware
- Demographic changes
- Changes in perception, mood, and meaning
- New knowledge—scientific and nonscientific

SKILLS AND KNOWLEDGE NECESSARY FOR INNOVATORS

Cianelli, Clipper, Freeman, Goldstein, and Wyatt (2016) developed a roadmap to assist nurse leaders who wish to foster innovative thinking and behavior. Activities to promote innovative thinking and action to build a culture of innovation should be deliberate and inclusive. The characteristics and components of innovation described by Cianelli, Clipper, Freeman, Goldstein, and Wyatt (2016) needed to embed innovation in our health care organizations are listed in Exhibit 14.2. Nurses are well positioned within our health care delivery system to lead interprofessional teams that design innovative products and services.

A mix of skills and knowledge is necessary to move your entrepreneurial career forward. The ability to innovate by inventing new products, services, or processes is a learned ability. Eight habits will help you expand innovator knowledge and incorporate new skills (Exhibit 14.3) into your leadership practice.

Scan the Environment

Establish the practice of regular environmental scanning. Social, economic, technological, competitive, and regulatory trends and changes (Meyer & Crane, 2015) all provide information that will inform your analysis. Pay attention to news sources, professional journals, and what you see and hear in your workplace and your community. Talk to the early adopters. Expand your scope

---

EXHIBIT 14.2 Aspects of Innovation Needed in Health Care Systems

Characteristics of Innovation

- Divergent thinking
- Risk taking
- Failure tolerance
- Agility and flexibility
- Autonomy and freedom

Components of Innovation

- Employee feedback
- Role filling
- Role modeling
- Employee engagement
- Education
- Protected time
- Technological support
- Rewards
- IDEO methodology
- Budgeting
- Leadership

Team Collaboration

- Unlikely and diverse team members
- Productive interaction
- Play
- Pauses and breaks
- Skill set development

EXHIBIT 14.3 Knowledge and Skills for Entrepreneurs

Scan the environment
Incorporate what you know
Determine what you do not know
Develop analytical thinking
Embrace ambiguity
Know when to take a risk
Manage change
Learn from failure

---

and time horizon and review successes and failures in other industries. Use trending to make predictions about the future. Consider things that do not fit or cannot easily be classified. These might be indicators of opportunity. Saffo (2007) outlines a process for forecasting that can be used by innovators or anyone wishing to take advantage of changes. Watch for things that do not fit and examine interesting failures or good ideas that did not "take off." Remember that change starts slowly and may move slowly and incrementally for a time. Watch for patterns and build that information into your environmental scan.

Successful entrepreneurs are always scanning the horizon for new information, new perception, and changes in the environment. And they do it on a regular basis. Steve Jobs, one of the most successful innovators of our time, was constantly assessing the way people used Apple products to predict the best innovations (Isaacson, 2010).

Incorporate What You Know

Your clinical background, incorporating knowledge of patient conditions, and the ability to use the nursing process to assess and determine an appropriate course of action are invaluable skills. Nurses are trained to work in complex systems where multitasking abilities are crucial to success. Your skill set and competency in managing these systems and your ability to problem solve give you unique insight into needs for improvement. Nurses have learned to communicate in chaotic and stressful situations. Think about how you can translate that expertise into opportunity. First, you need to identify constraints challenging our assumptions and acknowledge common limiting beliefs in order to innovate (Fisher, 2016). The American Hospital Association (AHA) Environmental Scan (2017) identifies current political and market forces that will affect the delivery of health care. New products and services that deliver the highest value will be in demand. The AHA Environmental Scan (AHA, 2017) calls for products and services that deliver the highest value. In order to innovate, we must discover unmet needs and develop valuable benefits to meet those needs. Nurses are in an excellent position to identify unmet needs and work with health care consumers to meet those needs.

Determine What You Do Not Know

Health care is a knowledge-intensive industry. Currency requires a life-long learning approach where the individual practitioner assumes responsibility for knowing—or knowing how to acquire—the latest in evidence-based practice information. If you do not know how to conduct electronic searches or do not have access to electronic library databases, remedial consultation is available. The reference librarian in your hospital or public library can help you get started.

Business, finance, and statistical knowledge are other areas that beginning nurse entrepreneurs may lack. Again, most health systems have experts in these areas who, given the right projects, would be willing to partner with clinical nurses on innovative projects. You must have a clear idea of your project with specific goals and measurable objectives before you meet with potential partners. Federally funded small business development centers, community colleges, and the many foundations that fund health care development are potential sources of money.

Develop Analytical Thinking

The ability to organize and analyze data is an important attribute in the entrepreneurial world. Identifying essential from nonessential data is a more important and difficult task. Analysis of trends using demographic, economic, and social change data will point the way toward needs for innovation (Ryrie, 2011). Statistical and financial data must be presented in an acceptable fashion to funders, evaluators, and sometimes clients. Chapter 9 reviewed the essentials of analyzing financial data, a skill that DNPs should have.

You need to use data in a number of ways: to demonstrate the need for your product or service, to define your population or customer base, to quantify the value of your business, or to define and measure outcomes. If you lack the skills to collect, manage, and display data, then you should consider hiring, partnering, or otherwise securing someone to assist in this critical area.

Embrace Ambiguity

There are no clear roadmaps into the future. When moving into a new area, clarity may not be possible, while uncertainty is definite. If you are particularly uncomfortable functioning in the "gray areas" while adopting and championing new things, entrepreneurship may not be for you. Health care is in an era of unprecedented uncertainty. Reimbursement and resource issues, new technology, and workforce changes will create areas of ambiguity and a need to function when penalties and rewards are not certain. The idea of disruptive technology and the ability to reconfigure business models in the health care industry by using new technology is rapidly changing the work of nurses and other professionals (Christensen, 2009).

Now, more than ever, we need to embrace ambiguity. You can adopt strategies to deal with ambiguity. Feedback loops, concept mapping, root cause analysis, use of forecasting techniques, and peer support are useful tools when moving into an uncertain future. Be aware, however, that the search for "perfect information" can doom a project to failure.

Know When to Take a Risk

All new ventures involve some element of risk. It is important to determine your ability to tolerate risk. How risk averse are you? Are you able to determine the nature of the risk and quantify how it might affect your new venture? Can you develop strategies to mitigate the risk? Should you avoid it altogether (Macko & Tyszka, 2009)? If you decide to accept the risk, you must develop a plan to control it or manage the effects of the risk.

Risks can come from internal or external forces. Risk drivers such as budgetary constraints, time compression, facilities, workforce pressures, and system failures must all be managed so that you are promoting the best use of the project and controlling the risks (Taleb, Goldstein, & Spitznagel, 2009). Methods for measuring risk by quantifying the frequency and severity of events can help you understand and manage the risks in your business. You will have to recognize two types of risk: risk financing, which deals with the uncertainty of revenue and capital, and risk control, which deals with the need to control the possibility of loss (Gaamangwe, Krivoy, & Kresta, 2008).

Manage Change

The nature of innovation or new concept/business development requires that change happen in a fashion that is acceptable to your organization, your clients, and your colleagues. Successful change is frequently a matter of perception; therefore, your ability to facilitate the process will determine the outcome. Building trusting relationships, neutralizing resistance, and influencing the power base are necessary steps to achieve change in any system. Your ability to achieve these steps will be dependent upon your formal authority. If your position allows access to decision makers needed to operationalize your ideas, develop a strategy to best communicate the need for your product or service.

Change is a natural state and managing change is a continual process. In the current health care environment, the DNP needs to embrace change and question the status quo. Change is part of your world.

Learn From Failure

The most successful business models are based on a philosophy that we learn from failure. Don Hewlett and Bill Packard, founders of Hewlett-Packard, were famous for promoting the idea that failure should be encouraged because we learn from it (Malone, 2009). Their philosophy was that failure is a sign that you are willing to try new things, to innovate. Many of the disruptive technological advances were outcomes of failed endeavors. The Newton was a tablet device conceived by Steve Jobs that did not resonate with consumers and was considered a failed product. It is the direct predecessor of other tablet devices. Sometimes, a good idea fails because it is ahead of the time, the technology, or the perceived need. Watch for those failed ideas and determine whether you can recycle them into innovations that will succeed.

Overcome Barriers

There are barriers to all new ideas. Before you embark on your innovation journey, it is wise to evaluate and prioritize the barriers. Gather all the data you have available and perform a SWOT (strengths, weaknesses, opportunities, and threats) analysis (Exhibit 14.4). What internal and external factors can impact your idea? How important are these factors—taken individually and as a whole? Once you have identified strengths and opportunities as well as weaknesses and threats, you must rank them in terms of the potential impact. Match strengths to weaknesses and opportunities to threats and develop a conversion strategy to maximize success and minimize failure. Common barriers are legal and regulatory issues, financial constraints, lack of infrastructure, and lack of special knowledge or skills.

Legal and regulatory barriers include scope of practice issues, copyright or trademark laws, licensing regulations, and the need for contractual agreements that specify what your rights and obligations are with regard to your innovation. The health care industry is a highly regulated and competitive one, requiring legal advice to navigate many of these barriers.

Financial barriers generally are caused by a lack of access to capital. You will need to have a business plan (addressed in the second part of this chapter). A market analysis will provide data to calculate start-up costs and construct a budget that allows sufficient time to develop, market,

---

EXHIBIT 14.4 SWOT Analysis

Strengths:
What features make it marketable? Why is it a good idea?

Weaknesses:
Do you have the resources? Do you lack institutional support?

Opportunities:
Any time of rapid change will present opportunities for innovation. This certainly is that time.

Threats:
Are there copyright or trademark considerations? Is there stiff competition?

and embed your product or service. Financial statements that project your expectations for profit-ability within an accepted time frame must be prepared (Finkler, Jones, & Kovner, 2013). It is not uncommon to read about entrepreneurs who have used credit cards, bank loans, home mort-gages, and other personal debt to finance a start-up; however, this is not recommended. Consider writing a grant proposal, seeking a small business loan, partnering with a larger company, or approaching a venture capital company to get the necessary funding.

The concept of "makerspace" can be instrumental in overcoming barriers to innovation. Administrative support to provide time, materials, and designated space for nurses and other health care workers to develop solutions and prototypes that address products and materials to improve care can be developed (Marshall & McGrew, 2017). Hospitals and health care systems that have distinct innovation laboratories for front-line workers to experiment with tools and support to explore and develop solutions will benefit, The MakerNurse website features tools, support and ideas for creating these innovation spaces (www.makernurse.com).

AONE GUIDING PRINCIPLES

Innovators and successful entrepreneurs are connected. They acquire information and ideas from professional colleagues and organizations. Membership in your national and local leadership organizations will provide a wealth of support for your career. The American Organization of Nurse Executives (AONE, 2010) developed a document that projects five major assumptions about the care delivery system of the future, with guiding principles and an action plan for each assump-tion. These assumptions (Exhibit 14.5) can help guide innovation in all areas of the health care system. Nurse leaders will need to understand health care and economic systems at a macro level. They will work within new structures such as accountable care organizations (ACOs) in which new methods of care delivery must be developed. The leader of the future will have strategic respon-sibilities related to internal and external forces driving cost, quality, and efficiency. Interdisci-plinary initiatives that partner with the health care consumer will create an increased need for transparency and a better educated workforce.

EXHIBIT 14.5 AONE: Guiding Principles for Future Patient Care Delivery

Assumption 1: The role of nurse leaders in future patient care delivery systems will continue to require a systems approach with all disciplines involved in the process and outcome models.

Assumption 2: Accountable care organizations will emerge and expand as key to defining and differentiating health care reform provisions that will impact differing care delivery venues.

Assumption 3: Patient safety, experience improvement, and quality outcomes will remain a public, payer, and regulatory focus driving workflow process and care delivery system changes as demanded by the increasingly informed public.

Assumption 4: Health care leaders will have knowledge of funding sources and will be able to strategically and operationally deploy those funds to achieve desired outcomes of improved quality, efficiency, and transparency.

Assumption 5: The joint education of nurses, physicians, and other health professionals will become the norm in academia and practice, promoting shared knowledge that enables safer patient care and enhancing the opportunity for pass-through dollars to apply to advanced practice registered nurse (APRN) residencies and/or related clinical education.

Incremental changes to the health care system are a thing of the past. Newly developed care delivery models and services will reflect the emerging technologies and the economic realities. Increasingly diverse populations and settings offer interesting possibilities for nurses with advanced practice and leadership skills to design innovative solutions.

MARKETING YOUR IDEA

Why is a marketing plan important? In today's economy, with competing agendas and the focus on health care quality, safety, and cost, the small entrepreneur must have a viable marketing strategy to promote a new concept. First, market research is necessary to define and understand your consumers. Who is your primary consumer? The patient? The physician? The hospital? Define your consumers, research their characteristics, and find out why your idea would provide value to them. An understanding of customer behavior will help you develop a concept that meets a defined need. You may need to segment your market, as patients, physicians, and hospitals would all have differing needs and values. Can you quantify the demand for your product? What is the total size of your market? Can you predict growth? Seasonality? Obviously you need data to answer those questions. Your marketing plan will be built on data.

You must determine your marketing mix, and there are four traditional variables, the 4 Ps, to consider: product, promotion, place, and price (Finkler et al., 2013). Your product may be related to equipment or a medical supply. It might be service, such as consulting, an educational program, or a method for process improvement. Once you have defined the product, you then must consider how to promote it. Where should it be positioned? What messages do you need to communicate to your target audience? What methods and media will you use to communicate? Promotion of your venture is key to success. Place designates where your consumer will access your product, and how available it will be. In an era of web-based products and services, being "online" might provide a great advantage to a beginning entrepreneur and allow a synchronicity to promotion and place. The message can be appropriately tailored to segments of your market and instantly delivered. Finally, price must be determined. This will be a critical decision and will relate to several factors: supply and demand, your cost to develop or provide the product, and the volume of sales that you must have to make a profit.

In addition, marketing models should include analysis of the 4 Cs: consumer wants and needs, cost to satisfy the consumer, communication, and convenience to buy (Schultz, Tannenbaum, & Lauterborn, 1993). They are integral and should be analyzed together (Exhibit 14.6). For example, when designing your product or service, you will analyze consumer wants and needs. You may consider whether to use focus groups, surveys, or other ways to show your product and let users give feedback. If your product is a medical device or piece of equipment, you will have to test it for safety and usability. Does your product provide the greatest solution for the end user? How can you test this?

EXHIBIT 14.6 Marketing Variables

4 Ps	4 Cs
Product	Consumer
Price	Cost
Place	Communication
Promotion	Convenience

Before you develop a price for the product, determine the cost needed to satisfy the consumer—what is the consumer willing to pay? If the cost of production is more than the consumer is willing to pay, the price needed for you to make a profit is then higher than the market will bear. You will have difficulty selling it at that price.

Marketing campaigns traditionally rely on promotion to move an idea or product, whereas the newer methods rely on communication strategies that involve a dialogue with the target consumer. Strategic messaging is used to promote new products. This involves a structured process in which communication is value driven, designed for specific groups, and is tied to a stated mission or set of goals. Generally, a core statement designed for all audiences is developed, then subset statements for specific groups, based on characteristics or shared needs, follows. The core message must capture the attention of the desired audience, and relate your product to their need. The messaging campaign creates an "identity" for your product, and can be further used to describe more complex ideas or product substrates, once the product identity is established. Your challenge will be to develop consistent messages, designed for specific audiences and available over several types of platforms. Choose your words for impact, clarity, and simplicity. Your messaging campaign is critical to marketing.

A variety of social media are employed to provide a forum for dialogue. Many of the behavioral treatment modalities related to weight loss, smoking cessation, and other life changes rely on social media platforms with interactive capabilities for dialogue. Products and services that allow online dialogue are rapidly being developed. Marketers have traditionally relied on defining a place where the product is strategically positioned for sale. Newer online methods emphasize convenience: 24-hour access from your home. As you analyze your product or service, consider the 4 Ps as well as the 4 Cs (Exhibit 14.6) to determine the best marketing strategy. The marketing plan then becomes part of the business plan.

▦ BUSINESS ACUMEN, PLANNING, AND BUILDING A SOLID BUSINESS CASE

BUSINESS SKILLS

As a DNP, having good business skills will enable you to not only negotiate for what you want for your patients and the organization, but for yourself and your career. Business planning is a process that DNPs will increasingly use as the businesses of providing health care expand to meet the demands of health care reform. One must build a compelling business case to obtain the funding and support necessary to move forward.

TALKING THE TALK

In nursing school, nurses are taught a vocabulary specific to the profession. To the untrained ear, this nursing language can seem confusing. It is the same with finance and accounting professionals; they use their own terminology to communicate. As a DNP, learning the language of finance will make your job easier and help you gain the respect of the financial team (Waxman, 2015).

Business planning skills are essential, whether you are writing a plan for your own business or building a business case within an organization. A business plan is a written document that summarizes a business opportunity (Vestal, 1988). The plan will outline what the team or organization will gain and the steps it must follow to actually benefit from the opportunity. Whether you are writing a business plan for your own business or pitching a product or program within the organization, there are specific components of a business plan that will need to be addressed. Depending on which model you use (and there are several), the components may be named differently but the basic framework is the same.

Many organizations are requiring a business plan or a business case to be written and presented for any proposed change in staffing, equipment, program, or service line.

For purposes of this text, we will outline seven key elements of a business plan. Each of the elements will be described and a brief sample will be provided at the end of each section.

CONSTRUCTING THE BUSINESS PLAN

Executive Summary

The executive summary is a one- to two-page document that summarizes the opportunity and its importance. Similar to writing an abstract for a publishable manuscript, the executive summary is usually written after the business plan or business case has been written. This section should include the goals and objectives of the program and ensure that they are in alignment with the organization's goals, objectives, and mission. It should include statistical information, a statement of need or external threat, the connection between the proposed idea and the organization's viability, a well-planned business solution, the projected benefits of the business, and the break-even point in terms of dollars (Johnson, 1990). This section should be no more than two pages, as busy executives need a document they can review quickly to understand the proposal and the cost–benefit.

1. *Description of the present situation and summary of existing conditions*—Your description of the current status and why change is needed goes here. Be thorough in your summary and explanation of the existing conditions. The executives need to know why they should adopt your suggestion, so you need to describe in detail what is not working. This can also be described as a "gap analysis," whereby the present state and the future state difference is considered the gap. Your proposal will, theoretically, close that gap.
2. *Description of the new program or proposed solution*—This section is designed to explain your solution to the existing problem or gap. Considerations in this section include ensuring that the solution is in line with the organization's goals and objectives, mission, vision, and values. If there is a gap in compliance or if it relates to patient safety, indicate that in this section and make sure to include it in the executive summary.
3. *Presentation of options*—This section provides the opportunity for you to present your proposed solution and other options to consider. Starting with the status quo enables the executive to understand what the ramifications will be if nothing is done. Will the organization lose money? Will patient safety be impacted?
   a. The second option should be your proposed solution. You should summarize what you wrote in Section 2.
   b. The final option should be a compromise—your backup plan. Because it is your second proposed solution, fully explain why it is not your first option and why you feel your original solution would be better. Do this by listing the pros and cons of each (Waxman, 2015). For example, you might indicate that your secondary solution is to hire a 0.5 FTE (full-time equivalent) rather than a 1.0. You would then need to include the advantages and disadvantages of adopting this solution.
4. *Market analysis*—If you are proposing a new program or service, this section is important. However, it may not be needed for business cases such as an additional FTE. This section is where the SWOT analysis takes place. As you recall from Chapter 11, the SWOT is a review of the program's strengths, weaknesses, opportunities, and threats. The administrative or executive team will appreciate the fact that you have a well-thought-out plan and a SWOT analysis can

help. This section should also include the data you gathered to back your analysis. Data such as physician practice patterns, volume projections, competitor information, and patient satisfaction scores and revenue projections are examples.

5. *Implementation plan, timeline, and schedule*—This section is where you explain how you or your team will implement the program into practice. Using project management tools such as a Gantt chart can be very useful depending on the amount of detail you wish to show. This section can be combined with Section 6 or separated depending on the detail and complexity of the business case. This is where you will describe whether job descriptions need to be written, ads need to be placed, informational meetings need to be held, supplies need to be purchased, and so forth. Identify why these tasks are important and who is going to take the lead on each. As the author of the business plan documents, this does not imply that you will be doing the bulk of the work. Your first task in this section may be to create a team and describe roles and responsibilities.

   Developing a clear, realistic timeline is critical. From a macrosystem perspective, what other changes have been implemented organizationally in the recent past? Is your project going to interfere with others that are in progress? Consider seasonality, scheduling, vacations, holidays, and budget cycles. These can impact your schedule, so be realistic. The timeline can be placed in a Gantt chart as mentioned earlier and combined with the assignment of tasks, milestones, and key deliverables.

6. *Evaluation plan*—Once your program is implemented, how will you know it is effective? This section reviews how you and your team are going to measure the effectiveness. The administrative team or executive will expect that you have thought this out and have provided an evaluation plan that best measures the return on investment (ROI) for the organization. Ways to measure include patient satisfaction surveys, employee satisfaction surveys, cost, revenue, length of stay, cost-avoidance, and so forth.

7. *Financials*—The final section is dedicated to the financial impact of the program. Is this a revenue-producing program or an expense-reducing program? Will this program help avoid costs? Perhaps it is actually a budget-neutral program but patient satisfaction is expected to increase. This section includes the budget and a pro-forma of when the program will actually make money or bring in revenue to the organization. It may also include a cost–benefit analysis. The narrative piece is included in the written document, and the budget, ROI, and pro-forma are usually attached as appendices.

Sample Executive Summary

Patient injuries from falls are an all-too-common and unfortunate occurrence within today's hospital environments. One frequently employed fall prevention strategy is the use of sitters for continuous patient observation. This labor-intensive approach to fall safety costs the average U.S. acute care hospital approximately $1.3 million per year (Spiva et al., 2012). Current literature reveals a growing body of applied evidence demonstrating how sitters can be effectively replaced by alternative fall safety strategies. An engaged nursing team supported by necessary education, tools, and resources is the foundation to an effective sitter reduction and patient safety improvement effort (Lang, 2014).

   The proposed sitter reduction program will coordinate the implementation of policy training, monitoring technology, and safety equipment to provide a new and broad inventory of alternative patient safety options for staff. The program targets nonpsychiatric sitter usage within the organization's adult acute care inpatient environments and will monitor sitter use, fall reports, and alternative strategy effectiveness in real time as a feedback loop for continual process improvement. Goals of the program are to reduce nonpsychiatric sitter utilization by 75% and decrease patient fall rates and harm from fall events by 25%. The labor savings achieved by this sitter reduction program, in conjunction with the initiative's supply cost savings, targets a cumulative 5-year positive net contribution to the organization of $943,656 (Bock, 2016).

Sample Description of the Present Situation and Summary of Existing Conditions

We currently are experiencing high overtime on many of our nursing units due to the use of sitters. Since sitters were not budgeted, we use our nursing assistants to sit with patients, and many of them work double shifts to cover this need. A growing concern for the organization is that although the internal rate of falls is below the national average, the rate remains essentially unchanged over the past 3 years despite a nearly fourfold increase in nonpsychiatric sitter usage over the same time frame. The trajectory in sitter utilization is driving a significant increase in costs without producing value for patient safety. Assuming a standard wage rate of $18.68/hour, these five units have increased spending on patient care sitters from $76,252 in FY13 to $249,616 in FY16 without a corresponding improvement in fall outcomes. However, considerations of overtime dramatically increase the budgetary impact of using sitters for fall prevention. Although the organization does not currently capture overtime hours used in the job code for patient care sitters, an assessment among frontline managers and the staffing department indicates overtime utilization for sitters is as high as 30% or more. When considering overtime, system-wide nonpsychiatric sitter costs for the organization likely exceed $500,000 annually (Bock, 2016).

Sample Program Description

The dimensions of the proposed sitter reduction plan include aligning best evidence with current practice, implementation of patient monitoring technology, and an expansion of new patient safety supplies for staff. The specific safety alternatives are based on the results of a gap analysis comparing current practices with best evidence identified by a literature review. Although a single policy guides patient safety practices for the organization, there is significant discrepancy across departments as to actual practice. In discussions with staff and unit leaders, the most significant contributors to patient fall safety are lack of visibility into a patient room and insufficient time to respond to unstable patients attempting to get out of bed. As a result, staff utilize patient sitters for continuous observation of high fall risk patients. To reduce the reliance on sitter usage, this program will engage select vendor partners to provide alternative safety measures that address the visibility and time deficiency concerns identified by the nursing departments. Working in collaboration with frontline staff, combining best practice with new patient safety equipment and technology will achieve the goals of the improvement project.

Recognizing the rationale behind sitter utilization and the need to effectively address these concerns, the improvement project will provide revised practice recommendations based on current evidence and top performers in the organization. Particular best practices identified by the gap analysis include an active fall safety huddle at the beginning of each shift that identifies all high-risk patients and the current efforts employed to maintain their safety. Another high-yield intervention is inclusion of a scripted safety education discussion with patients during a bedside shift report. Although other practices produce strong results, these two efforts appear to work consistently within the organization wherever they are employed.

The project will deploy a new patient monitoring technology for the organization. Utilizing an in-room camera mounted in the ceiling, the closed-circuit monitoring system is either actively or passively viewed from a central station to provide direct visibility into a patient room. Beyond simple visibility, the system employs a superimposed virtual rail system that in combination with a proprietary algorithm detects egress activity around a patient. This image, viewable only from the central station, is targeted on either a bed, chair, or other configurable location and serves as an invisible safety border around the patient. If the patient attempts to exit this zone, the camera system detects this motion and alarms the central monitoring station accordingly, thus providing staff with time to intervene before a fall occurs.

The final element of the program includes provision of a new formulary of patient safety equipment for staff. The new vendor provides an expanded set of tools and resources staff can utilize in managing patient safety in lieu of continuous observation. Particularly notable is the availability of a patient body belt. This nonrestraint device is designed to remind patients to call for help when assistance is required as opposed to impulsively exiting the chair or bed. The tool is easily removable by the patient; however, the time delay and tactile action required provide an opportunity to identify patient egress movements and to remind the patient to call for assistance (Bock, 2016).

Sample Presentation of Options

Option 1: Do nothing. If we choose not to move forward with this proposal, costs will continue to rise related to sitters. (In this section, you can note the current costs in terms of dollars and that if you continue, the costs will continue to be incurred or rise).

Option 2: Implement the nonrestraint device program hospital wide, which will avoid costs incurred with sitters and overtime, and will increase productivity.

Option 3: Implement on one unit and evaluate after 90 days to determine whether we want to roll it out house wide.

Sample Market Analysis

Comparing current evidence to best practice and the results of the gap analysis indicate several opportunities where the organization can reduce utilization of patient sitters for fall prevention. When combined with staff education and a comprehensive approach to fall safety, video monitoring technology has shown to reduce sitters by 50% without a negative impact on patient fall outcomes (Burtson & Vento, 2015). Other contemporary studies of continuous video monitoring technology show that both a reduction in patient care sitter usage and a decrease in patient fall events are achievable when specifically combined with staff training as well as patient and family education on fall prevention (Jeffers et al., 2013; Sand-Jecklin, Johnson, & Tylka, 2015). Though promising, a likely contributor to the reduction in patient falls observed with deployment of video monitoring is the increased attention realized by comprehensive efforts around fall prevention and patient safety (Hardin, Dienemann, Rudisill, & Mills, 2013). (In this section, you can also indicate if you know other hospitals that have implemented the program in your region to show a competitive edge.)

Sample Implementation Plan, Timeline, and Schedule

This could take the form of a Gantt chart as an appendix in Excel.

January: Meet with chief financial officer (CFO) to gain buy-in; establish committee, hold meeting. Committee should include managers, staff representatives, risk management, physicians, physical therapists, nursing assistant.

February: Meet with vendors to determine best products. Gather financial data, hold committee meeting.

March: Establish outcome metrics, committee meeting, order products.

April: Roll out program on one unit, followed by house-wide roll out after 30 days.

May–August: Continue to monitor program outcomes, which include financial data to show ROI.

Ongoing: Plan–do–check–act (PDCA) model of continuous quality improvement.

TABLE 14.1 Performance Outcome Metrics

Metric	Organizational Definitions	Collection Source
Patient care sitter utilization in hours used	• Patient care sitter—any job class assigned to the direct and constant observation of a patient. • Sitter utilization—the number of hours recorded by the organization's staffing office in which personnel are assigned by a patient care unit to the role of patient sitter.	• The central staffing office is responsible for tracking assigned patient care sitter hours for the organization. • Full-month data are available within 10 business days of the end of each month.
Rate of patient falls	• Patient fall—any unplanned, assisted, or unassisted descent to the floor by a patient. • Fall rate—the number of documented fall events per 1,000 patient days.	• All fall events, regardless of the level of harm, are recorded in the organization's incident report system. • Fall event data are available within 30 days of the end of each month. • The organization's finance department is solely responsible for tracking inpatient census. • Audited census data are available the next business day.
Rate of falls with injury	• Fall injury—diagnosed as moderate (sprain, deep laceration) or severe (fracture, change in mental status) harm or death resulting from a fall. • Fall injury rate—the number of qualifying fall injury events per 1,000 patient days.	• Fall injury data are recorded in the organization's incident reporting system. • The quality management team is responsible to identify all quality fall injury events. • Audited fall injury event data are available within 30 days of the end of each month. • The same census data collection and auditing processes apply as previously noted (rate of patient falls).

Sample Evaluation Plan

The evaluation plan could be expressed in tabular form (Table 14.1).

Sample Financials

The financial details could be expressed in tabular form (Table 14.2).

BUSINESS PLAN SUMMARY

Although the components of a business plan are essentially the same in all organizations, the templates may vary. The process of writing a business plan, or building a solid business case, coupled with the DNP's knowledge of the macrosystem of health care can easily result in ensuring success in initiating and operating successful programs.

TABLE 14.2 Overtime Reduction Model and Resulting Net Contribution to Organization

| | 50% Sitter Reduction | | | | | |
OT %	Y1	Y2	Y3	Y4	Y5	Total
Base (no OT)	$106,845	$115,549	$119,355	$121,089	$125,089	$587,927
15% OT	$176,783	$187,410	$193,192	$196,939	$203,043	$957,367
	75% Sitter Reduction					
OT %	Y1	Y2	Y3	Y4	Y5	Total
Base (no OT)	$174,783	$184,743	$190,452	$194,123	$200,150	$944,251
15% OT	$279,094	$292,535	$301,208	$307,925	$317,081	$1,497,843

Budget
90-Day Evaluation Budget[1]

Item	Cost/ (Savings)	Evaluation Quantity	90-Day Cost/ (Savings)	Assumptions
Staff training	$35/hour	1 hour/FTE	$4,200	60 FTE per department
IS project time	$100/hour	8 hours	$800	Time required validated by IS
Patient safety supplies	(20%)	90-day supply	($1,200)	Savings based on historical usage of $1,000/month per unit
Patient monitoring technology	$70/camera/month $130/monitor station/month	29 cameras 2 stations	$6,090 $780	Install in one third of patient care rooms, one monitor per central station.
Sitter reduction	($18.68/hour)	Unit 1 = 630 hours Unit 2 = 550 hours	($22,042)[2]	Based off of 50% reduction in FY16 average monthly sitter usage
	90-day evaluation total		($11,372)[2]	Savings

[1] 90-day evaluation budget based on a two-unit deployment as described at two hospitals.

[2] Conservative estimate of 50% reduction in sitter hours. Program targets a 75% reduction in sitter utilization. If target is achieved, sitter reduction savings would increase to $33,063, resulting in a net 90-day savings of $22,393 for the organization.

FTE, full-time equivalent; IS, information services; OT, overtime.

Potential programs that a DNP could be involved with or that he or she may lead include helping a nurse manager justify the need for a unit-based clinical educator, creating an outpatient program to increase revenue, creating a short stay program to decrease unit expenses, and developing a organization-wide back safety program to reduce employee injuries. DNPs are sought after as Magnet® coordinators, directors of centers of excellence, and chief nurse executives.

■ CONCLUSION

Nurse leaders moving into roles that require a DNP must demonstrate knowledge and skills that will help them be successful in advanced practice. This chapter has presented a number of topics related to business acumen. The ability to innovate as well as develop entrepreneurial proposals and solid business plans will prepare nurses to have a strong voice in the C-suite and the board room.

CRITICAL THINKING EXERCISES

1. Successful entrepreneurs are "made," not born. They have acquired a skill set that promotes the identification and development of new ideas. Rate yourself, using the following criteria, to determine where your ability to function in an entrepreneurial role can be improved.
   a. I have a low level of comfort with uncertainty.
   b. I find it difficult to "sell" my ideas.
   c. My inexperience with business procedures makes me unsure.
       An answer of "yes" to the previous questions should not be viewed as a barrier to your entrepreneurial effort. Instead, use this exercise as a tool to help you develop new skills. List five things that you can do to boost your chances of success in each of the previous areas.
2. As our country ages, the impact of baby boomers turning 65 every 7 seconds is significant. What does this mean to the DNP? How can the DNP help the organization develop a plan for succession planning?
3. Writing an executive summary should occur after the business plan is written. Think about a project or proposal that will either increase revenue or decrease expenses. Write a two-page concise executive summary outlining your proposal and the benefits.
4. In a small group, build a business case to add clinical nurse specialists (CNSs) to a nursing unit. What are the costs? What are the benefits? How would you build a case to add this additional 1.0 FTE? How would you measure the ROI?

REFERENCES

American Association of Colleges of Nursing. (2006). *The essentials of doctoral education for advanced nursing practice.* Washington, DC: Author.

American Hospital Association. (2017). AHA environmental scan. Retrieved from http://www.hhnmag.com/articles/7616-aha-2017-environmental-scan

American Organization of Nurse Executives. (2010). *Guiding principles for future care delivery.* Chicago, IL: Author.

Bock, T. (2016). Unpublished work: Sitter Reduction Business Plan. University of San Francisco Executive leader DNP course: Advanced financial management.

Burtson, P., & Vento, L. (2015). Sitter reduction through mobile video monitoring. *Journal of Nursing Administration, 45*(7/8), 363–369. doi:10.1097/NNA.000000000000216

The CMS Innovation Center, Center for Medicare and Medicaid Innovation. (2017). Retrieved from http://www.innovations.cms.gov

Christensen, C. M. (2009). *The innovator's prescription: A disruptive solution for health care.* New York, NY: McGraw-Hill.

Cianelli, R., Clipper, R., Freeman, R., Goldstein, J., & Wyatt, T. H. (2016). The innovation road map: A guide for nurse leaders. Retrieved from http://www.aone.org/resources/innovation-road-map-infographic.pdf

Drucker, P. (1985). *Innovation and entrepreneurship: Practice and principles.* New York, NY: Harper and Row.

Finkler, S. A., Jones, C. B., & Kovner, C. T. (2013). *Financial management for nurse managers and executives* (4th ed.). St. Louis, MO: Elsevier Saunders.

Fisher, S. A. (2016). Fresh ideas to foster true innovation in nursing. *Nurse Leader, 14*(4), 238–239.

Gaamangwe, T., Krivoy, A., & Kresta, P. (2008). Applying risk management principles to medical devices performance assurance program-defining the process. *Biomedical Instrumentation and Technology, 42,* 401–406.

Hardin, S., Dienemann, J., Rudisill, P., & Mills, K. (2013). Inpatient fall prevention: Use of in-room webcams. *Journal of Patient Safety*, 9(1), 29–35. doi:10.1097/PTS.0b013e3182753e4f

Healthcare Financial Management Association. (2016). Health care 2020: Transformative innovation. Retrieved from https://www.hfma.org/healthcare2020

Isaacson, W. (2010). *Steve Jobs*. New York, NY: Simon & Schuster.

Jeffers, S., Searcy, P., Boyle, K., Herring, C., Lester, K., Goetz-Smith, H., & Nelson, P. (2013). Centralized video monitoring for patient safety: A Denver Health lean journey. *Nursing Economic$*, 31, 298–306. Retrieved from http://0-search.ebscohost.com.ignacio.usfca.edu/login.aspx?direct=true&db=a9h&AN=92907333&site=ehost-live&scope=site

Johnson, J. (1990). Developing an effective business plan. *Nursing Economic$*, 8(3), 152–154.

Lang, C. (2014). Do sitters prevent falls? A review of the literature. *Journal of Gerontological Nursing*, 40(5), 24–33. doi:10.3928/00989134-20140313-01

Macko, A., & Tyszka, T. (2009). Entrepreneurship and risk taking. *Applied Psychology: An International Review*, 58(3), 469–487.

Malone, M. S. (2009). *Bill and Dave: How Hewlett and Packard built the world's greatest company*. New York, NY: Penguin.

Marshall, D. R., & McGrew, D. A. (2017). Creativity and innovation in health care: Opening a hospital makerspace. *Nurse Leader*, 15(1), 56–58.

Meyer, M. H., & Crane, F. G. (2015). *Venturing: Innovation and business planning for entrepreneurs*. Boston, MA: The Institute for Enterprise Growth.

Ramsey, D. (2011). *Entreleadership: 20 years of practical business wisdom from the trenches*. New York, NY: Howard Books.

Ryrie, I. A. (2011). Tool to assess the cost and quality benefits of nursing innovation. *Nursing Management*, 18(4), 28–31.

Saffo, P. (2007, July–August). Six rules for effective forecasting. *Harvard Business Review*, 1–10 (Reprint R0707K).

Sand-Jecklin, K., Johnson, J., & Tylka, S. (2015). Protecting patient safety. *Journal of Nursing Care Quality*, 31, 131–138. doi:10.1097/NCQ.0000000000000163

Sanford, K. (2011). The call for innovation. *Health Care Financial Management*, 65(9), 56–58, 60.

Schultz, D. E., Tannenbaum, S. I., & Lauterborn, R. F. (1993). *Integrated market communications: Putting it together and making it work*. Chicago, IL: NTC Business Books.

Spiva, L., Feiner, T., Jones, D., Hunter, D., Petefish, J., & VanBrackle, L. (2012). An evaluation of a sitter reduction program intervention. *Journal of Nursing Care Quality*, 27, 341–345. doi:10.1097/NCQ.0b013e31825f4a5f

Taleb, N. N., Goldstein, D. G., & Spitznagel, M. W. (2009, October). The six mistakes executives make in risk management. *Harvard Business Review*, 1–6 (Reprint R0910G).

Vestal, K. (1988). Writing a business plan. *Nursing Economic$*, 6(3), 121–124.

Waxman, K. T. (2015). *Finance and budgeting made simple: Essential skills for nurses*. Marblehead, MA: HCPro.

15 Teaching Financial Management and Program Development

Fay L. Bower and Anna Mullins

This chapter is dedicated to preparing nurses who have a doctor of nursing practice (DNP) degree about how to teach financial management to nurses in both practice and academic environments. All nurses need to understand health care economics because knowledge in this area promotes a better understanding of the nature and organization of the health care environment. In addition, appreciation and the use of economic theories and principles help advance the profession of nursing and assist nurses with advanced degrees to share this important information with others. Health profession education is an important "bridge to quality" as emphasized by Greiner and Knebel in *Health Profession Education: A Bridge to Quality* (2003).

This chapter also contains a discussion on the use of economic principles during program development and program evaluation, along with frameworks and teaching strategies that are important for teaching these economic principles and theories. For example, the implementation of a new academic program, regardless of the focus, requires many processes, procedures, and approvals. Thus, planning and allowing for adequate time must be considered early.

Teaching financial management requires the use of adult learning principles and critical thinking in order to maximize and enhance the learning experience. The use of a variety of teaching strategies such as case studies, role-play, the use of treasure hunts, and so forth, is very important in assisting the adult learner to experience and gain skills in the application of what he or she has learned about financial management.

The chapter is presented in two parts: The first part covers the issues, processes, and strategies needed to develop an academic program, and the second covers information about teaching financial management.

■ PROGRAM DEVELOPMENT FOR ACADEMIC SETTINGS

This part of the chapter discusses the necessary considerations for the development of an academic program. This process is presented and organized into five phases: needs assessment, approval, preimplementation, implementation, and evaluation. Each phase is discussed in depth and is provided for those who are interested in the development of a DNP program.

PHASE ONE: THE NEEDS ASSESSMENT

There are three steps in the needs assessment phase: development of a feasibility study, cost analysis of the program, and development of the curriculum for the program. Each step takes considerable time, as there are several activities to be completed in each.

Development of a Feasibility Study

One of the most important activities when developing a new program is to determine the need for the program. This activity is known as the feasibility study. During this study, a survey of the surrounding area is conducted to determine whether there are any similar programs being offered and whether they are public or private, if they are online, if they are offered in the classroom, or if they are hybrids (a combination of both). Knowing whether there are other programs provides information about the potential for enrollments in this new program. Whether the programs are public or private lets one know about the cost, which is a critical indicator of whether anyone will be interested in paying what it takes to enroll in the new program. The design of the curriculum is also very important, as it indicates whether potential students will be interested. Every program needs to have something special to offer to entice interest. A survey of what is currently offered elsewhere will provide valuable information that can be used when the design of the program is being considered.

It is also important to determine whether there are workplace positions where the graduates can find jobs, as students are not willing to obtain degrees that do not prepare them for a position in health care and/or education.

Not only is there a need to determine the outcomes for the graduate, but there is also a need to determine whether any changes in the college/university will be necessary to offer the program, such as space, resources, courses outside of nursing, and so forth. Thus, the feasibility study includes a survey of the college/university, as well as a survey of the opportunities for employment at graduation.

Cost Analysis of the Program

The very important next step is to determine the cost of the program. This would include the cost of administrators and faculty over a period of at least 5 years; the cost of new equipment, if needed; and the cost of services beyond what is currently available, such as remedial services, library hours, and food services if the program is offered on campus. If the program will be offered by interactive video, the cost of the hours being used to deliver the program to other sites would need to be estimated. This would also include the cost of a video assistant, who would be in charge of monitoring and managing the delivery of the program.

The cost analysis might also include monies for the rental of space if the campus cannot provide adequate classroom or lab space. Many DNP programs are offered at off-site locations, so the program is more accessible to students. If the program is offered online, there are other costs that must be determined.

Another important cost is the marketing of the program. Monies for the development of flyers and ads by radio and television (TV) can be very costly, so the selection of which venue to use becomes very important. The way to determine the best venue is to know something about the population to be sought; that is, are the nurses likely to listen to the radio, watch TV, or learn about the program as a member of a nursing organization? To gain this information, it is necessary to contact different nursing organizations, talk with nurses at nursing schools, or do a random survey using the names of nurses that can be purchased from a board of nursing or nursing publications, such as *Nurse Week*.

Along with the cost of items is the prediction of the revenue. Again, the feasibility study is used to determine the estimated number of students who would be attracted to the program. It is wise to have the number of projected students be enough to pay for the costs and to generate a profit for the institution. It is not enough to demonstrate the costs are covered. The projected number of students should not only be a guess, but should be supported by strong evidence. Many schools have conducted surveys of nurses using names by zip code to determine interest in a new program.

As can be imagined, the cost analysis in the feasibility study is very important and can be the determinant of approval or denial of approval; therefore, much time and energy should go into its development. Again, it helps to have input from various persons on campus who can help with the costs of services and the projected needs.

Curriculum Development

Another important area of the feasibility study is the curriculum, which is to be described and validated so that it is consistent with the mission and goals of the college/university. For example, if the mission of the university is (a) to support individual achievement; (b) to provide excellence and the use of creative, effective teaching; and (c) to serve the academic needs and interests of a diverse student body, these aspects must be reflective in the curriculum either as course content, classroom activities, or the way students are evaluated. Since each academic institution has a different mission and goals, it is very important that the curriculum developer seeks advice from others on campus who can help with the incorporation of the mission and goals into the program.

In addition, the curriculum must include the *Essentials* of a DNP program as described by the American Association of Colleges of Nursing (AACN, 2010). These essentials are:

- Scientific Underpinnings for Practice
- Organizational and Systems Leadership for Quality Improvement and Systems Thinking
- Clinical Scholarship and Analytical Methods for Evidence-Based Practice
- Information Systems/Technology and Patient Care Technology for the Improvement and Transformation of Health Care
- Health Care Policy for Advocacy in Health Care
- Interprofessional Collaboration for Improving Patient and Population Health Outcomes
- Clinical Prevention and Population Health for Improving the Nation's Health
- Advanced Nursing Practice

The curriculum elements, structure, and several other required aspects of the program can be found at the AACN website (www.aacn.nche.edu).

When designing the curriculum, considering the aforementioned criteria, it is also important the developer consider the potential enrollees—that is, the students. Since most master's and doctoral students are adults who are working, it is important to consider what, besides the content, should be considered to attract them. This is again where the feasibility study becomes important, for knowing what is currently available at other institutions and what the population of nurses might be looking for help in the design of the curriculum. Although the content is driven by the AACN *Essentials of Doctoral Education for Advanced Nursing Practice (DNP)*, the schedule of classes and the method for the delivery of the content can be determined using the data collected in the feasibility study.

Another aspect of the curriculum is the focus of the program. Many DNP programs are designed for nurse practitioners (NPs), whereas some are designed for educators or administrators. Again, it is the feasibility study and the AACN *DNP Essentials* that need to be used to determine the focus of the program. Determining the focus may also depend on the resources of the college/university. Since some of the courses might be outside nursing, it is important to determine whether the courses are already available on campus or whether new courses outside nursing will be needed. The feasibility study is the best source for this information.

PHASE TWO: THE APPROVAL

Department/School Approval

Once the feasibility study, which includes the curriculum, is completed, it usually is presented to the department or school of nursing faculty for approval. Although several faculty members may have been consulted during the development process, the usual next step is to present the new program to the entire faculty for approval. This might mean a presentation to the science faculty, as well as the nursing faculty, since there may be courses in the curriculum outside of nursing.

This presentation to faculty should not be done without previous discussions, so it is clear to the faculty exactly what is being asked for when the proposal is presented. Informal discussions are also helpful if there are questions. These questions could then be included and answered during the formal presentation.

Academic Senate Approval

Once the faculty approves the new program, the Academic Senate of the college/university is approached for approval. Again, the proposal must be clear, include the curriculum design, and be sent to the senate members prior to the presentation for approval. If approved by the senate, it usually must be approved by the college/university board of directors. Throughout this process, it is important to notify the college/university accreditation agency to keep them informed of any changes in the offerings of the institution.

State Board Approval

Dependent on the processes and regulations of the state, approval may be required from the State Board of Nursing. This is different for each state, so knowing the regulations of the state should also be part of the feasibility study. If there is a need for state approval by the Board of Nursing, an additional study might be required. The Commission on Collegiate Nursing Education (2009) provides an excellent reference for accreditation standards.

PHASE THREE: PREIMPLEMENTATION

Development of a Marketing Plan

An important aspect of the development of a new program is letting the public know about it. This means a marketing plan must be developed. The marketing plan includes at least three activities: a description of the identified population, the information to be disseminated about the program, and the ways this information will be delivered to the identified population.

Description of the Identified Population

Here again is where the feasibility study comes into use, as the population to be attracted to the program should have been identified in the study. In the case of the DNP program, the potential enrollees are usually master of science in nursing (MSN) graduates interested in a doctoral degree that focuses on the practice of advanced nursing. Surveys, email blasts to nurses in particular areas, and visits to schools of nursing to talk with the students are some of the strategies used to reach this population.

Information to Be Disseminated

The preparation of flyers, ads, and email blasts must be short, to the point, and attractive. Color is also important. The outcome of being a graduate of the program also needs to be emphasized, as well as what makes this program better or more useful than another. Evening courses, online delivery, and the location are often areas of interest to nurses. Since most nurses in a DNP program are employed, it is useful to design a program that addresses this issue.

One way to address these issues of what to say about the program is to ask, "Why would I choose this program? What do I expect after completion of the program, that is, what can it do to advance my career?" The answer to this question will provide data that can be used to promote the program. For instance, if the program meets one weekend a month for 4 days and is followed by online activities during the rest of the month, and I have a full-time job that includes three 12-hour shifts a week, I might be very interested in the program because I can fit it into my work week and can also enjoy the student-to-student activities once a month in the classroom. And if I know what this degree can do for my career in nursing, then I would probably be interested.

Another aspect of marketing is to use the right words, that is, words that attract attention, such as, "going to school while working fulltime," "advance your career with a DNP degree," or "join those who are preparing for the future."

Ways to Disseminate Information About a New Program

Mailed flyers, radio and TV announcements, and signs in public places, such as train and bus stations, city posters, and in areas where there is a lot of visibility are some of the ways to reach nurses. Information in professional publications is another useful way to reach nurses. Visits to nursing organizations are another way to promote a new program. Over time, a useful and very productive way to attract new students is by word of mouth, especially if provided by a satisfied graduate of the program.

Development of Admission Procedures and Policies

After the curriculum has been approved, the admission policies and procedures need to be determined. For example, what criteria will be used to admit students? What procedures will then need to be implemented to admit the students once the criteria have been defined? For example, if the criteria include a grade point average (GPA) of 3.00 in the master program, two letters of reference, and a statement of purpose, who will review the data and who will make the decision for admission? In many academic institutions, the admission staff makes the decisions, and at others, a committee of faculty makes the decisions.

Besides who, what specific issues will be expected in the reference letters and in the student statement of purpose? At some institutions, the specific issues to be addressed in a reference letter are included in the form sent to the person providing the reference. This could be a statement about the student's motivation, quality of communication, ability to relate to colleagues, and so forth. As for the student statement of purpose, usually this letter is about the student's reasons for seeking the degree and what the student expects to do after receiving the degree. This letter helps the persons evaluating the letter determine whether the applicant understands the purpose of the degree and whether the applicant is ready for advanced practice in nursing.

Lastly, it is important to determine a cutoff point when no more applications will be accepted. This deadline might also apply to when the reference letters are submitted.

Generally, the last day for an application is about 3 weeks before the beginning of the semester/quarter, which gives the staff time to process the late applications.

Preparation of the Syllabus

Preparation of the syllabi for the total curriculum involves a lot of time and many participants. In order to have a quality program, experts in various areas and levels must be involved in the preparation of the syllabi. For instance, experts in advanced pathophysiology, advanced health assessment, and advanced pharmacology will be needed, as not all faculty have expertise in these advanced areas, and these areas are required by AACN in a DNP program. Again, it is important to consult the AACN *DNP Essentials* document (AACN, 2006) to determine the areas that are needed in the curriculum. Additional resources regarding syllabi are provided by O'Brien,

Missis, and Cohen in *The Course Syllabus* (2008) and B. Rambur in *Healthcare Finance, Economics, and Policy for Nurses: A Foundational Guide* (2015).

Like any syllabus, the following areas should be included:

- A course description
- A statement about the purpose of the course
- The objectives that must be accomplished by each student
- A list of the required textbooks
- How the student will be evaluated, such as what activities will be graded and how the grade will be determined
- If the course will be offered in a classroom, a schedule that has a list of the dates of the classes and what will be covered during each session. If the course will be online, there should be a time frame for when the content will be offered and what the students are to specifically do on their own time
- Frequently, specific activities are described, such as an assignment about a review of the literature, or a scholarly discussion about a subject selected by the student that meets a specific course objective

Selection and Approval of Faculty

Another important activity is the selection of faculty. This process should begin way ahead of these other activities, as it is not easy to locate properly prepared faculty for a doctoral program. In most cases, the faculty should have a doctoral degree and expertise in the areas of the program. Online searches, ads in professional journals, and help from search companies will be needed and can be costly but well worth the expenditure.

Once information from applicants is received, a "teaching episode" should be scheduled so that the applicant can demonstrate his or her teaching style. Also, each resume should contain the names of persons the search team members can call for questioning. Although reference letters are helpful, a call to the applicant's present or former dean/director is very often more informative. An important aspect of a call to a reference person must be to include the same questions each time so there is consistency in the data acquired.

If the applicant has never taught before but is qualified by nursing practice and a degree that prepared her or him for teaching, a part-time position might be offered, giving her or him a chance to gain the level of teaching skills necessary for the program. If the program is governed by Board of Nursing regulations, there may be other procedures the applicant will need to meet.

Scheduling of Classes

The scheduling of classes depends on the design of the program. If the program will be offered online, the scheduling is more open, yet the students need to know when certain activities are to occur and whether there is any time allocated to the campus site. If the program is to be offered in the traditional classroom, the student needs to know the dates and the expectations for those dates. The expected dates for the submission of assignments must be clearly stated in the syllabus so that the student can arrange the necessary time to accomplish the tasks.

Classes or online activities are often scheduled during the late afternoons, evenings, and during the weekends because most of the students are employed while attending school.

PHASE FOUR: IMPLEMENTATION

Review of the Applications

This implementation phase begins with the review of the student applications. Again, there should be a consistent process used, so the selection is based on standard criteria. Generally, the committee that reviews the applications looks first at the GPA earned in the former completed program (usually a master's degree program) and then at the recommendation letters. Using standard criteria, the committee members look at the statements provided to determine whether they are what is needed to successfully complete the program. Such items as self-direction, motivation, good communication skills, and the ability to accomplish the objectives of the program will be expected. There may be other items offered in the reference letter than those the committee is looking for, but they need to be indicators of success to be considered.

If a letter is required that indicates the applicant's goals for the future, then the committee must agree on what they expect. They also often use this document to determine the applicant's writing skills. A problem often encountered with the applicant letter is that one never knows who really wrote the letter. To address this problem, some faculty have had the applicant write a statement at the time of the interview about his or her goals for the future. This way they know the applicant wrote the statement and they also can determine the applicant's writing skills.

A history of nursing practice will also be expected, as many programs offer a specialty in the DNP. If the program offers an NP focus, then the committee will be looking for a history of the applicant's practice in acute care. If the focus is nursing administration, then the nursing history of the applicant should be acute care or community care. If there has been a period of no employment, the applicant will probably be asked during the interview to explain this phenomenon.

Interviewing Applicants

A valuable way to determine the qualifications of a program applicant is to use an interview to collect data. However, the interview should be standardized, that is, be the same for each applicant so no bias enters the data. A list of questions that reveal in depth the applicant's understanding of the degree and what it will take to complete the program is very helpful in the selection process. A few of the questions that have been used are:

- What do you know about the DNP degree?
- How did you learn about the curriculum?
- What are your career goals after completion of the DNP program?
- Will you be working while attending the DNP program? If so, will you have support with your other responsibilities?
- How long has it been since you were in school, working on the completion of a degree?
- How would you describe your reading and writing skills?
- Have you ever attended an online program?
- Do you have any questions about this DNP program?

Selection of Students for Enrollment

Once the applications have been reviewed and the interviews have been completed, the selection process can begin. It is wise to wait until all of the applicants have been interviewed to make the decisions about who to accept into the program. The number of acceptances is contingent upon the predetermined first group. This group could be smaller than later ones in order to determine whether there are any program changes needed in the future. It is not uncommon for the first group to be a "pilot group."

Letters should be sent letting the applicants know of their acceptance to the program. In the letter, there should also be a statement about what the new student should do to register. It is not unusual for the registration to take place online with the help of a faculty person. However, some schools like to register new students in person so they can get to know them.

Registering New Students

During the registration process, the faculty members get to know the student and the student gets to know more about the curriculum. It is also a time for questions that were not addressed earlier, including new questions from the student that may have arisen during the registration process. It is also a chance for a review of the entire program and what the demands on the student may be. It is at this time the student learns about how to communicate with faculty and how to access the library, an important resource when registered in a doctoral program.

Where the classes will meet and at what time is also reviewed at this time; other topics, such as how to access the courses online, when the assignments are due, and where to get the syllabus, can be described by the faculty. If applicable, getting passwords, entry codes, and instructions to access the online site are also provided at this time.

Offering First-Year Courses

When the courses for the first semester/quarter are offered, the *implementation phase* has been completed. Although this could be considered the completion of the initiation of a new DNP program, there are several other important activities that must be addressed, and some of them begin with the implementation of the first courses. For example, the following activities must be considered as some of the ways an evaluation of a new program can be accomplished:

- Student evaluations
- Teacher evaluations
- Pre- and posttesting of students' critical thinking skills
- An annual program review
- Employer follow-up calls about graduates of the program

PHASE FIVE: EVALUATION

Student Evaluations

Evaluation of the program is extremely important in order to keep it current, relevant, and future focused. It is a common activity for a program to be evaluated by the recipients of the program (the students). Some educational institutions require students to evaluate each course, whereas others expect students to evaluate the program at its completion. Either or both is a good idea, as the information can be very useful with a new program to determine whether the objectives are being met, whether the teaching style of the faculty is considered helpful, and whether the AACN *DNP Essentials* are being implemented.

The evaluation tool should be easy to answer yet be complete so that the data collected can be used to make changes, if necessary. This tool has been used for many years at the end of every course, because it provides the data needed to determine the effectiveness of both the teacher and the coursework. Many changes have been made as a result of the findings gained from this tool.

Space should also be provided on the evaluation tool for comments, because this allows students to provide data that might not be realized with standard items. Students like the opportunity to offer concerns and ideas for change. They believe this acknowledges them as an important source of personal information.

Teacher Evaluations

Feedback from faculty about a new program is necessary, because they have a unique and close view of the successes and failures or problems that surface during the implementation of a new program. Whether it be content focused, a teaching strategy, or something about the students, it is important to hear from those who are actually implementing the new program. Sometimes, it is an issue of time, such as not enough time given the scope of the content; the numbers of students in a classroom; or access to the library from home. Being in the center of the action, the faculty members have a view no one else has and have the opportunity to bring to the attention of others what changes need to be made.

Pre- and Posttesting of Students' Critical Thinking Skills

Another useful strategy for measuring the outcomes of the program is to measure the students' critical thinking skills. The role of the DNP, as a leader, suggests that the graduates of the program need to be critical thinkers. One way to determine whether the program prepared them to be critical thinkers is to measure their critical thinking skills at the beginning and then again at the end of the program.

There are several tools to measure critical thinking, but one that is used by a local university department of nursing can be accessed online. It is a 25-multichoice question tool that presents a scenario for each question. It is not measuring nursing decisions, but simple situations that demand the consideration of options to answer the question. It truly demands that one think critically about the right answer.

If critical thinking is one of the objectives of the program, then being able to measure whether the students' critical thinking skills have improved is essential. The findings are then used to examine the program to determine whether critical thinking is a strategy used by the faculty in the clinical sites, in the classroom, or in the assignments the students submit for grades.

Annual Program Review

A very useful tool for measuring the effectiveness of a program is to conduct an annual review of the total program. The annual review is comprehensive and allows for a comparison among years. One format for an annual review is the following:

I. Centrality: Contribution to the mission of the university
   A. How do instruction and service contribute to the coherent whole of the mission?
   B. How does this program help to sustain and stimulate related work elsewhere in the university?
II. Program description and data
   A. Degrees offered
   B. Faculty–student ratio
   C. Average credit hours generated in the program
   D. Appropriateness and effectiveness of the admission requirements
   E. Appropriateness and effectiveness of the utilization of the existing human/physical/financial resources
   F. Recommended innovative changes in the program(s) that would address changes in:
      1. Discipline or field
      2. Student demand
      3. Occupational demand
      4. Societal need
III. Learning outcome assessment
   A. How is assessment information used in a systematic way to improve the curriculum, teaching, and learning?
   B. What is the evidence that feedback and adjustments have improved the curriculum, instruction, and student learning?
IV. Program strengths
V. Market attractiveness
   A. Accessibility
   B. Flexibility
   C. Reputation
   D. Alumni support
   E. Quality of faculty
   F. Cost
   G. Accommodating staff

      H. Partnerships
      I. Availability
  VI. Areas in need of improvement
 VII. Action plan

Employer Follow-Up Telephone Survey

Because employers are so busy, telephone calls arranged in advance with the approval of the graduate have proved to be very useful. The process begins with a call to the graduates to determine where they are working as a DNP and whether their supervisor or administrator would be willing to answer some questions in a 15-minute telephone call. When the list of those willing to take a call is long, a random selection of those names can be done to make the process possible.

    The questions to be asked of the employers should reflect the objectives of the program, so the data can be used to determine whether the program is accomplishing the goals set by the planners of the program.

▨ TEACHING FINANCIAL MANAGEMENT

USING ADULT LEARNING AND CRITICAL THINKING AS FRAMEWORKS

Learning is the act, process, or experience of gaining knowledge or skills. It helps us move from novice to expert, as described by Benner (2001) in her book *From Novice to Expert: Excellence and Power in Clinical Nursing Practice*. In order to work with adult learners, the following body of knowledge is helpful.

    Adults are usually motivated to learn in the following ways:

- Seeking learning experiences to help them cope with a life-changing event (e.g., a new job, promotion, divorce, retirement). The more life changes an individual experiences, the more likely he or she is to seek learning opportunities that will assist him or her in dealing with significant changes.
- Seeking a learning experience because they need the knowledge or skill being taught. Learning, for them, is a means to an end, not an end in itself.
- Being self-directed and expecting to take responsibility for their decisions and their learning.

    When working with the adult learner, there are key principles that are important to keep in mind:

- The learning program should capitalize on the experiences of the participants.
- Adult learners need to know why they need to learn something and to be involved in the planning and evaluation of their instruction. They also want feedback.
- Experience (including mistakes) provides the basis for the learning activities.
- Adults approach learning as problem solving so they need to be involved experientially.
- Adults are most interested in learning something that has immediate relevance to their job or their life.
- Adult learning is problem centered rather than content oriented and the instructor should act as a facilitator or resource rather than a lecturer or evaluator.
- Adults need to be able to integrate new ideas with what they already know so they can retain and utilize the new information more readily.
- Adult learners tend to take errors personally with a negative impact on their self-esteem; sometimes, as a result, they stay with tried-and-true solutions rather than taking risks.
- Adult learning opportunities must be designed to accept viewpoints from people in different life stages, cultural and ethnic backgrounds, and with different sets of values.

Rideout's *Transforming Nursing Education Through Problem-Based Learning* (2001) is a good reference.

LEARNING STYLES

Learning styles are different approaches or ways that people learn. Having an awareness of one's own learning style can help that person develop strategies to maximize his or her ability to learn in a given situation. Also, when serving as an instructor, by knowing the learning style of students and discussing similarities and differences, one can establish more effective ways to construct and deliver classes and classroom activities to promote greater comprehension learning.

Types of Learning Styles

Visual learners—These individuals need to see the teacher's body language and expressions in order to understand the material presented. One often finds these learners sitting at the front of the room to avoid any obstruction, such as people's heads. They learn best from diagrams, flip-charts, handouts, and other visual aids, and they often take very detailed notes.

Auditory learners—Auditory learners prefer verbal lectures and discussions. They like to discuss issues with others. These learners are particularly astute to tone of voice, pitch, speed, and so forth to assist them with their interpretation of underlying meaning. Written information is not as meaningful until it is heard, and the auditory learner often benefits from reading aloud and using a tape recorder.

Tactile/kinesthetic learners (TKL)—These individuals learn by doing, moving, and touching. They like a more hands-on approach and are eager to explore the physical world around them. TKLs often find it hard to sit for long periods of time and may become distracted by their need for activity and movement.

Few individuals have just one learning style. Most often, there are combinations with perhaps greater dominance in one area than another. For example, a person may be primarily an auditory learner who also absorbs materials better when they are listening and doing something at the same time. Table 15.1 is a tool that is very helpful in assessing one's own learning style as well as that of learners.

This chart helps determine the learning style. Reading the word in the left column and then answering the questions in the successive three columns determines how to respond to each situation. The answers may fall into all three columns, but one column will likely contain the most answers. The dominant column indicates the primary learning style.

Critical Thinking

The second framework that is very important in teaching financial management is that of critical thinking. Critical thinking is a vital problem-solving tool in every realm of nursing and is an integral component of clinical decision making. It is the ability to think in a systematic and logical manner promoting more comprehensive identification of problems/issues and therefore a better opportunity to identify the most appropriate actions and solutions. Critical thinking promotes adherence to intellectual standards for nurses as well as the proficiency to use reason and thinking skills for sound clinical judgments and safe decision making. It also guarantees the effective exercise of professional judgment. Scheffer and Rubenfeld (2000) provide a good reference in the article "A Consensus Statement on Critical Thinking in Nursing."

Critical thinking is necessary for:

- Problem solving
- Priority setting
- Decision making

TABLE 15.1 Assessment Tool for Learning Styles

When You . . .	Visual	Auditory	Kinesthetic and Tactile
Spell	Do you try to see the word?	Do you sound out the word or use a phonetic approach?	Do you write the word down to find if it feels right?
Talk	Do you dislike listening for too long? Do you favor words such as *see, picture,* and *imagine*?	Do you enjoy listening but are impatient to talk? Do you use words such as *hear, tune,* and *think*?	Do you gesture and use expressive movements? Do you use words such as *feel, touch,* and *hold*?
Concentrate	Do you become distracted by untidiness or movement?	Do you become distracted by sounds or noises?	Do you become distracted by activity around you?
Meet someone again	Do you forget names but remember faces, or remember where you met?	Do you forget faces but remember names, or remember what you talked about?	Do you remember best what you did together?
Contact people on business	Do you prefer direct, face-to-face, personal meetings?	Do you prefer the telephone?	Do you talk with them while walking or participating in an activity?
Read	Do you like descriptive scenes or pause to imagine the actions?	Do you enjoy dialog and conversation or hear the characters talk?	Do you prefer action stories or are not a keen reader?
Do something new at work	Do you like to see demonstrations, diagrams, slides, or posters?	Do you prefer verbal instructions or talking about it with someone else?	Do you prefer to jump right in and try it?
Put something together	Do you look at the directions and the picture?		Do you ignore the directions and figure it out as you go along?
Need help with a computer application	Do you seek out pictures or diagrams?	Do you call the help desk, ask a neighbor, or growl at the computer?	Do you keep trying to do it?

And, it includes:

- Attitude—the willingness to recognize a problem and go after the whole picture
- Knowledge—an ability to determine the accuracy of evidence presented
- Skills—the ability to put the above into practice

For example, when one applies critical thinking to nursing, he or she thinks of clarifying the meaning of data or a situation; to recognize a pattern and form a proposition that then leads to analysis in which the ideas are prioritized and examined to identify implications. Through inference one draws conclusions based on the evidence and analysis in order to generate a set of priorities, utilize available resources, and draw conclusions. A person can then explain the conclusion and make choices based on a rule, principle, or standard. One can then evaluate in order to assess and reassess the data and conclusions for ongoing relevance.

Rubenfeld and Scheffer (2010), in the book *Critical Thinking Tactics for Nurses*, describe the 10 key tactics for critical thinking as

- Confidence
- Contextual perspective
- Creativity
- Flexibility
- Inquisitiveness
- Intellectual integrity
- Intuition
- Open-mindedness
- Perseverance
- Reflection

For example, if a DNP is teaching aspects of financial management in an academic and/or practice environment to other nurses, it is important to determine the learners' level of knowledge in the field and how they will utilize the standards and guidelines in their area of practice. In the next section of this chapter, the authors will provide examples of activities that can be used with learners to improve their abilities in the area of critical thinking, building on the principles of adult learning, as well as how to use their various learning styles. Fink, in *Creative Learning Experiences* (2003), stresses the importance of providing different learning experiences when developing and implementing curricula.

TEACHING STRATEGIES

The process of teaching or the study of being a teacher is often referred to as pedagogy. The term generally refers to strategies of instruction, or a style of instruction. As a teacher, one creates an environment in which students can participate to the best of their abilities. For adult learners, that environment is where the adult learner can tackle a problem or issue, apply his or her experience and skills, and be actively involved in the learning process. The instructor acts as a facilitator or resource for the educational activity. The teaching strategies that will be discussed in this chapter are preparing a class, case studies, small group work, role-play, treasure hunts, and games.

Preparing a Class

When beginning preparation for a class, effective teachers systematically and carefully think about what content is to be taught so that they can make productive use of whatever instructional time is allotted. In other words, what financial principles are going to be taught and how one can use the time provided in an effective and meaningful manner that promotes the most effective use of the adult learning theories and critical thinking.

A primary role for an instructor is to design a lesson plan for class(s). Such plans are essential to aid in the organization and delivery of lessons. Lesson plans also need to suit the individual teacher's style of presentation and the type of content being presented. Important steps in preparing a class include:

- Class title and description, including date, time, length of class, and any continuing education hours
- Goals
- Learning objectives
- Type of student
- Content
- Instructional procedures/teaching strategies

- Evaluation procedures
- Supplementary reading, materials required

Preparing a class requires more than making arbitrary decisions about "what I'm going to teach today." As illustrated, a number of activities precede the process of actual delivery of the class content. The job is not complete until after the instructor has assessed both the learner's attainment of the objectives and anticipated outcomes and effectiveness of the class in leading learners to these outcomes.

An important note to remember is that instructors rarely adhere to highly structured and detailed class plans in lock-step fashion. Such rigidity would probably hinder, rather than help, the teaching–learning process. The steps for preparing a class, as outlined earlier, are guiding principles because the actual preparation must permit flexible delivery.

Case Studies

Case studies are an effective way to provide examples of situations that can be interpreted in many different ways and lead to a variety of conclusions by the participants. The use of case studies enables participants to apply learned concepts through either group discussion or role-play.

When explaining case studies, the instructor asks the participants to consider examples that may have occurred in their own personal/work environment. Second, he or she directs the participants to identify the issues in the case study and also think about their own "personal case study" and how it may or may not relate to each. At the conclusion of the case study activity, the instructor summarizes the issues addressed as well as the lessons and messages to be taken away by the participants.

Example: Evaluation of an Electronic Medical Record

As the nursing representative to your organization's electronic medical record (EMR) project, you are asked to consider financial issues associated with EMR implementation in your department. To do this, you must be very clear about how your department wants to use the EMR. Although vendors should be expected to provide measurement tools to help estimate costs throughout the planning, development, and implementation phase, purchasers of systems share the obligation of determining how the costs and benefits of the EMR will be evaluated.

1. Describe how your department will utilize this technology.
2. Suggest benefits you might expect the EMR system to provide, and the measures that could be used to describe those benefits.
3. Discuss ways your work as a nurse might be influenced by future EMR developments.

Small Group Work

Small group work and group discussion is not a debate. It is an effort to bring out a wide variety of ideas and understandings about an issue or topic. A major component of the group's work is to clarify the issues presented and to form a group opinion or recommendations concerning the issues or to formulate better questions, which might help find the answers. Important guidelines are the following:

- Select a person to be the recorder and one to be the spokesperson for the group
- Listen carefully to others and take notes of different perspectives presented by group members
- Watch for body language that may indicate what a group member is feeling
- Build on what others have said as a way of expanding and combining ideas in order to achieve the best possible end product
- Remember to be courteous and respectful
- Encourage each group member to share pertinent information or ask questions that will help accomplish the task

- Keep the group's task in mind at all times; all group members must help keep the focus on the task at hand
- Stay within the time limitations for accomplishing the task
- Do not let someone dominate the discussion; all should be encouraged and given the opportunity to participate

Example: Group Discussion

Emergency department (ED) use for nonurgent care is extremely costly in comparison to care in clinics or nonurgent care settings. Many ED users do not have access to health care other than the ED; therefore, monitoring resources is important.

1. Select a person to record the outcomes of the group discussion.
2. Select someone to facilitate the discussion and to encourage each member to participate and share his or her views and/or questions. Areas for discussion on this topic should include:
   a. Identification of the financial management role of the nurse as a manager and leader
   b. Determine the major issues in this situation and how they are being addressed
   c. Name three things you would suggest to address this situation
   d. Determine whether nursing is involved and, if not, should it be?

Role-Play

Role-playing as a teaching strategy offers several advantages for both teacher and student. First, a student's interest in the topic is raised along with his or her participation in the learning experience. Research has shown that integrating experiential learning activities into a class increases the learner's interest in the subject matter and his or her understanding of the class content. Secondly, the learner is more involved by engaging in a role-playing lesson. A third advantage to using role-playing as a teaching strategy is that it teaches empathy and understanding of different perspectives. Role-playing activities require a person to assume a role, acting as that individual would in a given situation.

Example: Role-Playing and Reducing Waste Without Impacting Quality of Care

Working in groups of six, identify one way that waste in the use of supplies/products could be reduced in everyday practice without impacting quality of care. Discuss an implementation plan and select a chairperson to act as a representative from the finance department. The remainder of the participants will be: two nurses, one housekeeper, one person from central supply, and one person from food services who will assume these roles for the deliberation. At the end of the activity, the chair will describe the idea and plan, as well as the process used for reaching a decision within the group.

Summary and concluding discussion:

1. Provide a time for participants to debrief and define what they have learned through the role-playing activity and emphasize the importance of the lessons learned.
2. Allow for all participants to have the opportunity to speak.
3. Summarize the purpose of the role-play scenario and add any additional feedback.

Treasure Hunt

A treasure hunt is a very effective tool for teaching nurses how to access and use resources within their organization. Even though nurses may work in an organization, they often lack the understanding of how things are done. This is particularly true in the area of financial operations within an institution. Many employees do not see financial statements, participate in the preparation of the budget, or know how financial operations work. A treasure hunt is a creative and iterative instructional activity that can enable a nurse to gain a better of understanding of a particular area and build relationships with those who work there.

Example: Treasure Hunt for Things Commonly Used in Patient Care

The following listed items are some of the commonly used activities to provide patient care. Also listed are resources that can be used during the daily practice. Time should be taken to not only locate the supplies, but also to thoroughly familiarize one's self with the contents of the resources listed. This is also a time to introduce one's self to the nurses and other staff on the unit. Unit staff can help find:

- Location of evacuation routes
- Location of fire extinguishers
- Emergency (code) cart
- Personal protective equipment
- Bathrooms
- Empty patient room:
  - Emergency power outlets
  - Emergency lighting
  - Wall O_2
  - Call light
  - Bed controls and brake
  - Side rails
  - Bathroom door light switch

Additionally, the process used for monitoring budgetary performance also needs to be identified.

Students will locate the following items and be prepared to give a verbal and written report on their findings:

1. Conduct an interview with a member of the health care management team in the organization. This individual should be one level higher than one's current position. For example, if you are a staff nurse, interview the nurse manager; if you are a nurse manager, interview the chief nurse executive to determine the processes used for:
   a. Developing the capital and operating budgets for the organization
   b. Developing the capital and operating budget for the specific nursing unit/department, service, and so forth
   c. Budget approval
   d. Budgetary monitoring and/or corrective action
2. Bring a copy of the operating and capital budget from the area where the interview was conducted, along with a description of the size and type of the area. Remove the name of the area or organization. Save this material because it will be used for a future activity in the class.
3. Bring a copy of the latest financial or variance report for the area that indicates the actual performance as compared to the budget. Remove any identifying factors about the organization.

Games

The use of games for instruction began thousands of years ago. For example, China used board games and war games for teaching purposes over 5,000 years ago. One of the greatest strengths of using games for learning is that they are excellent tools for connecting learners to knowledge, key concepts, facts, and processes in a way that is both fun *and* purposeful. They are an interactive method used by the instructor that engages and increases the participants' knowledge and awareness of a particular topic. The high level of involvement of the participants, the competition, and the pleasure of playing a game allows for the building of skills and competencies over time. El-Shamy, in the book, *Training Games* (2001), discusses how games are fun and reinforce learning, and how it takes careful reflection and facilitation of the game by the instructor to make it meaningful for the participants. Regardless of whether one is in an academic environment or corporate America, games can enhance the learning process.

Example: Jeopardy

Directions for the game would include:

- This popular television game is played with three contestants and a host.
- Contestants are presented with an answer and must provide the question that precedes it in order to win a round.
- The contestant who wins the most rounds is the winner.
- Responses must be phrased in the form of a question (e.g., capital of the United States; response is, "What is Washington, DC?").
- Four volunteers are selected from among the class participants; three to serve as contestants and one to serve as the timekeeper/scorekeeper.
- Each contestant will have 15 seconds to offer his or her response once the answer is flashed on the screen and read by the instructor, the host for the game.
- No more than eight to 10 answers should be included in the game.
- A contestant will shout out his or her response as soon as he or she knows it; the student to respond first is the winner of the round.

Sample Jeopardy answers in a game regarding financial management could be:

- Document for an organization that focuses on revenues, expenses, and profitability. Answer: What is a balance sheet?
- Money owed to the organization for services rendered. Answer: What is accounts receivable?
- Land, buildings, and equipment that won't be converted into cash within one year. Answer: What are fixed or long-term assets?

At the end of each round, the instructor/host may want to comment on the particular answer, its significance, points to remember, and so on, and the fact that the goal of this game was to familiarize participants with key principles in financial management relevant to their area of work. At the end of the game, the scorekeeper will announce the winner: the person with the most correct answers. It is suggested that the host offers a small prize to each of the four class participants.

■ CONCLUSION

This chapter contained a description of the essential components to assist nurses who are pursuing a DNP degree to teach financial management to nurses in both practice and academic settings. The reader should keep in mind the suggestions offered in this chapter have worked for others and can be used; however, since each practice environment and academic setting is different, other activities and strategies may be demanded in addition to those presented here. The information presented is not a recipe intended to be proscriptive, but rather assistive so that financial management principles are not shrouded in mystery for nurses. They can learn how to apply these principles to program development in an academic setting and teach other nurses how to understand and use these concepts and principles, as well.

And, as an advanced practice registered nurse (APRN) who will teach others, this quote is an important one to remember, "A good teacher is like a candle—it consumes itself to light the way for others" (author unknown).

CRITICAL THINKING EXERCISES

1. Take a moment and think about the benefits that budgeting provides. Then write one sentence in response to each of these questions:
   a. How can budgeting help planning?
   b. How can budgeting improve communication?
   c. How can budgeting facilitate coordination?
   d. How can budgeting improve motivation?
   e. How can budgeting help with control?
   f. How can budgeting contribute to assessing performance?

2. Generally, it is believed when quality improves, cost is reduced. What statements would you make to defend this position?
   a. Identify the basic factors that affect the cost of quality.
   b. How can you, as a nurse or nurse leader, influence this area?

3. Before you submit the budget for your unit or service, you decide to seek benchmarks from other organizations within the community.
   a. Describe the unit or service.
   b. How would you go about this undertaking?
   c. What indicators could be used to evaluate clinical and cost outcomes for comparison of agencies?
   d. How would you incorporate these cost outcomes into your budget presentation?

4. A variance report indicates the following:

Cost Center: Nursing Month: March				Unit: Intensive Care Unit Manager: Jenny Curtis
Item:	Actual	Budget	Variance	Prior Explanation Plan
Salaries Productive	85,670	76,243	(12.4)%	80,107
Salaries Overtime	4,547	6,701	32.1%	9,611
Salaries Contract	18,319	8,734	(109.7)%	13,919
Ed/Orient	8,279	9,184	9.9%	7,119
Total Salary Expense	117,715	102,932	(14.4)%	111,027
Supplies	19,760	17,355	(1.1)%	19,650
Units of Service (UOS)	680	655	1%	665
Revenue		Month		
	339,501	318,724	1%	286,985
		Year-to-date (YTD)		
	1,700,790	1,632,062	10%	1,488,463

   a. What are the major areas of variance?
   b. What issues do you see?
   c. What would be your plan of action?

REFERENCES

American Association of Colleges of Nursing. (2006). *The essentials of doctoral education for advanced nursing practice*. Washington, DC: Author. Retrieved from http://www.aacnnursing.org/DNP/DNP -Essentials

American Association of Colleges of Nursing. (2010). *The essentials of master's education in nursing.* Washington, DC: Author.

Benner, P. (2001). *From novice to expert: Excellence and power in clinical nursing practice.* Upper Saddle River, NJ: Prentice Hall.

Commission on Collegiate Nursing Education. (2009). *Standards for accreditation of baccalaureate and graduate degree nursing programs.* Washington, DC: Author.

El-Shamy, S. (2001) *Training games: Everything you need to know about using games to reinforce learning.* Sterling, VA: Stylus.

Fink, D. (2003). *Creating significant learning experiences: An integrated approach to designing college courses in higher and adult education.* San Francisco, CA: Jossey-Bass.

Greiner, A., & Knebel, E. (Eds.). (2003). *Health profession education: A bridge to quality.* Washington, DC: National Academies Press.

O'Brien, J., Missis, B., & Cohen, M. (2008). *The course syllabus.* San Francisco, CA: Jossey-Bass.

Rambur, B. (2015). *Health care finance, economics, and policy for nurses: A foundational guide.* New York, NY: Springer Publishing.

Rideout, E. (2001). *Transforming nursing education through problem-based learning.* Sudbury, MA: Jones & Bartlett.

Rubenfeld, M. G., & Scheffer, B. K. (2010). *Critical thinking tactics for nurses: Achieving the IOM competencies.* Sudbury, MA: Jones & Bartlett.

Scheffer, B. K., & Rubenfeld, M. G. (2000). A consensus statement on critical thinking in nursing. *Journal of Nursing Education, 39,* 352–359.

16 Financing Nursing Care Around the World: Global Health Care

Lisa Gifford

"It is all connected."

(Koodbe Eniwun, 2011)

The DNP role must only be filled/held by those who care about the who, what, when, where, how, what for, and who for of the "all connected."

THE QUESTION

In *The Autobiography of Alice B. Toklas*, Gertrude Stein, just before she died, asked Toklas, "What is the answer?" Toklas replied, "There is no answer." Stein laughed and said, "In that case, what is the question?" and then she died (Stein, 1990). The question is, how does the doctor of nursing practice (DNP) develop and deliver the knowledge, skills, and attitudes to uphold the art and science of professional nursing as the DNP meets the duties of the role of ensuring safe, evidence-based practice for patient-centered care? How does the DNP do this within the complex adaptive system (CAS) of health care, which is embedded in the complex systems of international trade, politics, and aid to foreign countries (as well as the national issues related to security, unemployment, increasing disparities in health care, and increasing use of technology), all embedded in the struggling business model orientation of managing sickness, disease, and disability for profit versus loss?

THE ESSENTIAL COMPONENTS AS AN ANSWER IS SOUGHT

Although this chapter is written with the responsibilities of the DNP foremost, the principles, concepts, and recommendations may be of interest and use to any and all associated with professional nursing and concerned with local and global application of social policy that honors the needs of all. The goal is to heighten the awareness and leadership responsibility of all readers to accept the interconnectedness of "all of us." The American Nurses Association's (ANA) Social Policy Statement is written for American nurses, by stating that, "Nursing is the protection, promotion, and optimization of health and abilities, prevention of illness and injury, alleviation of suffering through the diagnosis and treatment of human response, and advocacy in the care of individuals, families, communities and populations" (ANA, 2003).

The DNP, however, has a much wider biosphere than the bedside nurse, with reward and accountability that is justly awarded for the delivery of service at micro and macro levels. The ANA code of ethics is clear:

> "The nurse collaborates with other health care professionals and the public in promoting community, national and international efforts to meet health needs" (ANA, 2010, p. 164).

The DNP has a broader expanse of reachable influence than the bedside nurse, again with reward and accountability justly measured.

The Universal Declaration of Human Rights (1948), Article 25, states:

1. Everyone has the right to a standard of living adequate for health and well-being of himself and of his family, including food, clothing, housing and medical care and necessary social services, and the right to security in the event of unemployment, sickness, disability, widowhood, old age, or other lack of livelihood in circumstances beyond his control.
2. Motherhood and childhood are entitled to special care and assistance. All children, whether born in or out of wedlock, shall enjoy the same social protection.

Thus, the principles of distributive justice, the right to health as a means of attaining individual potential, and many principles in between are not secret and the author welcomes further "stretch" reading by clinicians, educators, administrators, and directors. These foundational statements of purpose, within the complex system of health care, fall to the role of the DNP. The DNP role meets bedside, organization, community, state, national, and international principles of distributive justice as well as principles of beneficence and nonmaleficence. The content of this chapter is written with global health in mind, yet application of the thoughts and concepts are applicable from the bedside to the boardroom and beyond, in any country. The intent is to move right behavior to an effective local behavior, which in fact may not lose sight of a responsibility of global health. The privileged knowledge of the global scene, by the DNP via education and academic recognition and award, is the major tool for accomplishment. The population of interest is "all of us," here and there, developed and underdeveloped country. The DNP has the opportunity and responsibility to effect local health, but not at the expense of others. Acquisition and allocation of resources are a primary concern to all who deliver health services. The DNP must approach this concern with a "there-is-room-for-us-all" mind-set and commitment.

Our focus so often is the "me" focus. Yet, nurses in undergraduate education for professional nursing admit to terminal values of happiness, self-respect, family security, equality, and true friendship. These same young persons identify instrumental values of being loving, honest, helpful, forgiving, broadminded, and ambitious. The tool for values assessment was that designed by Milton Rokeach (1973). This is not "me first" choosing. This is "we are all on this globe together" thinking. The way the nurse approaches all situations related to allocation of resources has room for the "all of us" perspective. Our humanity continues to enjoy the fruits of our intelligence and emotion, yet some on our planet have a life expectancy of 46 years and some others a life expectancy of 78 to 83 years. How does one spread the wealth of the collective human discoveries? How does one see the worth in each life and its potential? How does one think and enjoy the benefits of clear images of our fellow human beings through the new technologies? How does one think way beyond "the bottom line" and maximize the percent operating income? Who says that the latter should be 29%? What if resource use was pursued with a "tomorrow for all" commitment? The end recommendation will be to use a 3D-plus (3D+) framework to view the immediate patient–nurse interaction and the larger international nurse–world interaction. This new approach in no way intends to downgrade the wealth of frameworks, theories, and recommendations from our Florence to now, yet hopefully it will permit a comprehensive, immediate, valuable tool to make changes for the now, with an ongoing appreciation for the concepts in the many CAS on/in/with our global society.

■ FINANCING WITHOUT LOSING THE ESSENTIALS

The first responsibility, at a DNP level, is to sort through the woods and trees of words and terms to determine where equitable, effective, efficient effort should be exerted. The effort of the DNP must incorporate an appreciation of the local, national, and international pressures that impact his or her utilization of resources. Without such a diverse world/global knowledge base, the ethics of the DNP may in fact and deed support nonequitable, nonefficient, ineffective percent operating income-focused service instead of patient-centered care. Issues of nurse immigration related to international agreements, soft U.S.-aid return to countries by immigrant nurses, maintenance of diplomatic and military relationships, and balance of trade agreements all impact the supply of resources available to professional nursing supply. How does one ensure cultural sensitivity of all patients when hiring the ready supply of immigrant nurses is the trend? Who needs to be understood? The patients or the providers? Whose language is the dominant language? How is the immigrant nurse educated in the cultural beliefs of the diverse patient population that presents in the United States? African Americans, Caucasians, Hispanics, Asians, Eastern Europeans, and Native Americans? Where is the American-educated nurse? Why are there American-educated nurses who are not finding positions?

It all must be viewed from the perspective of complexity theory. We owe the impetus of our application of CAS to professional care to physics formulation of quantum theory (Polkinghorne, 2002). Each agent has a survival need that is being met in order to succeed in the business model and framework. How do these various relationships between and among agents support or not support the moral responsibility of the DNP? The DNP's expertise in ethics and economics must include identification of credible attractors, based on values embedded in both science and art. To partake in the privileges and responsibilities of a DNP role necessitates appreciation of the impact of globalization and global health. Some call globalization "monetization." Others refer to it as a Western-style smoke and mirrors produced and directed by multinational corporations. Globalization affects global health, now and tomorrow. Aginam (2005) maintains that global health futures are "directly or indirectly associated with transnational economic, social, and technological changes" (p. 32) across the planet. Slote (2011) purports that nurse leaders directly or indirectly are accountable for seducing the third-world nurse to the higher wage in the developed world. Idealists speak of one world. Watch and wait as the European Union resents and resists the single currency across nation states across national tradition and identity. Watch and wait as the Brexit vote of the 21st century creates some new chaos, calling for adaptations for survival of important relationships.

The effort of the DNP must incorporate an appreciation of the local, national, and international pressures that impact his or her utilization of resources in an ethical, sustainable manner, with caring that all is connected—this day is the future. M. Smith's (1992; as cited in Watson, 2005) five constituents of caring (Watson, 2005, p. 156) give reasonable, usable compositional framework for elucidation of the directive to DNPs. Their concern should include:

1. Manifesting intention
2. Appreciating pattern
3. Attuning to dynamic flow
4. Experiencing the infinite
5. Inviting creative emergence

The intention of the DNP must meet the ethical, just, efficient, effective goals of patient-centered care, using evidence-based practice. Understanding the pattern of the available resources on the intent is a duty to both institution and patient. The dynamic flow of recruitment, retention, migration, and emigration all need to be given their just due relative to concerns for global health, as all human beings are entitled to health care in order to maximize their potential. The relative placement of any DNP's immediate responsibilities must consider a universal balance, beyond the reactive stance of filling positions. The DNP must invite deviance, watch for emergence, and seek order with readiness for unpredictability and the ongoing understanding of relationships that change due to supply, demand, politics, and other socioeconomic agents.

The DNP will be educated in an appreciation of complexity science and view the attainment of positional duties within CAS. Although much in nursing literature (Neuman, 1994; Rogers, 1990; Swanson, 1993; Watson, 2005) and in complex science (W. E. Smith, 2009; Stacey, 2010; Waldrop, 1992) speaks of this as new, in fact, Buckley (1968) gives detailed understanding of CAS in his 1968 paper. The theorem presented by Buckley was the importance of the relationship of agents. He took the importance from the personal and cultural beliefs and placed the importance in the relationship between and among agents and environments. He moved from homeostasis and equilibrium being the desired goal states, conscious and unconscious, to the observation that the coevolution of human interactions was in fact the creating of new structures. Buckley's work clarified that the activity of an organism's mapping was to take self-regulation to a new level, out of chaos, to a restructure. And at the same time, Buckley reflected and upheld the point of Jules Henry (1959), that as the species in its development lacked the specificity of evolving lower animal species, "it [humans] must attempt to maximize social adaptation through constant conscious and unconscious revision and experimentation, searching constantly for social structure, patterns of interpersonal relations, that will be more adaptive, as he feels them" (p. 221). It is this constant search for the best relationship for all that becomes the social and professional learning so necessary to affect DNP leadership, to sort sense from nonsense, help from harm, and self-survival from global health.

COMMITMENT TO THE "MAGIS"

Leadership is vision, direction, and inspiration (Grossman & Valiga, 2005; Kouzes & Posner, 2010; O'Toole, 1996). Vincenzi, White, and Begun (1997) further load these concepts, incorporating three tasks: provide direction, inspire commitment, and face adaptive challenges. Accepting this would necessitate DNP competencies to include:

1. Sense making, looking at the interactions among people
2. Exploration, searching for new roles, opportunities, and answers to challenges
3. Connecting and establishing relationships

Specific strategies are offered to effect such leadership by these authors in language that can be embraced by the DNP: "abandon false notions of control, accept the reality of change, accept the unpredictability of the future, including the uncertainty of your own position, keep learning, build relationships, and change the world" (Vincenzi et al., 1997, pp. 28–30). These activities of sense making, exploration, and connecting would be with staff, communities, states, nations, and countries. These activities would take into consideration the socio–economic–political events guiding those same groups of persons as they attempt to maximize their potential in a world of varying kinds and supply of resources. Within these groups the DNP can apply principles and concepts of CAS, knowing that emergence is happening at all times, and that successful change can happen from any level in the complex array of control agents including immigration, certification, licensing, trade, taxation, insurance investment, education, professional associations, and political parties. The efficient, effective, ethical management of a patient population, hospital, or other health care organization requires the DNP to possess a base and ongoing knowledge cache related to all these aspects of society and societal interaction. The financial performance within current established interactions of stakeholders needs concerted change, creativity, and a return to dedicated attention to reasonable, safe outcomes for all who come with needs to the health care system. This should apply to urban and rural America and Africa, island villages, and nations struggling to find peace and productivity in the mangle of destruction from bombs dropped by major players. Bringing the know-how of democracy to such directly damaged communities needs the altruistic compassion of professional nursing led by the DNP, the academically prepared, clinically competent health systems change agent.

CREDIBILITY THROUGH COMPETENCE

The execution of DNP duties must be credible. DNPs must know their product. This includes formal postgraduate learning in finance, economics, international legal and governance affairs, religious studies, social policy, political persuasions, clinical outcomes, and human resources, all with particular attention to immigration and trade policies. In addition, the DNP needs knowledge of trade policy and the effect on supplies, disease transmission, public health, and balance of distributive justice. The DNP from this point forward requires knowledge of the energy challenges, including development of renewable and environmentally safe energy and the impact of the planet being released as the hostage of the fossil fuel industry. DNP leadership will require ongoing appreciation of information technology and the application to "health for all." The DNP will need to be informed of energy sources, as well as their sale, storage, transportation, and delivery and the resultant impact of each of those components of the industry on health needs and care. The DNP must understand the "asset" value of "oil in the ground" as it sits on our debts in the hands of other nations. The progress of humans in the new industries, and the collapse of the old resource industries (Rifkin, 2011), will present disease, disability, and discomforts that will need care. The DNP will be an active agent in the provision, direction, and creation of needed care. Provision of needed care will require assertive insistence on ethical distribution of available interventions. The DNP from today onward must participate in the restructure of amassed insurance wealth that up to now has not been available for the same needed care. The DNP must acquire knowledge of the real traffic of money around the planet and be an advocate for ethical distribution of available funds for effecting visible adherence to Article 25 of the Human Rights Declaration. The DNP must incorporate an appreciation of the local, national, and international pressures that impact his or her utilization of resources. The DNP holds a duty perspective that is now recognized and rewarded with academic award. Previously, the trend of nursing leadership in the practice arena was to be recognized with a terminal degree from another discipline or, for many, to arrive from the "rung below" to the higher position of clinical delivery, management, and administration without the required knowledge. For any nurse to do such now, simply arrive from the "rung below," now that we have the accomplished societal academic achievement defined and accepted for the DNP, would be to take from patients and persons their rightful standard of care.

A CAS-DEPENDENT APPROACH–FOCUS LOCAL TO ACHIEVE GLOBAL

The nursing profession as we know and love it came out of trauma and disease, which, if lucky, underwent some medical intervention. Florence Nightingale was concerned with abnormal mortality related to the wounds of soldiers. We started in or around 1854 with a nursing process consisting of assessment, planning, intervention, and evaluation. We have used that same formula, with a little SOAP (subjective, objective, assessment, and plan) and SBAR (situation, background, assessment, and recommendation), begged or borrowed, to become the right hand of medicine as it has progressed to improve and save lives. Nursing has completely made the practice of medicine livable. As persons became and become medicalized through diagnosis and labels, nursing has remained through to the person who exists in the now medicalized human. Yet these same persons/patients come to nursing via the clinical setting, and we apply our science and art to deliver clinical reasoning. Benner, Sutphen, Leonard, and Day (2009) encourages nursing to move from the critical thinking of old to the clinical reasoning of the new. Nursing is a discipline to assist persons to recover, adapt, or die from medical interventions applied to disease disability and discomfort. The nurse clinician needs a working framework to quickly yet thoroughly capture the needs of a person as a CAS. Although the full assessment as taught in nursing schools may remain as an educational tool, the clinician needs to move to an acceptance that the sum is more than the whole. The person in the patient is more than the sum of the diagnosis and interventions. Inherent in not doing this is the palpable frustration of at least the American patient in not feeling as if the medicalization process gives a rat's booty about the person who presents the problem of life/living. Inherent and deeper in this event is the patient not being able to access the person (the self) who could help with the recovery, adaptation, or death of the living organism.

The clinician is entitled to a knowledgeable progressive assessment tool to use repeatedly during the nurse–patient relationship, which is an ever-changing dynamic CAS. The CAS is understood, accepted, and honored as a single agent with multiple complex interconnecting systems within, and multiple relationships without, other CAS providing feedback and flow of energy to and from the person/patient. The progressive tool must commit to the fact that the person in the care of the nurse is more than the sum of the parts, with history, present status, and evolving future all relevant components of the care to be delivered.

The tool is called 3D+ and consists of seven departments within and without the CAS of our human person/patient:

Disease

Disability

Discomfort

Internal environment

External environment

Ability to participate

Ability to resist other illness

The tool is original in concept and arrangement and has been utilized over months and years of individualized practice. It is a compilation of experience, education, ethics, and energy, which has emerged as the necessity for rapid comprehensive assessment and the fast delivery of "productive" health care services. The tool has been used to educate hospice nurses as they transition from acute to home-based care, or another setting of the client's choice for care at end of life.

This framework can be used in 21st-century progressive times where practice behaviors need to be useful to clinicians in the very complex moment where macro and micro changes observed and understood by the clinician nurse impact minute-to-minute and hour-to-hour interventions. It is necessary for persons/patients to maximize the knowledge and technology of the experts for their (patient's) best recovery, adaptation, or death. The framework can be applied to all phase states of the DNP's purview, responsibilities, and duties, as well as the clinician faced with ever-changing dynamic individual patient human responses to disease, disability, and discomfort. The formula of 3D+ has emerged at the edge of chaos—the edge for nurses is the bedside, where the knowledge, egos, research, and politics all try to dance together and quiet the moaning patient while they lose not step or rhythm in the nurturing of their more important knowledge, egos, research, and politics. These latter can be called the real or the representative of the central currency. The subjects are weighty, they have many soldiers in each of their armies, and even the patient has begun to believe that "they" know better. The central currency of meeting the payments on borrowed capital is truly what is governing the flow of care. Can the DNP, through education and experience, and perhaps the "caritas" of Jean Watson (Davidson, Ray, & Turkel, 2011), apply human caring for human conditions, and caring as well for the caregivers and licensed operators, within truly human policies and procedures? Yes.

■ THE RESPONSIBILITY OF THE DNP

The DNP must understand the complete picture of what is governing the flow of resources. The DNP must not sell out to the already deep and powerful river of all systems being overspent and in debt, and needing to make payments to the central currency. What local currency might the DNP raise to the visibility of the caregivers and licensed operators under his or her leadership? The local currency must be of value to all the stakeholders. The DNP must lead to this end. The DNP has the privilege of perspective, which is far greater than an organizational "bottom line," "margin," or "percent operating income." The DNP by privilege and position knows that the sell-out of the governors and managers of national and international debt, assets, and payments and write-offs will continue for "anyone's guess" until the multiverse reveals more of the emergence in its multiconnected agents and relationships. It will be another of what we call disaster and catastrophe, when in fact it is the natural survival of the multiverse in its penchant for survival and procreation.

What is new local currency? What could possibly equal or perhaps supplant the ever-seductive quicksand of "the bottom" as recorded in dollars and cents, and the variance of the actual to the budgeted? Wherein might lie a heretofore untapped resource that might become the local currency, with sufficient human satisfaction for choosing local currency over central currency? What attractor could pull the physical, mental, spiritual, biochemical individual masses (other humans) toward the attractor? Is there such? Yes.

The stakeholders first are owed a share in the DNP knowledge, experience, and responsibility to ethics and morality of upholding the Declaration of Human Rights, which states that health care is a right (Article 25, 1987). The DNP knows the "big picture," the relationships of supply related to national, international debt and agreements to balance those debts. The DNP shares at every interaction, never misses an opportunity to inform the stakeholders of the real picture of "why" we are being asked to meet certain "percent operating income" goals. The DNP must embrace and pass to others the knowledge that the sickness and need before them can be cared for in a caring, competent, compassionate, efficient, effective, equitable, safe, patient-centered fashion. This is indeed the deep and "doctoral" responsibility of the DNP, with expert clinical knowledge and experience. The DNP has committed to systems change leadership. The DNP has been awarded a terminal degree for demonstrating the ability to understand, design, implement, and record outcomes of a system's final change project, or capstone project. This, in fact, is the ticket and now duty for the DNP to enter or reenter the circle of directional, administrative, and clinical responsibility with new vision and tools to lead stakeholders to the human care that is nursing's professional responsibility, by code and contract.

So what local currency could emerge? Wherein will the DNP facilitate the self-regulation necessary for the local currency that in practice will be useful to the local stakeholders? The DNP must see what is before him or her in the local environment. The DNP can use the 3D+ as a framework. The stakeholders can use the 3D+. Nurses, physicians, administrators, vendors, and ancillary service providers can use 3D+ and thus serve patients and families to meet the challenges of disease, disability, discomfort, and understanding of their internal and external environments with multiple interconnecting articulations, all within their ability to participate in the prescribed care (not necessarily cure) and their ability to resist other illness. The strength of the 3D+ is that its design fosters focus on the local, with ever-improved awareness of the relationships of agents.

The 3Ds draw the energy to the local. The 3D+ enables local observation, local application of expertise, and local evaluation of locally desired outcomes. The disease (trauma) is the entry point of all into the multiverse of other agents. The variables of disability and discomfort ensure forever attention to the dynamic phase of illness and recovery. The internal and external environment assessment and appreciation ensure inclusion of all visible interconnections that may affect survival and procreation. The ability to participate in one's own care, and ability to resist illness, ensures that the observations stay within this patient's "whole," which is more than the sum of its, her, or his parts.

CONCLUSION

The author resists the old urge to draw the model on the paper. Have we not seen the abuse of imposing one model, designed for one population, on another population, with or without war? The art and science of 3D+ is the simplicity of the formula that will ensure incorporation of any and all relationships relevant to the center of the care, the patient. May we all continue to respect, enjoy, and truly love the privilege and responsibility of professional nursing at all levels, and support the DNPs as they deliver the duty of their degree.

CRITICAL THINKING EXERCISES

1. The details:

Setting	Ambulatory surgery hospital
Problem	Losing $200 per case per Medicare payer
Payer mix	One third each: Medicare, charity/self pay, managed care
Strategic plan	Grow business to valuable asset in the community hospital, enhancing its marketability in the larger hospital purchase/merger environment, for when it hangs out the "for sale" sign in 5 to 7 years.
Decision team	Chief nursing officer (CNO; DNP)
	Ambulatory surgery RN
	Human resources director
	Union representative
	Quality management director
	CFO (chief financial officer)
	Marketing/community outreach director
	Rehabilitation director
	The team is internal. The team would eventually extend to or include external players, surgeons, and other contract services.

Solve for local and global success relative to the payer mix, the cost, and the culturally diverse Mexican American community.

Include understanding of fixed and variable costs, margin, length of stay, average daily census, average time for unit of service, quality care, professional growth, and introduction of Institute of Medicine (IOM) direction that pushes professional nursing practice to its highest level of training and education.

Sample	$3,000 Medicare reimbursement	
Expenses	Outpatient nurses	760 45/hour × 2 RN
	OR/PACU nurse	760 excludes benefit pkgs
	Supplies, IV, irrigation, equipment	500
	Medications, intra op and OP	60
	Allocation of fixed overhead	200
	Contract anesthesia	400 $100/15 minute UOS
	Arthroscopy sterile package	600
Loss/UOS		−200

Solving for current and future financial success should include the DNP using previous information related to understanding of fixed and variable costs, assets and liabilities, variance, and depreciation. For added complication—which would occur in the natural environment—ethnic association, level of education, and length of time in the position may be added by individual readers and/or instructors. This exercise may be used as a simple discussion exercise or a detailed assignment. The exercise is meant to use 3D+ as the tool for arriving at the best local and global impact decision.

The disease of interest would be joint disease and/or trauma requiring arthroscopic surgery in an outpatient ambulatory surgery setting.

The disability of those who require surgery will be significant, with pain and loss of mobility taking them to this point of arthroscopic repair.

The discomfort, preop (in the community), and postop will need support, durable medical equipment, education, exercise regimens, and recovery from general anesthesia.

The internal environments to be assessed are the various physical states that come with need for the procedure.

The external environment includes community sports, farm worker soccer leagues, and other sports; church involvement by sportists; large ranches with or without insurance for the field workers; goodwill and donations by/from larger ranchers to a hospital foundation, and being the facility of choice for this local medical intervention with limited complications.

The ability of the patient population to participate in the plan of care, with professional guidance and education, will entail hours of care estimates for units of service (UOS).

The ability to resist other illness, anesthetic reactions, nausea and vomiting, pain not managed, and falls needs to be weighed into assessments.

The DNP needs to be skilled in the fixed costs of the unit, the variables, the allocation of hospital overhead as spread to the unit, the scope of practice and impact on cost of nursing service with a skill mix, bundled or unbundled charges, excluded costs, medications for perioperative events, anesthesia reimbursement, community wages of populations coming for uninsured service, dates and persons who negotiated managed care contacts, outreach to community sportists of all ages, the payer mix of the usual patient population, willingness of community large ranches to support injury to workers, relationships of the hospital to other social organizations, and many other contributing factors in order to maintain at least a cost-neutral operation. The DNP efforts do not rest with delivery of service, bottom line, and supply of "men, materials, and money." The DNP needs to know all of the previously noted items plus additional creative components in order to ensure a sustainable ongoing arthroscopy service to a community with high rate of disease and/or traumatized joints, treatable by arthroscopic intervention. The narrative given is not intended to be inclusive, but rather to encourage 3D+ clinical and administrative reasoning.

2. Nurses around the globe are following the better wages. So-called marketing and recruiting companies are seeking to provide thousands of nurses to the growing modern medicine in the

Middle East (e.g., The Hamas Medical Center in Qatar). How might the DNP apply ethics and principles of the "common good" to this business activity? Looking at the relationships—political, military, and economic—what interactions might the DNP review? What searching might the DNP explore looking for new roles, opportunities, and answers to the challenges? The countries from which the nurses are recruited are themselves experiencing a nursing shortage (e.g., Serbia and Ireland). How might the DNP foster connections and relationships that benefit "the Magis?"

Suggestions for utilizing the global nurse recruitment exercise might be further broken down by financial, economic, political, and military concentration. Certainly the DNP, with basic concern for quality patient care, supported by an extensive comprehensive education related to systems management, would be the ideal leader in this current global environment. Onward!!

3. Still in keeping with the DNP's role and responsibilities, the DNP is called to the gynecology unit to intervene in a dispute between a female patient requesting a voluntary interruption of pregnancy, a physician practitioner who has a professional relationship with the patient, and the husband, a practicing Muslim who wishes to prevent the female from her choice of procedure. All parties appear to be operating within their rights. How would the DNP proceed, knowing that his or her professional perspective will influence the outcome? What community agents might assist? The patient is insured.

4. Another use of the same scenario would be, "the patient is uninsured." How will the decision-making process of the DNP proceed?

In proceeding with Exercises 3 and 4, the DNP will identify all agents legitimately involved in the challenge. Will the insured/not-insured status enter into the decision? If so, why? If not, why? How does the respect for individual choice of husband and patient play into the DNP's process?

As the DNP role is designed, the DNP should be prepared for these situations and other equally complex experiences. It is hoped that the DNP will always rise to the occasion, attempting to facilitate the evolution of new moral order from the inevitable chaos of global traffic and migration.

REFERENCES

Aginam, O. (2005). *Global health governance: International law and public health in a divided world.* Toronto, ON, Canada: University of Toronto Publishing.

American Nurses Association. (2003). *Nursing's social policy statement* (2nd ed.). Silver Spring, MD: Nurses books.org.

American Nurses Association. (2010). *Guide to the code of ethics for nurses: Interpretation and application.* Silver Spring, MD: NursesBooks.

Benner, P., Sutphen, M., Leonard, V., & Day, L. (2009). *Educating nurses: A call for radical transformation.* San Francisco, CA: Jossey-Bass.

Buckley, W. (1968). Society as a complex adaptive system. In W. Buckley (Ed.), *Modern systems research for the behavioral scientist* (pp. 86–112). Chicago, IL: Aldine.

Davidson, A. W., Ray, M. A., & Turkel, M. C. (2011). *Nursing, caring, and complexity science.* New York, NY: Springer Publishing.

Grossman, S. C., & Valiga, T. M. (2005). *The new leadership challenge: Creating the future of nursing.* Philadelphia, PA: F. A. Davis.

Henry, J. (1959). Culture, personality and evolution. *American Anthropologist, 61,* 221–222.

Kouzes, J. M., & Posner, B. Z. (2010). *The truth about leadership.* San Francisco, CA: Jossey-Bass.

Neuman, M. (1994). *Health expanding consciousness* (2nd ed.). New York, NY: National League for Nursing.

O'Toole, J. (1996). *Leading change: The argument for values-based leadership.* New York, NY: Random House.

Polkinghorne, J. (2002). *Quantum theory: A very short introduction.* New York, NY: Oxford University Press.

Rifkin, J. (2011). *The third industrial revolution*. New York, NY: Palgrave MacMillan.

Rogers, M. E. (1990). Nursing: Science of unitary, irreducible, human beings: Update 1990. In E. A. M. Barrett (Ed.), *Visions of Rogers' science-based nursing* (pp. 5–11). New York, NY: National League for Nursing.

Rokeach, M. (1973). *Understanding human values, individual and societal*. New York, NY: Free Press.

Slote, R. J. (2011). Pulling the plug on brain-drain: Understanding international migration of nurses. Retrieved from http://www.findarticles.com/Health/MedSurg

Smith, M. (1992). *Caring science as sacred science* (p. 156). Philadelphia, PA: F. A. Davis.

Smith, W. E. (2009). *The creative power, transforming ourselves, our organizations, and our world*. New York, NY: Routledge.

Stacey, R. D. (2010). *Complexity and organizational reality* (2nd ed.). New York, NY: Routledge.

Stein, G. (1990). *The autobiography of Alice B. Toklas*. New York, NY: Vintage.

Swanson, K. M. (1993). Nursing as informed caring for the wellbeing of others. *Image: Journal of Nursing Scholarship, 25*(4), 352–357.

United Nations. (1948). Universal Declaration of Human Rights, Article 25, (1) and (2). Retrieved from http://www.un.org/en/universal-declaration-human-rights

Vincenzi, A. E., White, K. R., & Begun, J. W. (1997). Chaos in nursing: Make it work for you. *American Journal of Nursing, 97*(10), 26–32.

Waldrop, M. M. (1992). *Complexity: The emerging science at the edge of order and chaos*. New York, NY: Simon & Schuster.

Watson, J. (2005). *Caring science as sacred science*. Philadelphia, PA: F. A. Davis.

Glossary

3-F Framework An approach for capital projects and expenditures vetting in organizations that includes three equally essential components: finances, fit, and feasibility.

Accountability Acceptance for the responsibility and the outcomes for staffing for the performance of a task, department, and unit with the authority to lead the work and with the expectation of being evaluated on the performance according to recognized standards.

Accountable Care Organization (ACO) Groups of providers and hospitals that jointly provide coordinated care.

Accounts Payable (AP) During the normal course of business, debts can be due for services rendered. Bills for materials received or obligations on an open account may be accounts payable. This kind of liability usually arises from a purchase of merchandise, materials, or supplies.

Accounts Receivable (AR) Money owed by patients or others to an entity in exchange for services that have been delivered but not yet paid for.

Accrual Basis Accounting principle wherein transactions and events are recognized for financial purposes when they legally occur, regardless of an exchange of cash.

Activity The accumulated patient traffic admissions, discharges, and transfers in and out of the unit by a 24-hour period.

Activity on Arrow (AOA) Method of mapping a project network; activity is shown as an arrow.

Activity on Node (AON) Method of mapping a project network; activity is on the node.

Acuity A measurement of patient severity of illness that is related to the amount of resources required to care for the patient.

Admission, Discharge, and Transfer (ADT) Admission is a new patient admitted into the hospital. Discharge is an existing patient discharged to leave the hospital. Transfer is an existing patient that is moved from one unit to another within the hospital.

Advanced Practice Registered Nurse (APRN) A registered nurse with at least a master's degree who is also licensed as a nurse practitioner, certified registered nurse anesthetist, certified nurse midwife, or clinical nurse specialist.

Agile Project Management Iterative process to create a product or service.

Aim Drift An attempt, unconscious or deliberate, to back away from stretch goals that requires team corrective action.

Aim Statement A form of SMART goals recommended by the Institute for Healthcare Improvement (IHI) that emphasizes numerical stretch goals and direct measurement to create more accountability in the quality improvement process.

Allowance for Bad Debts The portion of debts owed to the organization that are assumed to be "uncollectible."

Alternative Payment Models (APMs) Value-based reimbursement options.

Amortization The process of retiring a debt, usually by equal payments at regular intervals over a specific period of time.

Analysis/Design Phase The project management phase that explores the factors necessary to ensure the project goals and outcomes are aligned with the organization's strategic plan, delineates project specifications, performs financial analyses, and builds a team capable of completing tasks and accepting responsibilities.

Appreciative Inquiry A discussion technique that focuses on shared goals and includes four phases consisting of discovery, dreaming, designing, and delivering the project.

Assets Resources that are possessed by the organization that have an economic benefit. Most assets are tangible in that they can be measured, such as cash, goods, or services, or intangible in that they are difficult to measure, such as reputation.

Available Bed A bed that is equipped but not staffed for patient admissions.

Balance Sheet (BS) A comprehensive financial statement that is a summarized assessment of a company's accounts specifying its assets and liabilities.

Bed Cleaning Interval The amount of time required for the unoccupied bed to be cleaned and readied for the next admission, which contributes to the bed turnover interval.

Bed Turnover Interval The amount of time beds are unoccupied until the next patient admission following a patient discharge.

Bed Turns How frequently a given hospital bed changes occupancy over the reporting period.

Bed Utilization The actual number of bed turns compared to the maximum possible number of bed turns to determine, expressed as a percent.

Benchmarking A method that assists in comparing outcomes of two or more entities.

Benefit The amount the insurance company pays when the insured suffers a loss.

Benefit Period The amount of time involved in an individual claim. In the case of hospitalization, the first day of the hospital stay through the day of discharge and often up to 60 days after release from the facility.

Best Practices Techniques or methodologies that, through experience and research, have proved to reliably produce results. Committing to use "best practices" is a commitment to using all the knowledge and technology at one's disposal to ensure success. A best practice tends to spread throughout a field or industry after a demonstrated success. According to the American Productivity and Quality Center, the three main barriers to adoption of a best practice are a lack of knowledge about current best practices, a lack of motivation to make changes involved in their adoption, and a lack of knowledge and skills required to do so.

Break-Even Point The point at which revenue covers cost.

Break-Even Time Length of time before break-even volume will be reached.

Break-Even Volume Number of units needed to break even on a specific project.

Budget A plan that provides a formal, quantitative expression of management's plans and intentions or expectations.

Budget Coordinator Identifies all costs related to the project, determines what funding mechanism will provide the right resources, and tracks responsible spending of the funds.

Budget Types:

> **Expense** Comprised of salary and nonsalary items.

> **Revenue** Total amount of income anticipated during a defined period of time. Manager rarely controls revenue, but can control variable expenses, usually payroll and supplies for nursing.

Cost Types:

> **Amortization** Predicting the rate of obsolescence of a given product and assigning a dollar value to that rate.

Capital Includes equipment and renovation expenses needed to meet long-term goals. Usually have life span of more than 1 year or more and exceed a certain dollar amount.

Fixed Remain constant despite fluctuations in activity levels.

Operating An annual budget based on anticipated revenues and expenses for the organization's fiscal year (12 months—not always calendar year).

Variable Fluctuate in response to internal or external changes, that is, census, patient acuity, staffing mix, and product cost.

Budgeting A process whereby plans are made and then an effort is made to meet or exceed the goals of the plans.

Bundling Including additional services such as laboratory tests in with an office visit.

Cafeteria Plan Offers a choice between two or more benefits or a choice between a benefit or cash.

Capital Assets Buildings or equipment whose utility is expected to continue more than a year beyond their purchase.

Capital Expenditures Budgetary entries for items outside of the day-to-day operations realm, usually with the total outlay of $1,000 or more, commonly abbreviated as CapEx.

Capitated Rate A rate per member per month.

Capitation An organization is paid a fixed, negotiated rate per member per month. The entity receives payment whether or not the member uses the services of the organization in a given time period. A business model calls for the risk to be spread within the group for the array of services that are agreed upon ahead of time.

Case Mix Combination of types of patients served; defined by diagnosis, payment source, and so forth.

Case Mix Index (CMI) A mathematical calculation that indicates the costliness of a hospital's case mix in relation to a national average case mix.

Cash Burn The monthly cash cost of new operations in the period prior to any revenue being generated.

Cash Flow A stream of money into (inflow) or out of (outflow) a project, an investment, or operations.

Cash Flow Statement A financial statement that shows how changes in the balance sheet accounts and income affect cash and cash equivalents, and breaks the analysis down to operating, investing, and financing activities; also referred to as a statement of cash flows or funds flow statement. Essentially concerned with the flow of cash in and cash out.

Census The number of patients occupying beds at a specific time of day. At a minimum, it is midnight and often includes the day, evening, and night shifts.

Centers for Medicare and Medicaid Services (CMS) Federal government agency overseeing Medicare and Medicaid programs.

Change Agents Individuals who influence others' decisions to accept change in the direction deemed desirable by the change agent.

Chi Squared A statistical calculation to determine whether the difference between an expected and actual distribution is significant; used primarily with nominal data.

Claim A request to the insurance company to pay benefits for a loss.

Clinical Significance Not a calculation but an application of clinical reasoning and sound clinical judgment, coupled with business sense. For example, a more expensive medication reduces the systolic blood pressure by only 1 mmHg; the decrease could be statistically and practically significant, but an expert understands that this is probably not clinically significant to the patient's disease process or well-being.

COBRA A federal law (Consolidated Omnibus Budget Reconciliation Act) that allows employees to continue their coverage, through self-pay, after they leave employment.

Co-Investigator (Co-I) Works with the principal investigator (PI) to identify and prepare drafts; provides formative and summative reviews in specific sections.

Community Foundations Their name usually alludes to the area they serve (e.g., Glendale Community Foundation), and they wish to see their community members somehow served in the scope of the grants funded. Community foundation grants generally support replication projects rather than groundbreaking research or experimental approaches.

Comparative Effectiveness Research Properly informs health care-related decisions. Defined as the comparison of one diagnostic or treatment option to one or more others.

Complexity Theory Mathematically demonstrates the unpredictable nature of living systems and the continuous effort to adapt toward a better "natural fit" over time.

Concluding Phase The project management phase that consists of final testing and deployment, training the end user, sign-off by appropriate parties, and transfer of key documents related to the projects.

Consultant Provides expertise and experience in one or more focus areas.

Contingent Workforce Temporary staff; includes traveler staff.

Continuous Data Answers the question "How much?" The precision of continuous data collection is, by definition, dependent on the accuracy of the measuring instrument.

Contractual Allowance A discount determined between a provider and a third-party payer for a given service. For example, the difference between billed charges and the amount paid by Medicare for the diagnosis-related group (DRG) is the contractual allowance for Medicare.

Contribution Margin Portion of the charge to a patient or payer for a procedure or supplies that are over and above the actual cost (does not include indirect costs).

Coordinator Assists with the grant application and coordinates all required sections and materials to be included in the application. Manages and coordinates personnel and procedures of a funded grant.

Co-Payment A small charge the insured pays at the time service is received.

Core Values Statements Declarations of the individual organizational value components.

Correlation A statistical calculation that gives a number that represents the amount and direction of the relationship between two variables; most common is Pearson's product moment correlation coefficient, used with ratio and interval data.

Cost–Benefit Analysis The analysis of health care resource expenditures relative to possible medical benefit.

Cost–Benefit Ratio Numerical relationship between the value of an activity or procedure in terms of benefits and the value of the activity's cost to the entity that could be a service line or a patient. Expressed as a fraction; if fraction is greater than one, benefits outweigh the cost.

Cost Center or Unit The financial unit or code from which wages are paid and costs can be identified and controlled by a specific nurse leader. Accounting practice is to assign all labor costs to the home cost centers and to allocate to all other cost centers the hours worked on those units. May also be called cost center, cost unit, or department number.

Cost/Cost Plus The provider organization is reimbursed for actual costs plus an additional percentage of those costs to generate a margin.

Cost-Effectiveness Analysis (CEA) Compares the costs and the values of different health care interventions in creating better health and longer life.

Cost of Care per Day or Cost per Unit of Service A mathematical calculation of the cost of care per day or unit of service using average salary costs by category of employee and HPPD (hours per patient day).

Cost per Encounter The product of intensity of services, productivity/efficiency, and resource prices/salaries and wages.

CPT Code Common Procedure Terminology.

Crashing Shortening an activity or project.

Critical Path The longest possible continuous pathway from the start to the completion of the project. A delay along the critical path will create delay reaching the project completion by the same amount. A series of delays along the critical path will have a cumulative effect on the delay.

Critical Quality and Operating Targets (CQOT) Goals set for the key indicators of an organization's overall health.

Cultural Alignment Degree to which employees subscribe to, accept, and model their employer's mission, vision, and values.

Cumulative Percent/Cumulative Relative Frequency Reports the percentage of occurrences as an additive measure.

Current Assets Organization's cash resources or other resources that can easily be converted into cash within a year or resources that will be depleted within a year.

Current Liabilities Obligations that the organization expects to pay off within a year.

Data The basic element by which many critical decisions are based.

Data Analysis The interpretation and application of statistical results, including types of numerical data, organizing and tabulating results, distinguishing differences, and interpreting and applying results.

Decision Innovation Process A description of the phases of adoption that networks of individuals undergo before incorporating a change in practice; it includes five stages: knowledge, persuasion, decision, implementation, and confirmation.

Deductible The amount of covered expenses the insured must pay out of pocket before the insurance company pays.

Deliberately Developmental Organization (DDO) A company dedicated to the personal and professional growth of its employees as the central premise of its organizational and business strategy.

Deliverables Major products or results that must be finished before a project can progress to the next step.

Denying the Claim When an insurance company does not pay a bill because the service was not covered, or because preapproval or other conditions were not met.

Departmental Operating Report Contains relevant information about the particular department or cost center; also referred to as cost center report, profit and loss statement, trend report, or another term, depending on the organization.

Depreciation Accounting for the cost of an asset across all of its years of useful, revenue-generating life. In accounting, depreciation is an operating expense that must be included in the price of the goods or services sold. It is the loss in value the organization anticipates for its buildings and equipment.

Developmental Alignment An employee's level of satisfying his or her needs in relation to the Maslow's hierarchy of needs.

Diagnosis-Related Groups (DRGs) A taxonomy of codes describing diagnoses in alphanumerics, used for reimbursement.

Direct Care Hours The number of hours of direct labor used in making a product or providing a service. In acute care, it is the hours of all staff providing direct care (hands-on caregivers) to patients. If your hospital does not separate direct and indirect hours, the total worked or productive and direct hours are the same.

Direct Costs Costs specifically incurred by the department over which the manager has responsibility and potentially authority to make changes.

Director of Strategy Head of the strategy committee; a full-time position reporting directly to the president/CEO, or a member of the management team in smaller organizations.

Discount Rate The reciprocal value of the interest rate that correlates the present and future values of an investment or a cash flow.

Discrete Data Answers the question "How many?" These data are frequency or counting values. There are no "in-between" values for discrete data.

Disproportionate Share The U.S. government provides funding to hospitals that treat indigent patients through the Disproportionate Share Hospital (DSH) programs, under which facilities are able to receive at least partial compensation (www.healthcarepayment.com).

Double-Loop Learning Process of questioning; reflecting on why a certain response is made, then shifting to a new response; paradigm shift.

Dysfunctional Conflict Conflict that hinders group performance and requires the project manager to intervene to get the project team back on course.

Earnings Before Interest, Taxes, Depreciation, and Amortization (EBITDA) Is the difference between a firm's operating revenues and expenses; could be positive (profit) or negative (loss). Represents how much money a company earns if it did not have to pay interest, taxes, or take depreciation and amortization charges. EBITDA is intended to be an indicator of a company's financial performance without consideration of debt, tax, or asset base. This is becoming a much more common way to determine earnings.

Economic Market A structure that allows sellers and buyers to exchange goods, services, or information.

Economics The study of how resources are allocated.

Editor/Proofreader Expert in the use of the English language and effective grantsmanship. Polishes the application before submission.

Efficiency The cost associated with a specific level or quality of care.

Endowments Resources contributed by a donor, which are used to generate additional, consistent income for the organization.

Entropy A term used in systems theory for a disorganization, which threatens the balance of complex systems such as those found in the health care setting.

Environmental Evaluation Broad assessment process performed to pinpoint an organization's standing in regard to the stated mission, vision, and existing strategic objectives and inform ongoing strategy formulation.

Equilibrium or Homeostasis The balance of a complex system into an organized and functioning whole.

Executive Sponsor Person who lends administrative support, expertise, or credibility to the project.

Expendable Supplies Supplies that are consumed as usable for one time use.

Failure Mode Evaluation Analysis (FMEA) Each potential risk is assessed in terms of severity of impact, probability of the event occurring and ease of detection.

Family Foundation Grants Reflect the values of the family members whose interests have been memorialized by the creation of the foundation. This creates significant variability in funding purposes, criteria, and patterns among family foundations. Although family foundations represent the largest subset of private foundations, their asset base and subsequent funding amounts are generally quite small, and they typically fund on a local level.

Federal Poverty Level (FPL) Poverty thresholds are the dollar amounts used by the U.S. Census Bureau to determine poverty status. Each person or family is assigned one out of 48 possible poverty thresholds, which vary according to the size of the family and the ages of the members. The same thresholds are used throughout the United States. Poverty thresholds are updated annually for inflation by the U.S. Bureau of Labor Statistics, using the Consumer Price Index for All Urban Consumers (CPI-U). Although the poverty thresholds in some sense reflect the family's needs, they are intended for use as a statistical yardstick, not as a complete description of what people and families need to live.

Fee for Service When the scope of work is clearer, this is a method most common for the Other Professional Services category in the National Health Expenditures data. A set fee is billed at the risk of additional services being required at the time of treatment. The local market drives the rates that patients are willing to pay.

Filled Position An allocation in the position control assigned to an employee in the unit based on the budgeted full-time equivalents (FTEs) for full- and part-time work agreement.

Financial Models Computerized tools for evaluating financial feasibility of investments and projects or forecasting and monitoring financial performance.

Five-Stage Model of Group Development A model of group development developed by Tuckman and Jensen to shed light into the phases of group activity and how to manage the group process.

Five Whys A questioning method of asking the question "Why?" five times to obtain more information about the problem and reduce the number of false assumptions made during evaluation.

Fixed Assets Assets that cannot be converted to cash within a year (also referred to as long-term assets). Examples are land, building, and equipment.

Fixed Bed Capacity An acute care facility may have more beds licensed for operation than are equipped to be available. Licensed and equipped available beds represent the hospital's fixed capacity, which remains constant over a fiscal year.

Fixed Budget Budgeting style based on a fixed annual level of volume that does not allow for variation.

Fixed FTEs Also referred to as permanent staffing or indirect staffing; they represent staff hours scheduled regardless of patient volume.

Fixed Price This approach focuses on a fixed price for treating a certain disease condition. This is the category in which the DRG system falls. The provider is rewarded for efficiency.

Flexible FTEs Staff hours scheduled based on actual or projected patient volume.

Float Also known as slack; the amount of time that a project task can be delayed without causing a delay in subsequent tasks.

Force Field Analysis Restraining and driving forces acting simultaneously to compete for and against goal achievement.

Forecasting The approximation of the time and cost it will take to complete project deliverables.

Frequency The number of times a given value occurs.

Frequency Distribution A table that shows how many times each given value occurs. It is the most common reporting format for frequency data.

Full Cost Sum total of all direct and indirect costs.

Full-Time Equivalent (FTE) Number of hours of work for which a full-time employee is scheduled for a weekly period; for example: 7-day (8 hour shift) period—needs 1.4 FTEs.

Full-Time Hours (FT Hours) The number of hours at or above which a person is considered to be working full-time. On average, it is usually between 69 and 72 hours per pay period.

Functional Conflict Conflict that supports the goals of the group and is a productive part of the group process.

Future Value (FV) The worth of a cash flow or an investment at a specified point in the future.

Gains Sharing Cash or equity bonuses that are a common method for motivating employees to achieve and exceed set financial, strategic, quality, and other goals; also known as profit sharing.

Gantt Chart A bar chart used during the monitoring phase of a project to break the project down into activities with distinct start and finish times.

Governing Board A committee responsible for the authoritative direction and control of an organization; frequently referred to as a board of directors or board of trustees.

Government Federal, state, and local entities participating in health insurance programs.

Gross Income Income before expenses are deducted.

Gross Margin The difference between sales revenues and manufacturing costs as an intermediate step in the computation of operating profits or net income; net sales minus goods sold.

Groupthink A phenomenon in which members of a group strive to be in agreement with each other, even though some members privately disagree.

Health Maintenance Organization (HMO) The passage of the HMO Act occurred in 1973. The principles underlying HMOs are cost-effectiveness based on productivity, population management with a focus on preventive care, a predetermined and agreed-upon array of services including both ambulatory and inpatient care, prepayment in the form of dues, and assumption of risk by the provider to meet the requirements of the promised care and service.

Heterogeneous Highly varied, when there is a lot of spread between and among the scores.

Hiring Plan The position control budget for the unit defining open positions by FTE or work agreement requirement, full- or part-time status, shifts and planned weekends for human resources, and recruitment.

Holding Hours per Patient A standard financial unit for the hours of care provided for the number of patients being held in the emergency department, postanesthesia recovery unit, admissions, or other units during the hours the unit is operational.

Homogeneous Condition of little variation among the data points; they are all closely clustered about the mean.

Hours/2 Weeks Defines the regular hours scheduled for a given 2-week pay period, including tenth-of-an hour fractions (i.e., 80, 40, 37.5). See Work Agreements.

Hours Classification A distinct grouping used to classify hours, correlated with financial industry standards. Standard hour classifications include direct, indirect, total worked or productive hours, nonproductive hours (benefit and, at some hospitals, education, meeting, and orientation), and total paid or annual hours.

Hours per Delivery A standard financial unit for the hours of care provided for the number of deliveries in the obstetric units during the hours the unit is operational. Census is reported as "couplets" meaning one mother and one baby.

Hours per Patient Day (HPPD) The hours of nursing care provided per patient per day by various levels of nursing personnel. HPPD is calculated by dividing the total paid hours for nursing personnel for a specific time period by the total number of patient days in the same time period.

Hours per Procedure A standard financial unit for the hours of care provided for the number of procedures completed during the hours the unit is operational.

Hours per Surgical Case A standard financial unit for the hours of care provided for the number of surgical cases completed during the hours the operating rooms or same day surgical units are operational. Time is tracked in surgical minutes or other increment based on minutes (e.g., 1 unit = 6 minutes or 1 unit = 10 minutes).

Hours per Unit of Service (HPUOS) A standard financial unit for the hours of care provided for the number of patients served during the hours the unit is operational.

Hours/Patient Day (HPPD) A standard financial unit for the hours of care provided for the number of patients in the hospital at midnight.

Hours per Visit A standard financial unit for the hours of care provided for the number of patient visits in the emergency department, outpatient clinics, pain clinics, and so forth, during the hours the unit is operational.

Hours Worked The actual hours worked for a given period, including regular hours and overtime.

Human Capital The economic value of an employee's skill set; recognizes that all employees are not equal.

Hurdle Rate Organization-specific minimum acceptable rate of return on investment or a project.

Implementation Phase The longest and most labor intensive phase of project management in which the project is built, implemented, and then monitored to verify costs and schedules meet baseline projections.

Incentive Compensation A variety of approaches for motivating employees; does not need to be monetary to be effective, as long as perceived to carry meaningful value.

Incident to Billing A Medicare rule requiring the doctor to be in the suite and immediately available in order for a service to be billed. The service provided is reported as if the billing provider provided the service.

Incremental Cost-Effectiveness Ratio (ICER) The ratio of the change in costs of a therapeutic intervention (compared to the alternative, such as doing nothing or using the best available alternative treatment) to the change in effects of the intervention.

Independent Practice Association (IPA) Open panel system in which individual physicians contact to provide care for enrolled members.

Indicators Measure conditions, performance, or results, and can be used to help find the root causes of problems.

Indirect Costs Costs that cannot be attributed directly to a specific area and are usually spread over several areas, that is, housekeeping and administration.

Indirect Hours Hours of staff (e.g., manager, health unit coordinator, monitor tech, and others) providing service to the unit, but *not* directly with patients or taking a patient assignment. Also include other worked and paid hours but *not* directly with patients such as education, orientation, and classes.

Institutional Research An organizational function responsible for collecting, aggregating, and interpreting internal and external data.

Insurance A system for the collective, long-term prepayment of the costs of health services.

Internal Rate of Return (IRR) The discount rate at which the net present value of a project or investment equals zero.

Level of Measurement Determines which statistical techniques can be used to analyze the data.

Leveling Method used to examine a project for overallocation of resources and making adjustments.

Liabilities The financial obligations of an organization, that is, bills to be paid.

Long-Term Liabilities Obligations that will be paid off within the following year.

Maintenance Expenses Expenses related to the upkeep and ongoing preventative care of the organization and its equipment.

Map of Dependencies Conceptualizations of the network of individuals who can potentially cooperate, approve, or oppose the project.

Margin Revenue less specified expenses.

Marginal Costs The additional costs related to providing one extra unit of a specific item.

Marginal Utility The value of one more, given that a certain amount has already been consumed.

Market Penetration How well the organization has exposed its services to potential users/buyers in a particular area.

Market Segmentation Dividing a particular market for potential services into subsections with separate, measurable needs.

Mean Also known as the average, a very common statistical test used to summarize a group of data. The mean is calculated by dividing the sum of each individual value by the total number of values.

Measure A standard, a basis for comparison, a reference point against which other things can be evaluated.

Median The midpoint of a group of results, indicating that 50% of the scores are above the median and 50% are below the median.

Medicaid Established in 1965, implemented in 1966. A federal program that pays for certain mandatory health services provided to low-income children and their caretakers. Amendments have been made to include people with developmental disabilities and other low-income groups, including the elderly, children, and pregnant women. Medicaid is jointly funded by the federal and state governments. A particular state's per capita income determines the amount of federal matching funds.

Medicare Created in 1965 under Title XVIII of the Social Security Act. Expanded in 1972 to include people of any age with end-stage renal disease. In 1973, it was expanded again to include people of any age who meet Medicare's definition of disability.

Milestones Groups of deliverables that represent a significant event or accomplishment.

Mission Organization's reason for existing.

Mission Statement Succinct and precise present-oriented passage that describes what the organization is and does.

Mode The most frequently occurring value in a distribution.

Monitoring Compilation of organizational systems and processes designed to promote outcomes visibility, targets achievement, and strategy execution.

National General Purpose Grants Made on the basis of a broad scope and impact across the nation and even world. These foundations may use professional consultants as reviewers; like to create change; and generally prefer creative, innovative, or model projects that others can replicate.

National Health Expenditures Payments to hospitals, providers, vendors, and long-term care agencies as a proportion of the gross domestic product.

Net Fixed Assets Determined by subtracting depreciation from the total fixed assets.

Net Income Income that exists after expenses have been subtracted from total revenues.

Net Loss Loss sustained when expenses exceed total revenues.

Net Present Value (NPV) Present value of predicted future revenues minus present value of predicted future payments.

Net Worth Value of an organization after paying off all its debts and/or liabilities.

Nominal Group Technique A group technique in which members document their opinions anonymously to reduce influence from others on the team.

Nominal Variables Classifications of variables into mutually exclusive categories. By definition, this means that the number used for a nominal variable is arbitrary and functions as a label rather than a quantity amenable to computation.

Nonparametric The results of measurement of a variable, when plotted on an x–y graph, are not distributed along a standard normal curve.

Nonproductive Hours A term used for all hours the hospital defines as "nonproductive." Always includes benefit time for paid time off (e.g., vacation, sick, holiday). Some organizations may also include education, meeting, and orientation hours as nonproductive time, although the employee is working and paid.

Normal Curve Symmetrical graphic in which the mean, median, and mode share the same point on the curve. The standard normal curve incorporates the measurement of standard deviation and defines the parameters for each standard deviation unit.

Observation Hours per Patient A standard financial unit for the hours of care provided for the number of patients being observed in the emergency department, obstetric unit, or other units during the hours the unit is operational.

Operating Budget Financial projections that guide day-to-day functions at every level of an organization.

Operating Expenses The daily costs required to maintain and run an entity.

Operationalizing The process of translating environmental evaluations, SWOT analyses findings, strategic objectives, and substrategies into concrete, executable tasks and projecting the costs associated with these undertakings.

Opportunity Cost of Capital The magnitude of the best-return investment alternative of the same risk.

Ordinal Measurements Also known as rankings. Ordinal data are ranked against some defined criterion.

Organizational Culture The shared values, beliefs, and assumptions of employees within an organization.

Out of Network Care Medical services obtained by managed care plan members from noncontracted health care providers.

Outliers Any situation in which outcomes are outside the normal pattern (i.e., patients who have an atypical care experience that extends their length of stay).

Overhead Operating costs not directly associated with revenue generation.

Overhead Allocation The amount charged per unit due to indirect costs, that is, administration, finance, and marketing.

Paid Claims Ratio or PCR What hospitals bill and what they actually collect.

Parametric The results of measurement of a variable are distributed normally; that is, if the individual results are plotted on an x–y graph, the spread resembles a standard normal curve.

Passion Skills Convergence of technical expertise and enthusiasm for performing specific duties.

Patient Classification A measurement of patient severity of illness that is related to the amount of resources required to care for the patient. The severity of illness measurements is grouped into "classes" or levels (between 1 and 20), which are mapped to a formula for calculating the required hours of care by direct caregivers for the patients in the unit. May also be called patient acuity.

Patient Classification System A standardized method of determining patient severity of illness. Classification systems assign patients to defined categories by care intensity, care level, assumed or average utilization of resources, or other variables. One example is that of California, where these systems are required by Title XXII.

Payback Model A common criterion for selection of business projects, which measures the time it takes for the project to recover its investment.

People Outcomes Subset of broader organizational strategic outcomes focused on cultural, role, and developmental alignment of employees.

Performance Appraisal Formal organizational process for evaluating an individual employee's achievements and compensation as well as setting goals, performed at predetermined time intervals.

Performance Improvement Plan Formal, individually tailored program targeted toward uncovering the root causes of objectively assessed underperformance and creating concrete, timed tactics for course correction.

Performance Management Organizational systems and processes established to control the progress toward achievement of individual, departmental, and firm-wide goals, including performance appraisal, periodic feedback, and performance improvement programs.

Periodic Feedback Semiformal organizational process that requires managers to check-in with direct reports from time-to-time and provide feedback, both positive and constructive, while inviting every employee to solicit and welcome such feedback.

Personal Dashboards Widely used tools for intradepartmental communication and progress monitoring, focused on individual performance targets.

Plan–Do–Check–Act (PDCA) A successive cycle that starts off small to test potential effects on processes, but then gradually leads to larger and more targeted change.

Plan–Do–Study–Act (PDSA) A process improvement model promoted by the Institute for Healthcare Improvement (IHI), originally developed by Shewhart and subsequently modified by Deming, to guide continual improvement processes by tracking the stages of the improvement process. Stages include the Plan Stage of data gathering, Do Stage of experimentation, Study Stage of evaluation, and Act Stage of adoption. The PDSA cycle is continual and once completed begins with testing and evaluating another potential improvement.

Planning Phase The project management phase that includes preparation of schedules and budgets with accompanying resource allocations, identification, and mitigation of risk.

Position Control A report showing the actual number of positions based on full- or part-time work agreements or FTEs filled on a unit as opposed to the number of positions budgeted.

Position Control Plan A plan for staffing requirements that determines how many FTEs are required to deliver the amount of care identified as being necessary.

Potential Patient Days The maximum number of patients who would occupy all staffed beds.

Practical Significance Calculating the significance of two different variable scores using an approach that will return a result in standard deviation units; this is used frequently for meta-analysis in evidence-based practice, because it allows research with different measurement approaches to be standardized and then compared.

Practice Management The continuum of processes, often unique for each practice, that impact the provision of patient care. These processes include staffing, scheduling, billing, and quality improvement practices.

Preapproval The requirement set forth by an insurance company to approve certain care before it is provided.

Preferred Provider Organization (PPO) Physicians, group of physicians, hospital, or other health care facility that has contracted with a private insurance company or business to provide health care services to a select group of patients.

Present Value (PV) Adjusted for the timing and risk, the current monetary worth of a future cash flow or an asset.

Principal Investigator (PI) In research projects, it is responsible for all aspects of the grant.

Procedures Specific activities carried out for or to patients in units that typically do not have inpatient census such as the emergency department or outpatient clinic at a specific time of day. At a minimum, it is midnight and often includes the day, evening, and night shifts.

Productivity Average measure of efficiency of production, often expressed as a ratio of output to inputs.

Professional Liability Insurance premiums that need to be paid to cover potential lawsuits.

Profit Margin Percentage difference between expenses and revenue.

Pro-Forma Predictive financial statement for a project or organization.

Pro-Forma Income Statements Tools that forecast revenues, expenses, and profits and/or losses resulting from future operations.

Project Short-term effort to give rise to a unique product, service, or end result.

Project Evaluation and Review Technique (PERT) A statistical analysis tool used to represent project tasks that shows the critical path.

Project Manager Writes the grant, manages the execution and deliverables, and submits final reports.

Prospective Payment System (PPS) Mechanism for prospectively transferring funds to hospitals based on the facility's DRG profile.

Psychological Safety Occurs when individuals believe that change can be made without harm to their personal values or integrity; encourages participation.

Quality-Adjusted Life Year (QALY) A measure of disease burden, including both the quality and the quantity of life lived.

Range The simplest measure of dispersion or variation. It is the difference between the largest and the smallest values in a given data distribution.

Ratio/Interval Data The most common type of variable that can be mathematically and statistically manipulated. Interval data are ordered and the distance between each number is identical.

Readmission Rates Measured 7, 15, or 30 days following discharge, the readmission rate is a quality indicator under increasing scrutiny by CMS and other payers.

Reimbursement Payment for health care goods and services, often made by a third party.

Reliability The consistency and dependability of the data.

Resource-Constrained Budget Assumes resources are fixed; a shortage of resources is compensated by adjusting time.

Restricted Resources The financial contributions to a foundation that have restrictions placed on their use by the donor.

Return on Investment (ROI) A formula that quantifies a project's value by determining the ratio of dollars gained by completing the project divided by dollars invested.

Revenue Gross amount of earnings received by an entity for the operation of a specific activity. It does not include any deductions for such items as expenses, bad debts, or contractual allowance.

Risk The likelihood that an insured event will occur.

Risk–Benefit Analysis Weighs the potential for undesirable outcomes and side effects against the potential for positive outcomes of a treatment and is an integral part of the process of determining medical necessity in the delivery of quality medical care.

Risk Breakdown Structure Tool used in risk mitigation; developed in conjunction with a work breakdown structure; aligned with the organizational hierarchy identifying risks and potential risks.

Role Alignment Extent to which an employee's job matches his or her passions and the level of skills and knowledge he or she possesses to be successful in the job.

Roster Duty list or work schedule.

Salary Costs per Patient per Day Divide total payroll expenses for nursing personnel for a specific time by the total number of patient days in the same time frame (more sensitive measure than HPPD in that it accounts for the staff mix).

Scrum An iterative process of developing a product or service characterized by flexible scope, short-term design process, embracing stakeholder feedback, and change.

Sensitivity Analysis Recalculations of financial results with a variety of different underlying suppositions and projections.

Simple/Absolute Frequency Distribution A table that reports the value and number of times that each value occurs.

Skill Mix A grouping of job positions or categories most often used to group caregivers into "direct" care and "indirect" care. Direct caregivers are usually grouped into four groups or classifications: RNs, LPN/LVN/LVNs, nursing assistants or unlicensed assistive personnel (UAPs), and other direct caregivers not included in the previous three groups. Indirect caregivers include all other job positions paid for by the unit that support the direct caregivers but are not included in the staffing plan ratio of caregivers to patients.

SMART Goals A method of developing goals that are specific, measurable, attainable, realistic, and time bound.

Snapshot Review A formal process for keeping the critical quality and operating targets as well as other strategic indicators continually visible throughout the institution and for driving performance to reach goals.

Special Purpose Foundations Very large organizations, usually funded by large asset bases, that define their area of concern quite specifically.

Staffing Distribution Number of personnel allocated by shift; for example, % for days, % for evenings, % for nights.

Staffing Mix Ratio of various types of personnel to one another; that is, RNs 40%, LVNs 40%, and others 20%.

Standard Deviation The positive square root of the distribution's variance.

Statement of Cash Flows Reports on a company's cash flow activities, particularly its operating, investing, and financing activities.

Statement of Comprehensive Income A report on an institution's income, expenses, and profits over a period of time; also referred to as profit and loss statement (P&L).

Statement of Financial Position Reports on a company's assets, liabilities, and ownership equity at any given point in time; also referred to as a balance sheet.

Statistical Deviation The amount by which an individual score differs from the group mean.

Statistical Significance A statistical calculation (p) that compares the probability that the observed p value is less than the significance level defined for the study. It tells us whether we should reject or accept the null hypothesis.

Statistician Works with the Pi and Co-I to develop the specific aims, determines the plan of analysis, assists in developing the database, and supervises the analysis.

Statistics The formal mathematical procedures used to organize and comprehend data.

Strategic Goals (Objectives) Broad, high-level statements that set targets for and describe how an organization progresses from the state of its present mission to the state of its desired vision.

Strategy Committee The body responsible for driving the strategy process in an organization.

Strategy Process Systematic, cyclical, dynamic, and broad-based framework for organizational management, consisting of four equally important stages—formulation, operationalizing, execution, and monitoring.

Substrategies Methods implemented to achieve the broad strategic goals.

Sunk Costs The resources previously expended on a project or investment that should be disregarded when evaluating the net present value.

SWOT Analysis Commonly used tool for analyzing an organization's strategic capabilities and positioning, referring to its *strengths, weaknesses, opportunities,* and *threats*.

Synergistic Effect The phenomena in which the group produces more knowledge than each of the members working on their own.

Systems Theory A theory that is useful in a complex setting such as health care because it analyzes processes by breaking them down into parts and then reassemble them to show how the parts work within the system.

Systems Thinking A method of root cause analysis looking at the interrelationships of the individual parts; problem solving by investigating the cause-and-effect actions between systems.

Tactical Map A document illustrating the tactics to be performed by units, departments, teams, and individual employees within an organization.

Tactical Planning Part of operationalizing; the process of deriving strategy execution tasks, assigning them to responsible parties, and establishing completion timelines.

Tactics The planned activities undertaken in order to meet the stated strategic objectives.

Terminal Value A method for determining the final worth of a project or an investment, which estimates the overall value of a mature enterprise by applying an industry-comparable earnings multiplier to the EBITDA.

Time and Materials An hourly payment method often used when the scope of work is not clear to either party.

Time-Constrained Project When time and schedule are not flexible, and resources are added to compensate for a project with a fixed schedule.

Total Paid Hours The actual number of hours paid per employee, which includes total worked and total nonproductive (e.g., time not spent in assigned duties such as education time) time.

Total Worked Hours Total worked and paid hours. If your hospital does not separate direct and indirect hours, then direct and total worked will be the same. This does not include any benefit time (e.g., paid time for no work) or education, meeting, and orientation if your hospital classifies these hours as nonproductive.

Turnover Rate Rate calculated by dividing the number of employees leaving by the average number of workers employed in the unit/facility during the year and then multiplying by 100.

Uninsured Those people who have no health insurance, either by choice or due to cost or other barriers.

Units of Service (UOS) The number of activities performed in a unit associated to revenues measured against the labor and other expenses. For example, census is the units of service for inpatient units, whereas visits or procedures are the units of service for units such as the emergency department, outpatient clinics, or other units that do not have inpatient census for a specific time of day. It is reported as hours, dollars, or FTEs per unit of service.

Utilization Rate Required hours of care divided by nursing hours paid.

Vacant Position An allocation in the position control in the unit based on the budgeted FTEs for full- and part-time work agreements. A position is vacant if it is *not* assigned to an employee.

Validity The level of certainness that the collected data actually represent the concept of interest.

Value Value is the payment model in which the organization providing the services is rewarded for the value delivered.

Value—Quality/Cost Quality includes compilation of outcomes, experiences, and safety.

Values A framework that serves as criteria for prioritization, problem solving, conflict resolution, and strategy development and allows all within an organization to evaluate decisions, take pride in their work, and make commitments.

Variable Costs Costs that vary with the volume; that is, payroll costs.

Variance Difference between planned costs and actual costs.

Variation The variability of a group of data points; how spread out or close together the values are from the other values within the group. Variation is a measure of the sameness of a group of data points.

Vision Statement Forward-looking pronouncement that describes what a firm aspires to be and do.

Visits The number of visits made by patients to the emergency department, outpatient clinics, or other units that do not have inpatient census for a specific time of day. At a minimum, it is midnight and often includes the day, evening, and night shifts.

Wage Index A value associated to the office of management and budget's core-based statistical area (CBSA)-based geographic designations by which the base rate may be adjusted.

Weighted Average Cost of Capital (WACC) Form of a discount rate that represents the combined risk-adjusted opportunity cost for company's debt and equity holders, or organization's cost of accessing cash for investment.

Work Agreements The specifications of the contract under which an individual was hired. Work agreement is a generic term that includes such things as number of hours to be worked each week or pay period, job code or position, hourly or nonexempt or exempt from overtime and benefits expected, and so forth. See Hours / 2 weeks.

Work Breakdown Structure (WBS) A diagram that outlines a project's work elements.

Working Capital Organization's current assets and current liabilities.

Workload Index Weighted statistic that reflects acuity level of patients, census, and productive hours: unit's acuity index × workload/productive hours.

Zero-Based Budgeting (ZBB) The type of budget system that starts at zero each year.

Index

CPSIA information can be obtained
at www.ICGtesting.com
Printed in the USA
BVHW082122161020
591226BV00007B/88